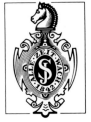

U. Heim   K. M. Pfeiffer

Small Fragment Set Manual

Technique Recommended by the ASIF Group

ASIF: Swiss Association for the Study of Internal Fixation

Second Revised and Enlarged Edition

Translated by R. L. Batten and K. M. Pfeiffer

With 215 Figures in more than 500 Separate Illustrations

Springer-Verlag
Berlin Heidelberg New York 1982

Priv.-Doz. Dr. URS HEIM
Thunstraße 106, CH-3074 Muri/BE

Professor Dr. KARL MARTIN PFEIFFER
Chirurgische Universitätspoliklinik, Kantonsspital,
Petersgraben 4, CH-4031 Basel

Translator:

R.L. BATTEN, F.R.C.S.
The General Hospital, GB-Birmingham B4 6NH

Translation of the German edition:
Periphere Osteosynthesen, second edition
© by Springer-Verlag Berlin Heidelberg 1972 and 1981

ISBN 3-540-11143-3 2nd edition Springer-Verlag Berlin Heidelberg New York
ISBN 0-387-11143-3 2nd edition Springer-Verlag New York Heidelberg Berlin

ISBN 3-540-06904-6 1st edition Springer-Verlag Berlin Heidelberg New York
ISBN 0-387-06904-6 1st edition Springer-Verlag New York Heidelberg Berlin

Library of Congress Cataloging in Publication Data
Heim, U., 1924–   Small fragment set manual. Translation of: Periphere Osteosynthesen. Bibliogra-
phy: p.   . Includes index. I. Internal fixation in fractures. I. Pfeiffer, K.M. (Karl Martin), 1927–   .
II. Arbeitsgemeinschaft für Osteosynthesefragen. III. Title.
RD103.I5H4413   1982   617′.3   81-23207
                        AACR2

Reproduction of figures: Gustav Dreher GmbH, Stuttgart

Typesetting, printing, and bookbinding by Universitätsdruckerei H. Stürtz AG, Würzburg

2121/3130-543210

Preface to the Second Edition

The rapid development in the surgical treatment of fractures during the past 9 years has necessitated considerable modifications to the first edition of this book. Numerous new implants and instruments are presented in this, the second edition. In 4.0-, 3.5- and 2.7-mm screws the hexagonal socket has definitively superseded the Phillips head, while mini-implants have been modified and a 1.5-mm screw introduced. A number of new plates and implants have been introduced and have long since proved their value. At the same time new techniques, described here, have been developed and applied.

The tension-band wire is included, despite the fact that it does not consist of specific AO implants, and use of the Kirschner wire is also illustrated and emphasized whenever the authors consider that this simple method is still the best available.

Alterations in the organization of the book have been necessary: the shoulder, the forearm and the knee are treated in separate chapters, and other sections have been extended.

With regard to clinical-radiological examples, new typical situations are described and documented. The case studies from the first edition have been recontrolled in all instances in which it was feasible to do so. In this way many valuable late results, 9–12 years after internal fixation, were obtained. We found that almost all joints had remained stable after healing of an articular fracture; so-called late arthrosis is rare in the peripheral skeleton.

Once again, we wish to express our thanks to many colleagues and friends for their help, advice and constructive criticism vis-à-vis this new edition. We especially wish to thank Mr. OBERLI, the artist, for the splendid new drawings he has produced, and also Mr. KELLER of the AO Documentation Centre in Berne for the perfect reproduction of the X-ray films. Our secretaries, Sister GISELA and Miss SCHAUB, again had to cope with mountains of paper. Many other helping hands were active in dealing with a large number of details. Finally, we would like to thank Springer-Verlag for their cooperation and for the outstanding presentation of the book.

Muri-Bern and Basel, Spring 1982
U. HEIM
K.M. PFEIFFER

Contents

I. Introduction and Objektives

Practical experience has shown the need for adding smaller implants to the standard instrument set of ASIF (AO). In certain situations there were clear deficiencies in the technical equipment developed between 1958 and 1960. This applied first of all to the fixation of thin, loose fragments detached from large cylindrical bones; the wide drill holes in these small fragments endangered their vitality and the conical screw heads threatened to split them (Spycher). The prominent screw heads also proved occasionally to be disadvantageous, particularly over diaphyseal crests.

The thick inflexible plates of the basic set were too large to apply to the metaphyses of the upper limb and the lower tibia, leading to disproportion between bone and implant, which was detrimental to the soft tissues, especially the skin. Comminuted fractures involving smaller joints such as the elbow and the ankle, in which the long-term prognosis depends very much upon exact reduction and fixation, were unsuitable for fixation with bulky cancellous screws. Kirschner wires were often used instead, but could not give enough stability. Clinical experience and experimental work (Schenk, Perren) have often shown that completely separated and loose fragments of cortical bone can be rapidly revascularized, provided an exact and stable reduction holds them in contact with living tissue. This has led to the introduction of special small implants for use in complex internal fixations. Thus the painstaking and precise reassembly of comminuted fragments, for a time derided as "radiological cosmetics" has received a fresh impetus.

Standard methods of internal fixation have little application to the narrow, short and cylindrical bones of the hand and the foot. In 1946 Kilbourne, impelled by functional considerations, was the first to perform internal fixation with small screws and plates. His results in 17 cases were published in 1958. Stable internal fixation and plaster-free postoperative treatment of the hand looked very promising, since prolonged immobilization often results in stiffness. In 1959 ASIF developed the "scaphoid screw" for cancellous bone. Later it was modified for wider application and renamed the "small cancellous screw". For the scaphoid fracture, however, it is only used in special situations. Yet in order to cope with the smaller and variable dimensions of the peripheral skeleton, a complete instrument set with the largest possible diversification seemed desirable. The credit for the development of this set is due to Dr. Robert Mathys of Bettlach. The early types of small cortex screws had smooth shanks without threads to allow interfragmentary compression, but their removal was often almost impossible. In 1964 the small fragment set of instruments was completed and made available for clinical testing.

The ASIF small fragment set (hereafter abbreviated to SFS) has been developed by practical use, partly following the principles of the Swiss watchmaking industry. All instruments and implants are so delicate that their handling calls chiefly for skill rather than force. In fact, the screws have considerable strength and provide remarkable stability, though there are limitations. They should never be applied in places where, for mechanical or anatomical reasons, standard size implants are required. The existence of such small implants should never induce the surgeon to jeopardize rigidity. Errors of the past, resulting from the use of excessively short or weak implants, should be avoided in the future. Small screws and plates should not be

1

used to obtain a feeble hold on fragments in an open reduction but should, like implants from the standard set, facilitate functional postoperative treatment. To emphasize this aim is one of the purposes of this book.

The basic problems of the indications and the technique of internal fixation have been solved for most fractures and pseudarthroses by animal experiments and clinical studies. The SFS enables the surgeon to treat skeletal injuries of the hand and the foot, as well as small fragments of larger bones, securing rigid internal fixation.

Over the past 10 years many supplementary instruments and implants have been developed. Of prime importance are: (a) the introduction of the hexagonal socket head for screws of 4.5-, 3.5- and 2.7-mm diameter; (b) the introduction of screws with diameters of 2.0 and 1.5 mm, which have cross-slots in their heads; (c) the development of the dynamic compression plate (DCP) to fit the small screws; and (d) the introduction of many special plates. All plates now have oval holes to allow more accurate setting of the screws and the possibility of self-compression in an axial direction.

Special instruments have been designated and introduced to supplement the standard set but will not be described or illustrated in this manual. The full range can be found in the revised catalogue of the SYNTHES company where they are shown in detail. There are also specific instruments and implants for use in veterinary and maxillofacial surgery.

All the small implants are now dealt with in the *Manual of Internal Fixation* (2nd edition published by Springer-Verlag Berlin-Heidelberg-New York 1979).

Literature on stable internal fixation in hand surgery includes work by Burri, Durband, Heim, Koob, Pannike, Pfeiffer, Rüedi, Segmüller, Simonetta, Wilhelm and others. A fuller bibliography can be found at the end of this volume.

Statistical data have been assembled from clinical work using these techniques and have helped to define more exactly the indications for the specific techniques over a period of 15 years. As there have been so many modifications of the method a thorough revision of the *Small Fragment Set Manual* was seen to be imperative.

As in the first edition, the material that follows must be understood to be the result of clinical study, and its aim is to serve as a guide to operative technique.

General Section

II. Implants and Instruments of the SFS

Experience has shown that the diversity of implants can lead to confusion and mistakes, so it seems imperative to furnish details of their sizes and to show which instrument is required for the application of each implant.

1. The SFS Screws (Fig. 1)

There are five different types of SFS screws:

a) The Small Cancellous Screw

The outer diameter of the thread is 4.0 mm, the shaft diameter between the head and the thread is 2.3 mm, and the core of the thread is 1.8 mm. The length of the thread increases from 5 to 15 mm in proportion to the screw length, which begins at 10 mm and increases by 2-mm stages up to 30 mm, then by 5 mm stages up to 50 mm.

Application (Fig. 2). To apply this screw a 2.0-mm drill bit is used with a drill guide and a 3.5-mm tap, using a tap sleeve.

Indications. This screw can obtain a good hold in cancellous bone because of its deep broad thread. It can also be used in the one-third tubular plate, the small dynamic compression plate (DCP) and in special plates. It has partly replaced the malleolar screw of the standard set.

b) The 3.5-mm (Small) Cortex Screw

This screw has an outer diameter thread of 3.5 mm, with a core of 2.0 mm. Each screw is threaded over its whole length, which begins at 10 mm and increases by 2-mm stages to 28 mm, after which it goes up in 4-mm stages to the longest at 40 mm.

Application (Fig. 2). These screws are applied with a 2.0-mm drill bit using a drill guide, and a 3.5-mm tap with the appropriate sleeve. To make a gliding hole, a 3.5-mm drill bit is used. When this screw is used with a plate, a 2.0-mm drill bit is still used with the appropriate guide and a 3.5-mm tap with the appropriate sleeve.

Indications. The 3.5-mm cortex screw has a broad thread and a narrow core, so it provides a very good bite. It is suitable for cortical bone as well as for strong cancellous bone and is used to fix the one-third tubular plate and the small DCP. It may occasionally be used to fix small plates in the hand and foot. It can be used together with a plastic spiked washer to reinsert an avulsed ligament into its bone (Fig. 1).

c) The 2.7-mm (Small) Cortex Screw

The outer diameter of the thread of this screw is 2.7 mm, the core is 2.0 mm and each screw is fully threaded. Screw lengths begin at 6 mm, increasing by stages of 2 mm to 24 mm.

Application (Fig. 2). These screws are fixed with a 2.0-mm drill bit and an appropriate drill guide. The tap measures 2.7 mm with its sleeve and the 2.7-mm drill bit is used for the gliding hole. With a plate the 2.0-mm drill is again used, with a guide and a 2.7-mm tap with sleeve.

Indications. The 2.7-mm screw is suitable for strong cortex in metacarpal and metatarsal bones and sometimes for larger proximal phalanges. It can be used to fix plates in the hand and foot, with the quarter-tubular plate and the DCP designed for 2.7-mm screws. It can also be used with the spiked plastic washer to refix avulsed ligaments (Fig. 1).

d) The 2.0-mm (Mini) Cortex Screw

The outer diameter of this screw is 2.0 mm; it has a core of 1.4 mm and is threaded throughout. The lengths begin at 6 mm and increase by 2-mm stages to 20 mm.

Application (Fig. 2). This screw is fixed using a 1.5-mm drill bit with its guide, and a 2.0-mm tap set in its special handle with a quick dental coupling, with a 2.0-mm drill guide as a tap sleeve. A 2.0-mm drill bit is used for the gliding hole. When employed with a plate, a 1.5-mm drill bit with its guide and a 2.0-mm tap with a 2.0-mm drill guide are used.

Indications. The 2.0-mm cortex screw is suitable for proximal and middle phalanges of hand or foot and sometimes for especially fragile metacarpals. It is also used for fixing the mini plate.

e) The 1.5-mm (Mini) Cortex Screw

This screw has an outer diameter of thread of 1.5 mm, with a core of 1,1 mm. It is fully threaded and lengths range from 6 to 16 mm (increasing in 1-mm increments between 6 and 12 mm and in 2-mm increments thereafter).

Application (Fig. 2). This screw is fixed with a 1.1-mm drill bit used with its guide, a 1.5-mm tap mounted in the small chuck with a mini quick dental coupling using a 1.5-mm drill guide as a tap sleeve. A 1.5-mm drill bit with a drill guide of the same dimension is used for the gliding hole. Because of the small difference between the diameter of the thread and the core of the screw it may be used in strong cortical bone without tapping the thread.

Indications. The 1.5-mm cortex screw is used in proximal and middle phalanges and in the distal phalanx of the thumb. It may also be used in the radial head or in the fixation of very small butterfly fragments.

Special Screw Lengths

For the fusion of finger joints, screws of additional length in the 3.5-, 2.7- and 2.0-mm sizes are available on request. For use in maxillofacial surgery 3.5-mm screws with specially small heads have been provided.

The Screw Heads (Fig. 3)

In the small screws, the heads are slightly vaulted but not too prominent. The heads of the 4.0-, 3.5- and 2.7-mm screws are provided with a hexagonal socket like the standard size screws.

The heads of the 2.0- and 1.5-mm screws have cross-slots with a central hole which is useful for applying and removing these screws with a special screw driver.

The lower surface of the head is spherical to give a better purchase in the plate holes. It also allows axial compression when the screw hole is drilled eccentrically, as with the DCP.

When screws are used alone in thick cortical bone, a countersink is recommended. In very thin cortical bone, a washer (Fig. 1) is used to prevent the screw head breaking the cortex.

The same screw driver can be used for the 4.0-, 3.5- and 2.7-mm screws (Fig. 9) but a smaller screw driver is made to fit the cross-slot of the 2.0- and 1.5-mm screws. This has to be mounted in the small chuck with the mini quick dental coupling (Fig. 9).

In the diagrams the new screw heads are shown but in some of the clinical cases, Phillips heads are shown as these were the only ones available for patients treated before 1972.

Washers

In order to prevent the screw head from (a) sinking into thin cortical bone and (b) splitting off small fragment points, small metal washers are available for the screw sizes 2.7, 3.5 and 4.0 mm (Fig. 1f).

Spiked polyacetal resin washers are available for the fixation of an avulsed ligament to the bone, or for the compression of small avulsion fractures or small areas of comminution. They have a fine built-in metallic ring for X-ray detection. Larger washers are fixed with the 4.0- and 3.5-mm screws, and a smaller one with the 2.7-mm screw (Fig. 1g).

2. The SFS Plates

These plates are made in different shapes so as to fit special sites. They are slightly concave to make them fit the bone diaphysis and to strengthen them. The holes in the plates are oval so that axial compression can be obtained by drilling the bone at the end of the oval holes away from the fracture. Oval holes also allow the screws to be inserted obliquely whilst still gaining a good purchase on the plate. The flat plates are flexible enough to be contoured with bending pliers and a bending iron, and are thin enough to be shortened with the special cutting pliers for finger plates. The 3.5-mm DCP needs to be shaped by two bending irons or the bending press.

a) The 3.5-mm Plates
(which can be used with 3.5- and 4.0-mm screws)

Straight Plates

One-third Tubular Plate (Fig. 5a). This is the most widely used plate in the SFS. It is slightly concave and is 10 mm wide. It comes in lengths of 26 mm with two holes up to 97 mm with eight holes. The oval holes allow the plate to be placed under tension by eccentric drilling, which compresses the fracture. Compression may also be applied by the use of the tension device at the end of a plate (Fig. 12a). This plate is most commonly used in the lateral malleolus, the metatarsals, the distal ulna and the olecranon.

The 3.5-mm DCP (Fig. 5b). 3.5 mm refers to the diameter of the screw used with this plate; its length, width, and number of screw holes are the same as in the one-third tubular plate. It is, however, 3 mm thick, which makes it much stiffer. Recently it has been used more widely, e.g. on the forearm bones and the clavicle.

Shaped Plates

Small T-plate (Fig. 6a). This plate is slightly concave and is of the shape shown. The shaft is 10 mm wide. It is provided in lengths of 50 and 57 mm with three and four holes respectively in the cross piece and shaft. It was originally designed for application to the palmar surface of the lower radius but it is also useful in the olecranon, the outer end of the clavicle, the ankle joint, the first metatarsal etc.

Small Oblique T-plate (Fig. 6b). The holes of this plate are deepened from both sides and its oblique part has an angle of 120°. It can be used on the dorsum of the distal radius, where it fits better than the right-angled T-plate. It is equally effective on the right or left radius.

Cloverleaf Plate (Fig. 6c). This plate takes 4.0 or 3.5 screws in its broad part, but in the shaft of the plate, normal 4.5-mm cortex screws are used. It was designed for the medial malleolus but has also been useful in the head of the humerus etc.

Special Plates

Reconstruction Plate. This plate comes in different lengths with lateral notches so that it can be bent in any direction, especially in the long axis using special pliers.

H-plate. This is intended for use in the cervical spine and also comes in different lengths.

Y-plate. This is intended for use in comminuted fractures of the distal end of the humerus.

b) The 2.7-mm Plates

(which are for use with the 2.7-mm and occasionally 3.5-mm cortex screws with the small head)

Straight Plates

Quarter-tubular Plate (Fig. 7a). This concave straight plate is much stronger than the small straight flat plate. The lengths are from 25 mm (three holes) to 65 mm (eight holes). It is chiefly used in metacarpal and metatarsal fractures.

The 2.7-mm DCP. This plate takes 2.7-mm screws, and is chiefly used for maxillofacial and veterinary surgery. Because it is 2.5 mm thick, it is used only occasionally in the hand, and then chiefly in secondary reconstructive surgery for delayed union or pseudarthrosis. Its length varies from 20 mm with two holes to 100 mm with 12 holes. The thickness of the plates up to the six-hole length has been reduced recently to 2.0 mm, which is appropriate for use in metacarpal bones.

Shaped Plates

Small T- and L-plates for use in the Hand and Foot (Fig. 7b). These plates are 3.5 cm long with five oval screw holes. The neck of the small T-plate has been widened to give more strength. The right-angled L-plates are very seldom used and are therefore not illustrated. These plates are appropriate for metaphyseal fractures of metacarpals and metatarsals.

Special Plates

H-shaped and Reconstruction Plates for use with 2.7-mm screws have been developed for special situations. As they are so rarely used they are not shown in the figures.

c) Plates for use with 2.0-mm Screws, the So-called Mini Plates

Straight Plates (Fig. 7c). These are made in lengths of 21 mm with three holes up to 37 mm with five holes.

Mini T-plates and Mini L-plates (Fig. 7c). These plates are 25 mm long and they are all fixed with 2.0-mm diameter screws though sometimes 1.5-mm screws may be used. They are only used in phalanges of the hand and foot.

3. SFS Instruments

Special instruments have been developed for the application of small implants, some of which are smaller copies of those in the standard set (drill bits, drill guides, small Hohmann retractors etc). Another group of instruments (reduction forceps, cutting forceps, small chuck, etc.) have been designed and are used for their individual functions.

The number of instruments and implants has increased considerably during recent years. In the book the standard instruments are described and illustrated. A number of additional instruments have been developed, only some of which are described and the manufacturers catalogue should be consulted for details. Instruments are shown in groups according to their functions. Each instrument is numbered to match the technical and functional drawings in the text.

4. Instrument Cases

a) The complete SFS, including mini instruments and mini implants, is contained in two cases. In the first are all the standard instruments, and in the second the implants, additional Kirschner wires, and cerclage wire of standard diameters (Fig. 8a, b).

b) The reduced SFS: This is provided as an addition to the standard set (Fig. 8c). The instruments included are for the treatment of fractures of the malleoli, the fibula, the distal radius and the elbow, and for the fixation of small fragments of larger bones. It contains the 4.0-, 3.5- and 2.7-mm implants and the appropriate instruments. The 2.7-mm implants can be omitted on request.

Instruments for Reduction and Temporary Fixation (Fig. 9a)   18

– Reduction forceps (No. 1) with pointed end (towel clips)   20, 21
– Reduction forceps (No. 2) (small ASIF forceps)
– Self-centering bone-holding forceps for small fragments (No. 3)   24
– Holding forceps for finger plate (No. 4) for reduction of fractures and temporary holding of small plate.
– Small Hohmann retractor (No. 5).

Drill Bits (Fig. 9b)

The 3.5-, 2.7-, 2.0-, 1.5- and 1.1-mm drill bits are available for attachment   17, 18, 19
to the quick coupling of the small air drill. The 3.5-, 2.7- and 2.0-mm drill bits are also made for use with the universal chuck. The 2.7-, 2.0-, 1.5- and 1.1-mm drill bits are made for use with the mini compressed air machine. The diameters and applications of the drill bits are as follows:
– The 3.5-mm drill bit (No. 6) for drilling the gliding hole for the 3.5-mm   17
cortex screw when used as a lag screw.
– The 2.7-mm drill bit (No. 7) for drilling the gliding hole for the 2.7-mm   18
cortex screw when used as a lag screw.
– The 2.0-mm drill bit (No. 8) for making the thread holes for the 4.0-mm   18, 19, 20
small cancellous screw, and the 3.5-mm and 2.7-mm cortex screws when   21
used as lag screws or for fixing a plate. It is also used for the gliding hole for the 2.0-mm cortex screw.
– The 1.5-mm drill bit (No. 9) for drilling the thread hole of the 2.0-mm   19
cortex screw and the gliding hole for the 1.5-mm cortex screw.
– The 1.1-mm drill bit (No. 10) for making the thread hole for the 1.5-mm   19
cortex screw.

Drill Guides (Fig. 9c)

Drills must always be used together with drill guides and tap sleeves as follows: 16, 17
– Drill guide for the 3.5-mm drill bit (No. 11), also used as a tap sleeve for the 3.5- and 2.7-mm taps.
– Double drill guide for 3.5-mm DCP holes (No. 12). The double drill guide   21
for 2.7-mm DCP holes is an additional instrument.
– Double drill guide for a 2.0-mm drill bit (No. 13). One side is for centering   16, 19, 22
the screw hole of a plate, the other side serves as a drill guide in pure screw fixation. It is also used as a tap sleeve for the 2.0-mm tap.
– Drill guide for 1.5- and 1.1-mm drill bits (No. 14), also used as a tap   19
sleeve for the 1.5-mm tap.
– Drill sleeve (No. 15). This has an outside diameter of 3.5 mm, and an   10, 17
inside diameter of 2.0 mm, is used inside the 3.5-mm gliding hole and guides the 2.0-mm drill bit for a thread hole. It corresponds to the small C-clamp, the 3.5-mm drill guide or the small pointed drill guide (Fig. 10).

Taps (Fig. 9d)

The 3.5- and 2.7-mm taps are provided with a quick coupling and can be mounted in the tap handle or the handle with the quick coupling (Nos. 22,

33). The 2.0- and 1.5-mm taps are provided with an attachment to the handle with the mini quick coupling (No. 25).

- The 3.5-mm tap (No. 16) is used for 4.0-mm cancellous screws and 3.5-mm cortex screws.   16, 17
- The 2.7-mm tap (No. 17) cuts the thread for 2.7-mm cortex screws.   18
- The 2.0-mm tap (No. 18) cuts the thread for the 2.0-mm cortex screw.   19
- The 1.5-mm tap (No. 19) is used for cutting the thread for the 1.5-mm cortex screws.

Screwdrivers (Fig. 9e)

- The small screwdriver with a hexagonal 2.5-mm socket (No. 20) fits the 4.0-, 3.5- and 2.7-mm screws.   16, 17, 18
- Sleeve for the small screwdrivers (No. 21). This holds the screw onto the screwdriver and may be used for picking up screws from the rack.   4
- The small 2.5-mm insert screwdriver (No. 23) is used like the previous one but has to be inserted in the handle with the quick coupling (No. 22).   19
- Phillips screwdriver (No. 24). This is only used for removing the old Phillips screws.
- The small cross-slotted screwdriver (No. 26) is provided with a sleeve and fits 2.0- and 1.5-mm screws. It needs to be mounted in the handle with the mini quick coupling (No. 25).

Other Instruments (Fig. 9f)

- Depth gauge for the 4.0-, 3.5- and 2.7-mm screws (No. 27).   17, 18
- Depth gauge for the 2.0- and 1.5-mm screws (No. 28). In the case of the 1.5-mm screws, the hook of the instrument is quite large and the depth sometimes has to be measured with a Kirschner wire.   19
- Small countersink tool (No. 29) with quick coupling, which is used with the appropriate handle. It is used for the heads of the 4.0-, 3.5- and 2.7-mm screws.   17
- The mini countersink tool (No. 29) needs to be mounted in the handle with the mini quick coupling and is used for the 2-mm screw heads.   19
- Handle with quick coupling (No. 25) accepts the 3.5- and 2.7-mm taps, the small screwdriver (No. 26), and the small countersink tool (No. 29).
- Cross handle with the quick coupling is an additional instrument and serves the same purpose as the straight handle.
- The handle with the mini quick coupling (No. 25) is used for the 2.0- and 1.5-mm taps, the cross-slotted screwdriver, and the mini countersink tool.
- Bending pliers (No. 30) are used for bending small plates.   24
- Small bending iron (No. 31) is also used for bending small plates.   24
- The sharp hook is for reduction of small fragments and for clearing soft tissue from the screw heads before their removal.

Recommended Additional Instruments (Fig. 10)

- Small chuck (No. 34): holds Kirschner wires of 1.2–1.6 mm in diameter.
- Open ended wrench (No. 39): fits all ASIF nuts.   13a

- Small bone spreader (No. 37): useful for revision of small bone fractures.
- Cutting forceps (No. 35): used for shortening and shaping small plates as well as for nipping off Kirschner wires.
- Small tension device (No. 38): for use with the plates with 3.5-mm holes.   12
  In difficult situations it helps with accurate reduction and axial compression of the 3.5-mm DCP and the one-third tubular plate.

Fig. 1 a–g. The small ASIF screws, enlarged (measured in millimetres)

– The screw heads with hexagonal sockets. SW = diameter of the 2.5-mm screwdriver.
– The shortest and longest screw of the different types
– The core and thread of the screws (in the cancellous screws ascending from 5 to 15 mm)
– Detail of thread with scale, below

a The 4.0-mm small cancellous screw

b The 3.5-mm (small) cortex screw

c The 2.7-mm (small) cortex screw

d The 2.0-mm (mini) cortex screw

e The 1.5-mm (mini) cortex screw

f Metal washers for the 4.0-, 3.5- and 2.7-mm screws

g Spiked polyacetal resin washers with built-in metallic ring: large model for 4.0- and 3.5-mm screws, small model for the 2.7-mm screws

Thread ∅	4.0	3.5	2.7	2.0	1.5 mm
Core ∅	1.9	1.9	1.9	1.3	1.0 mm
Shaft ∅	2.3 mm				

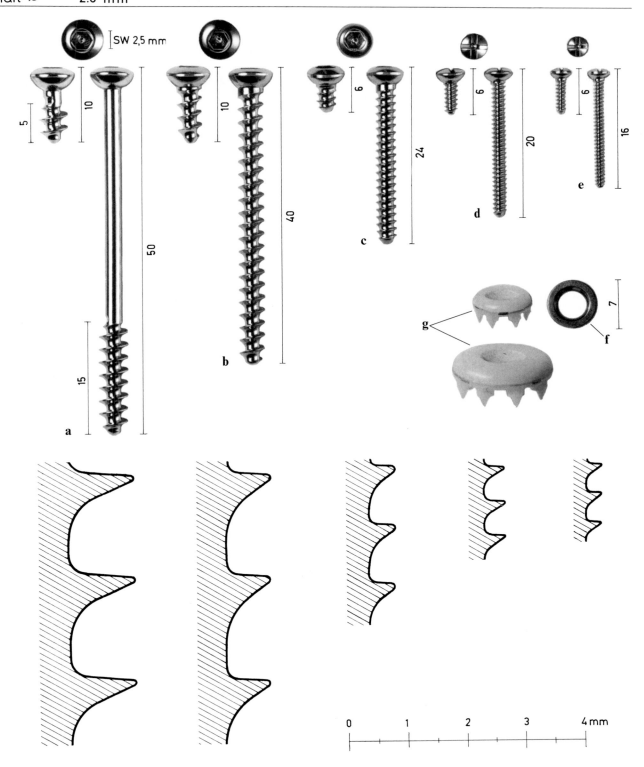

Thread ⌀	4.0	3.5	2.7
Core ⌀	1.9	1.9	1.9
Shaft ⌀	2.3 mm		

⌀	2.0	3.5		2.0	3.5	3.5		2.0	2.7	2.7

a   b   c

14

2.0	1.5 mm
1.3	1.0 mm

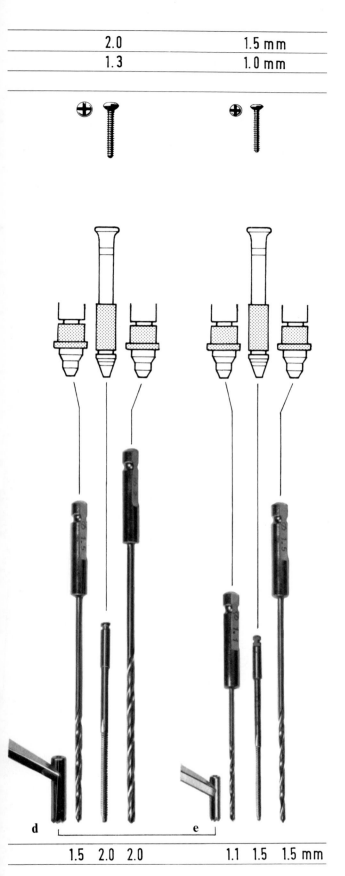

d   e

1.5   2.0   2.0   1.1   1.5   1.5 mm

Fig. 2a–e. The small ASIF screws together with the instruments needed for their insertion

The five small ASIF screws (Fig. 1a–e) with the instruments needed for their use (drill guide, drill bit, tap, tap sleeve). The dimensions are indicated at the margin. The drill bits are drawn to show the quick coupling end. The 1.1-, 1.5-, 2.0- and 2.7-mm drill bits are available for use with dental mini quick coupling chuck of the mini compressed air machine. One end of each of the double drill guides No. 13 and No. 14 is illustrated. It may be used as a tap sleeve as well, depending on the dimension. All the instruments are described and illustrated in Figs. 9 and 10

15

Head ⌀	6.0	6.0	5.0	4.0	3.0 mm
Thread ⌀	4.0	3.5	2.7	2.0	1.5 mm

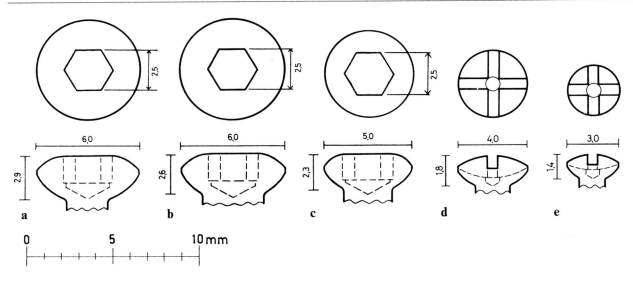

a b c d e

0   5   10 mm

Head ⌀	8.0	8.0 mm
Thread ⌀	4.5 / 6.5	4.5 mm

f

0   5   10 mm

16

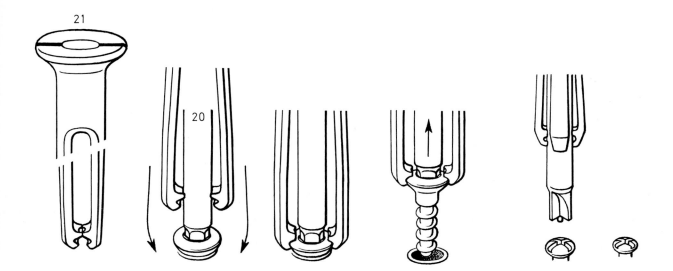

Fig. 4. Screwdriver with sleeve

The screwdriver for the hexagonal socket head (No. 20). The screw may be lifted from the rack with the aid of the sleeve (No. 21) and then the screwdriver engages the screw head. Alternatively the screwdriver first may be inserted in the screw head and then the sleeve slipped down to the head to lift the screw from the rack.

The procedure is identical with the screwdriver for the cruciform recess of the mini screws. The guide-pin of the screwdriver makes the insertion within the screw head easy and keeps it steady within the recess

◁ **Fig. 3a–f. Details of the ASIF screw head enlarged** (scale indicated)

a–e Upper half: The heads of the small ASIF screws with hexagonal socket. Their neck is spherical. The mini screw is provided with a cruciform recess and a central hole for the guide pin of the screwdriver

f Lower half: The heads of the large screws are illustrated for comparison: the standard screw head (4.5-mm cortex and 6.5-mm cancellous) at left, the malleolar screw at right

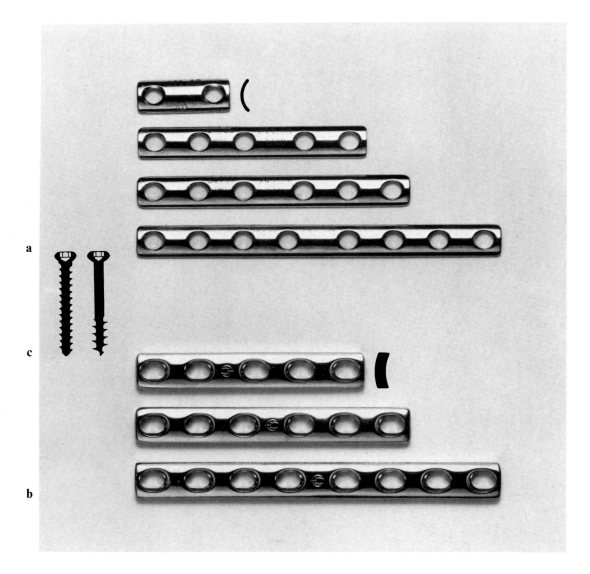

Fig. 5a–c. The straight standard SFS plates, 4.0 and 3.5 mm dimensions (sizes refer to **screw diameters**) (scale 1:1)

a The one-third tubular plate of various lengths (two to eight holes) shown in plan and in cross-section

b The 3.5-mm dynamic compression plate (DCP) (five to eight holes) in plan and in cross-section

c The corresponding 3.5- and 4.0-mm screws

Fig. 6a–c. The shaped 4.0- and 3.5-mm plates (scale 1:1) ▷

a The small T-plate for the distal radius in two different sizes (plan and cross-section). Corresponding 3.5- and 4.0-mm screws

b The oblique T-plate (120°) in different lengths. Since the screw holes are deepened from both sides, the plate may be used on either side

c The clover-leaf plate with the corresponding screws (4.0, 3.5, 4.5 mm).

Shown on a smaller scale are four different adaptations that may be made to the plate with the help of the cutting forceps: the side leafs or the end leaf may be removed and the whole plate may be shortened

Since they do not belong to the standard set, the reconstruction plates and the vertebral plates are not illustrated

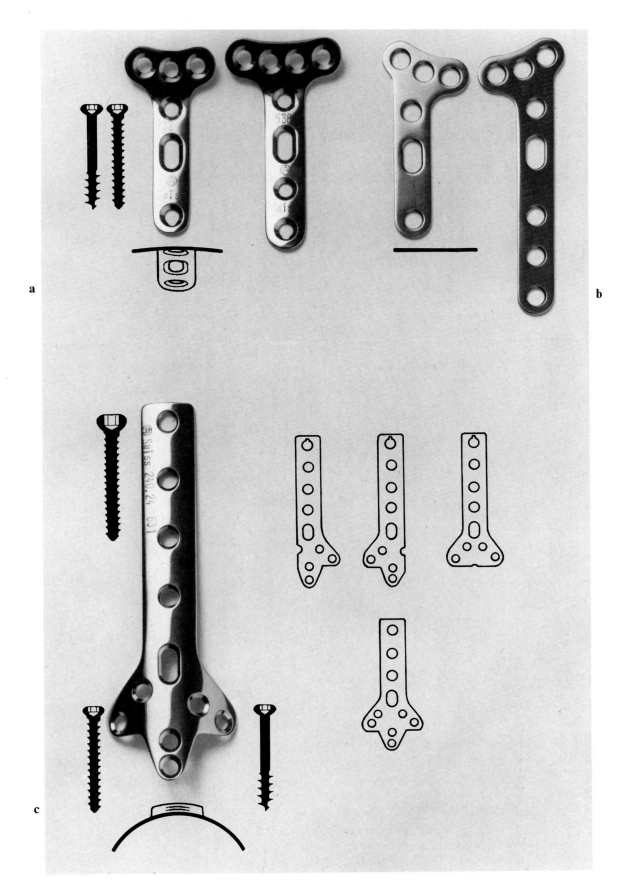

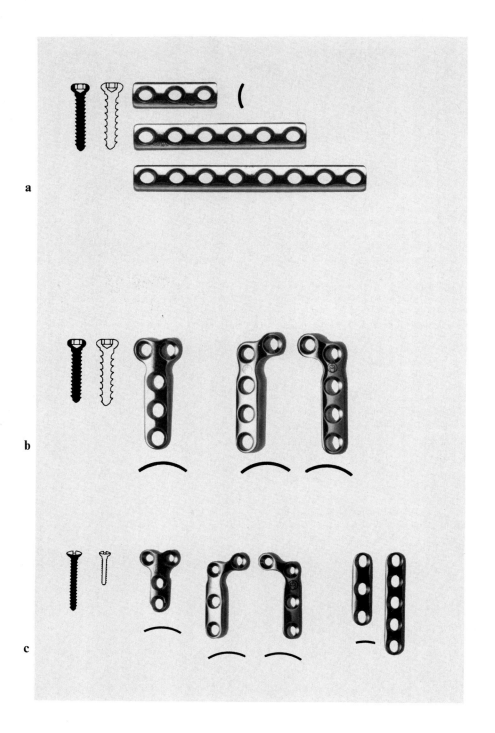

Fig. 7 a–c. The standard 2.7- and 2.0-mm plates

a The one-fourth tubular plate of different lengths in the plan view and in cross-section. The corresponding 2.7-mm screws (and exceptionally, 3.5 mm)

b The small T and oblique L-plate (plan view and cross-section) with its 2.7-mm screws (and exceptionally 3.5 mm)

c The mini plates: straight, T- and oblique L-plate. Corresponding 2.0-mm screw (and exceptionally 1.5 mm)

The 2.7-mm DCP is not shown, since it is not a part of the standard set

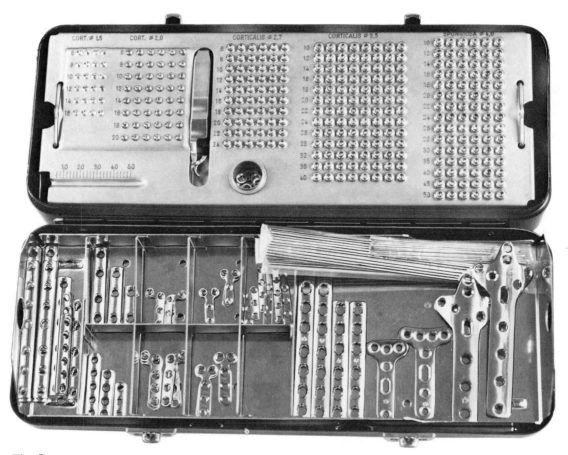

Fig. 8a

Fig. 8a–c. The cases for SFS instruments and implants

a Complete set: Case for implants

b Complete set: Case for instruments

c The reduced SFS with the 4.0, 3.5 and 2.7 mm dimensions. Implants and instruments are assembled in one case

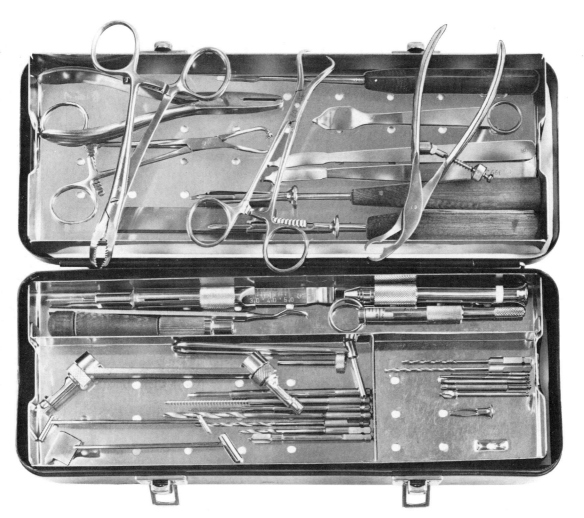

Fig. 8b [1]

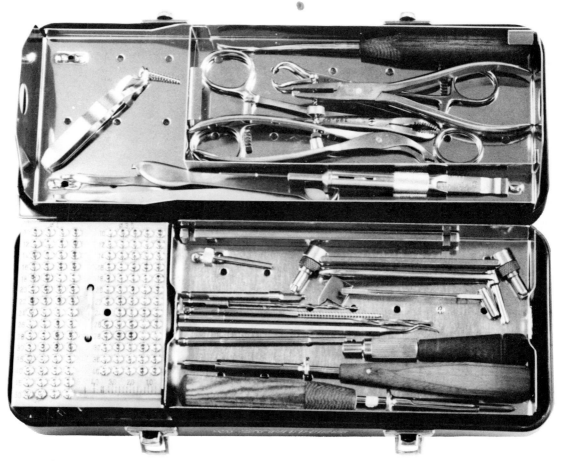

Fig. 8b[2]

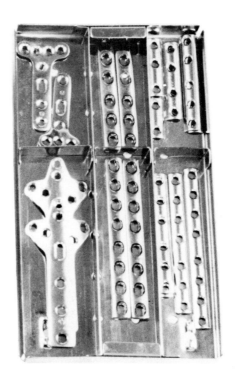

Fig. 8c

Fig. 9a–f. The standard SFS instruments
(reduced size, scale indicated)

a Instruments for reduction (Nos. 1–5): reduction forceps, holding forceps for small plates, small Hohmann retractors

b Drill bits in the 3.5-, 2.7-, 2.0-, 1.5-, and 1.1-mm sizes (Nos. 6–10) with flange for the quick coupling chuck. Drill bits of 2.7–1.1 mm are also available to fit the mini quick coupling of the mini compressed air drill

c Drill guides and tap sleeves (Nos. 11–15): 3.5-mm tap sleeve, double drill guide for the 3.5-mm DCP, 2.0-mm drill guide/drill sleeve, 1.5-/1.1-mm mini drill sleeve, 3.5-/2.0-mm insert drill sleeve

d Taps with flange for the quick coupling (Nos. 16–19) 3.5 – 2.7 – 2.0 – 1.5 mm

e The screwdrivers (Nos. 20–26):
– Screwdriver with sleeve for 4.0-, 3.5- and 2.7-mm hexagonal socket heads.
– The same screwdriver without sleeve with flange for quick coupling.
– Corresponding handle with quick coupling chuck.
– Phillips screwdriver with sleeve for the removal of old Phillips screws.
– Mini screwdriver with sleeve for the 2.0- and 1.5-mm screws with flange for mini quick coupling.
– Corresponding handle with mini quick coupling

f Other Instruments (Nos. 27–31):
– Small depth gauge for 4.0-, 3.5- and 2.7-mm screws.
– Depth gauge for 2.0-mm screws.
– Countersink tools for screws with hexagonal socket heads and for mini screws.
– Bending pliers.
– Bending iron for small plates.
– Small periosteal elevator

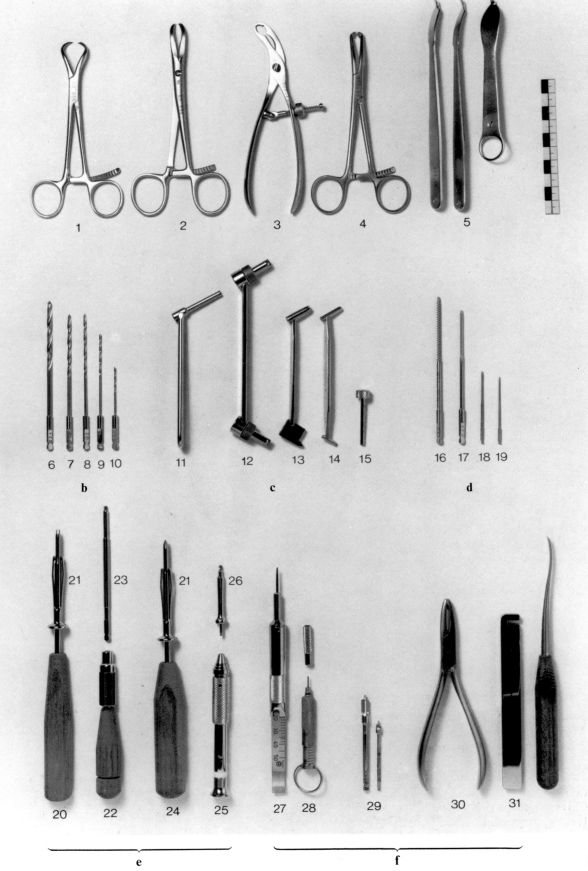

a

1   2   3   4   5

6 7 8 9 10   11   12   13   14   15   16 17 18 19

b   c   d

21 23   21 26   27 28   29   30   31

20   22   24   25

e   f

25

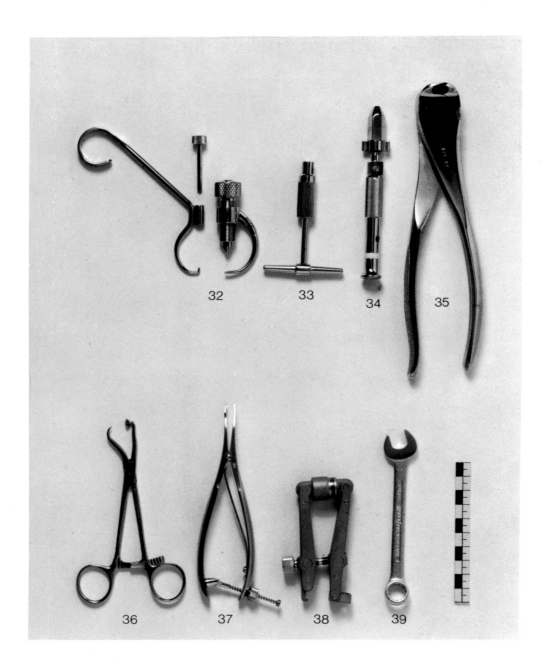

Fig. 10. Recommended additional instruments (reduced size, scale indicated)

– Small pointed drill guide with insert sleeve 3.5/2.0-mm (32)
– T-handle with quick coupling for tap and screw driver (33)
– Small chuck which holds larger Kirschner wires (34)
– Cutting forceps (35)
– Holding forceps for small plates (36)

– Bone spreader (37)
– Articulated tension device (38). It belongs to the standard instrument set for large implants but may be used for 3.5-mm plates as a tension device or as a distractor
– Openended wrench (39)

Other additional instruments which are frequently used are not illustrated

26

III. General Techniques of Internal Fixation Using the SFS

1. Fundamental Principles

The fundamental techniques of ASIF are laid down in detail in the *Manual of Internal Fixation* (Müller et al., 2nd edn, Springer 1979).

Extracts of this book appropriate to the use of the SFS are given here:

Rigid internal fixation is the prerequisite for rapid and economic healing, as well as for functional postoperative treatment. It may be achieved in different ways, depending on the nature of the fracture and the loading of the bone. The fundamental aims are to provide splinting and interfragmentary compression together with buttressing. In practice these principles are combined, seldom being used individually. Splinting chiefly involves medullary nailing or wiring or simple adaptation using Kirschner wires.

Interfragmentary compression may be applied by lag screw fixation, axially by using the tension device, or by the tension band principle, which acts by converting the asymmetrical loads of the skeleton into symmetrical loads by applying a plate or wire under tension.

Simple lag screw fixation, using cancellous screws, is ideal for large metaphyseal fractures and avulsions. In the diaphysis this technique is only applicable in very long spiral or oblique fractures, using a cortex lag screw. Optimal interfragmentary compression can then be achieved and thus shearing and bending stresses are neutralized.

It is very important to place the screws in the best biomechanical manner in respect to the fracture plane. The whole of the fracture interface should be uniformly compressed to obtain maximal rigidity. Screws therefore need to be inserted in different rather than parallel directions (Fig. 11). At least one screw should be placed at right angles to the axis of the bone; the others should be inserted so that they bisect the angles between the perpendicular to the long axis of the bone and the perpendicular to the fracture plane.

The commonest technique for stabilization nowadays is to use lag screws combined with an additional protection plate. This plate neutralizes shearing and bending stresses and adds to the interfragmentary compression by axial tension (Fig. 12).

Pure axial compression of a fracture plane is achieved by use of the tension device or a screw applied at the end of an oval hole away from the fracture (DCP principle: Perren 1969, Allgöwer 1970). The DCP principle (Fig. 13) has been adopted everywhere. Using this technique, neutralization plates as well as tension-band plates can be placed under tension and there is less need to use the tension device itself.

The tension-band wire, with or without Kirschner wires for splintage is gaining in popularity. It will be described in a later section of this book (Fig. 14).

In brittle comminuted fractures or in large defects, buttressing can be provided by a plate or an external fixator. The combination of a buttress plate with lag screws is widely used (Fig. 15).

In bony defects and loss of blood supply, cancellous bone grafts are often used in combination with internal fixation for their mechanical and biological effects.

The general techniques of the ASIF apply equally to the SFS since they all rely on biomechanical principles. The small implants call for a number of additions and modifications because of the topography of the peripheral skeleton or the smaller size of the bones. The three rules of stabilization are now explained.

2. Interfragmentary Compression with Lag Screws

a) Fixation with the Small Cancellous Screw

The deep thread and the large flat screw head can provide considerable compression of the fragments. The thread should only bite in the far fragment. The hole is drilled with a 2.0-mm bit and tapped with a 3.5-mm tap. In the presence of osteoporosis there is no need to cut the thread for the hole depth, as a 4.0-mm diameter screw can quite comfortably be driven in.

Example: Oblique fracture of the medial malleolus (Fig. 16).

b) Fixation with the Small Cortex Screw

In a relatively wide cylindrical bone the standard ASIF technique is used, though with a smaller gauge implant. The gliding hole in the near cortex is drilled with a 3.5-mm bit. The 3.5-mm drill guide is then inserted and the thread hole made in the far cortex with the 2.0-mm bit. The thread is made in this hole with the 3.5-mm tap, using the tap sleeve.

Example: Oblique and spiral fractures in the lateral malleolus in which individual small screws are used lag-wise in the lower fibula as in other long cylindrical bones (Fig. 17).

In small cylindrical bones both cortices are first drilled with a 2.0-mm bit and tapped with the corresponding 3.5- or 2.7-mm tap.

The gliding hole is then made by widening the near cortex hole with a 3.5- or 2.7-mm bit. Where the distance between the cortices is small, the screw easily engages in the far thread hole.

Example: Long oblique fracture of the metacarpal (Fig. 18).

Analogous procedures can be used with the 2.0- and 1.5-mm screws. The 1.5- and 1.1-mm drills are employed, the thread being tapped with a 2.0- and 1.5-mm tap after which the near cortex is over-drilled with a 2.0- and 1.5-mm drill bit.

Example: A small articular fracture or a spiral fracture of a phalanx (Fig. 19).

When the near cortex is very thin, the use of a washer is recommended to prevent the screw head from sinking in. If the far cortex is very brittle, the thread hole may be stripped, which can be felt while drilling or tapping. In such cases the over-drilling in the near cortex for a gliding hole should be omitted. Some interfragmentary compression can then be achieved by firmly tightening the reduction forceps before inserting the screw. With the 2.0- and 1.5-mm screws, very good stability is achieved by this method.

The countersink tool should only be used when there is a thick cortex or a very prominent screw head.

Stabilization Rule 1: Screw Fixation Rule

The rigidity of screw fixation depends upon the following principle: The fixation of spiral and long oblique fractures can only be accomplished with at least two screws placed in different planes. Resistance to tensile and shearing forces obtained by two screws fixing the fragment ends is considerably higher than that of a single screw placed in the centre of the fracture line. When a fragment is too small, two screws of the next smallest diameter should be used instead of a single broad screw. This rule applies to all sizes of screws (Fig. 26a, b).

Guiding principle: *Two small screws obtain a better fixation than one large screw.*

Exception: Perfect stabilization of articular fractures with serrated fracture lines can be achieved with a single lag screw (Fig. 26c).

---

3. Axial, Interfragmentary Compression with a Plate
(Using the Tension Band Principle)

Whenever the biomechanical situation is favourable (asymmetrical tensile forces), a plate should be applied on the tension surface of the bone, e.g. on the dorsum of a metacarpal.

If possible a lag screw should be placed in a second plane (Fig. 24b), or, in a short oblique fracture, one of the plate screws should traverse the fracture line as a lag screw (Fig. 22). It has been shown that much higher rigidity is achieved by this technique.

The One-Third Tubular Plate. After reducing the fracture and contouring the plate, drill holes are made. The first are drilled using the plate holes nearest the fracture. The drill is inserted at the end of the oval hole farthest from the fracture on each side, so that when the screws are tightened the plate is pushed axially away from the fracture and corresponding compression is applied to the bone (Fig. 20). The tension device (Fig. 10) may also be applied to increase compression of the fragments.

The 3.5-mm Dynamic Compression Plate. This thicker plate needs to be contoured with the bending press or with two bending irons.

Axial compression is again achieved by drilling eccentrically in one of the plate holes nearest to the fracture. To do this the special double drill guide is used, the ends fitting exactly into the oval plate holes. The green guide is first used and makes sure that the hole in the bone is exactly in the middle of the plate hole. This is known as the neutral guide (Fig. 21). The yellow drill guide ensures that the bone is drilled at the end of the plate hole farthest from the fracture if the arrow on the top of the guide points to the fracture. When the screws are tightened the fragments are pushed towards each other over a distance of 1 mm and the bone is therefore brought under compression. Theoretically the tension can be increased by eccentric drilling of one hole on each side of the fracture giving a total movement of 2 mm. If the screws are driven right home, however, friction between the plate and the bone is such that compression cannot be fully obtained. The small core of the 3.5-mm cortex screw is not strong enough to resist the bending stress of the plate, so it is better to use the small tension device if there is need to increase the compression distance (Fig. 12a). This instrument is also very useful for really accurate reduction.

The 3.5-mm DCP can also be used as a protection plate, as will be shown later. In this case all the screw holes are drilled with the neutral green coloured drill guide.

The oval screw holes and the spherical screw heads allow screws to be introduced obliquely to some extent – a possibility which is more pronounced in the longitudinal than in the transverse direction. In this way it is possible to put screws through fracture lines or to avoid separate lag screws (Fig. 21d).

Whenever possible the fracture itself should be compressed by inserting a lag screw through the plate at the hole nearest to the fracture. This greatly adds to the rigidity of the fixation.

Axial compression with the small plates in the hand and the foot is rather more difficult to obtain, especially using shaped plates. This is for two reasons: firstly because though reduction is quite feasible, temporary fixation with a reduction forceps or a thin Kirschner wire is difficult; secondly because the plate covers so much of the bone that the reduction cannot be easily seen. Secondary displacement may then occur after a good primary reduction.

As a rule we adopt the following procedure (Fig. 22):
- The open reduction is held in place by the assistant with his fingers.
- The plate is bent to fit the bone accurately, especially in the metaphysis.
- The first hole is drilled in the smaller fragment in the long axis of the bone. The position of this hole is decisive.
- The plate is fixed to the smaller fragment with the first screw.
- The plate, now having a firm grip in the small fragment, can be used to help with the reduction and can then be held to the shaft with a reduction forceps. The axial alignment can now be checked, and altered if necessary.
- The second screw is then inserted in the smaller fragment. Control of rotation may be obtained either by bending the plate or changing its position on the longer fragment.
- The eccentric hole can now be made in the large fragment and compression applied.

The screw being driven home, the forceps can be removed.

- The remaining screws can now be inserted into the larger fragment.

The purpose of this procedure is to avoid two of the commonest faults of this type of internal fixation, which are:

- Malposition of the axes when finger T-plates are applied. This is due to the action of eccentric tensile forces when the fracture is compressed before insertion of both screws in the cross-piece of the plate (Fig. 23a).

- Rotational deformity when the oblique L-plate is used. This occurs if the second screw in the L part of the plate is inserted after compression of the fracture by an eccentrically placed screw in the shaft fragment, which applies a torque to the smaller fragment (Fig. 23b). If in spite of all precautions rotational deformity develops, this should be recognised after inserting the third screw. The plate should then be removed and twisted to counteract the deformity. It can then be fixed with the same screws, and the last screw should only be inserted when the deformity has been fully corrected.

4. Neutralization or Protection Plate

The use of a plate for this purpose is common in peripheral parts of the skeleton, and any plate can be used (Fig. 25). The holes should be drilled eccentrically to give better rigidity.

Two different procedures are used for oblique and spiral fractures:

- If it is not clear where the plate should be placed, the fracture should first be reduced and fixed with a lag screw. The plate can then be bent to fit the bone and fixed with screws (Fig. 24b).

- If the point of one fragment lies below the plate, displacement of the fragment may not be recognized while the plate is fixed. This difficulty can be overcome by the following procedure (Fig. 24a):

- The fragments are reduced and temporarily fixed with reduction forceps.

- The appropriate plate is selected and contoured.

- An interfragmentary lag screw is placed in a hole which will come to lie in the middle of the plate (Fig. 24a). This screw has to be rather too long.

- The reduction must be checked, as well as the appropriate position of the joints, which must be flexed for this purpose.

- The screw is removed and reinserted through the plate but is not tightened fully. The plate should now lie snugly on the bone but if it does not, it should be removed and contoured more precisely and then fixed again with the lag screw to the reduced fracture.

- The remaining screws are only inserted when the plate has been found to lie accurately on the bone. This prevents secondary displacement and protects the plate against any bending and shearing stresses.

Mini plates are applied according to the technique for the small plates in the hand and foot.

5. Buttress Plates

In comminuted fractures and bony defects, plates may be used as buttresses. For this purpose a plate must have a solid hold on the main fragment (stabilization rule 2, Fig. 27). In such a case, cancellous or corticocancellous bone grafting is obligatory. The plate prevents any impaction of the bone ends.

When employing internal fixation with a plate, the screws should fix the main fragments with several cortices. As bending and shearing forces increase with body weight, the number of cortices that must be gripped to provide effective stabilization increases from the distal to the proximal parts of the skeleton. In phalanges three cortices held in each fragment are sufficient, while in metacarpals and metatarsals four cortices should be gripped. In oblique fractures in larger bones, five cortices in each fragment should be captured, while in transverse fractures six cortices should be held, as they are exposed to greater shearing forces (Fig. 27).

Guiding principle: *Distal bones, three–four cortices; proximal bones, five–six cortices.*

Exceptions:
- In transverse fractures with serrated bone ends in which perfect interfragmentary compression can be obtained, the length of the plate is more important than the number of cortices held in countering bending and shearing stresses.
- If there is cortical bone under the end of a plate, a short screw is sufficient, gripping one cortex only.
- When the concave section of the plate is acting as a splint on the diaphysis, stability is achieved by using the three-point fixation principle (Fig. 27 c), even with the smaller number of screws.

6. Combined Internal Fixation with Small and Large Implants

The transitional zone between "large" and "small" parts of the skeleton often calls for the simultaneous use of different operations and different implants, as in the distal tibia, the malleoli, the elbow or the distal part of the forearm. The SFS may be used on its own or as an accessory in achieving rigid internal fixation. The combination methods are mostly used in the tibia, where it may be necessary to fix small wedge fragments to larger fracture components without producing damage. Small fragments have to be replaced exactly in order to receive their blood supply from the adjacent bone. Experimental work has shown that completely separated small fragments, if exactly replaced, can be revascularized and incorporated as long as mechanical stability is guaranteed (Schenk, Perren).

7. Multiple Fractures

Multiple fractures are common in the peripheral parts of the skeleton. They can be mechanically independent ("autonomous fractures") or interdependent. When one fracture is predominant, we call it the "*dominant fracture*"; the other one, which is less conspicuous and depends on the first for stability, is labelled the "*vassal fracture*". This chiefly occurs in fractures of the second and fifth metacarpals, in the forefoot, in the malleoli and in the distal forearm. It is also applicable in some segmental fractures. A good example is the oblique fracture of the lower fibula in combination with a spiral fracture of the lower tibia (Fig. 28). Treatment should be concentrated on the dominant fracture, as all stresses must be eliminated in treating multiple fractures. The time factor is important in this type of internal fixation to minimize interruption of blood supply, development of infection and damage to soft tissues, and the technical performance may often be rather difficult. This leads to:

Where there is mechanical dependence between two fractures, the types of internal fixation should be differentiated. The dominant fracture should be reduced first, after which the vassal fracture will reduce spontaneously or can be reduced easily. Stabilization of the dominant fracture is obtained by a "load bearing beam" which also prevents any secondary displacement of the vassal fracture. Its fixation can be achieved by the simplest means, as with a single screw or an axial Kirschner wire and sometimes even this fixation proves unnecessary (Fig. 29).

Guiding principle: *Only the dominant fracture requires a plate.*

8. The Tension-Band Wire

"The tension-band wire provides dynamic compression and is indicated if it is able to neutralise all tension forces acting on the fracture, and if all the bending and shearing forces are excluded either by interfragmentary friction alone or by additional splintage with Kirschner wires" (*Manual of Internal Fixation,* Muller et al., 2nd edn. Springer 1979, p. 42).

Tension-band wiring is chiefly indicated for avulsion fractures and the fusion of joints. The Kirschner wires make reduction and provisional fixation easy. When the Kirschner wires are inserted parallel to each other, a better grip in the bone is provided and rotational stability achieved. The tension-band wire is passed around the ends of the Kirschner wires. A small loop should be placed in the middle of the tension-band wire

on one side and twisted up at the same time as the ends of the wire are twisted up on the other side, so that symmetrical compression of the fracture can be achieved. Flat-nosed parallel-bladed pliers are useful for this.

Typical examples are: Fixation of a fracture of the patella with a cerclage wire alone; combination of a tension-band wire and two parallel Kirschner wires for fixation of fractures of the lateral malleolus or olecranon.

9. Open Fractures

It has become accepted that skeletal stability and rest for the wound are essential for healing of open fractures without complications.

Selection of the implant depends upon the damage to the soft tissue and the contamination of the wound. In the periphery of the skeleton, choice of extension of incisions on the dorsa of the hand and foot is often limited by consideration of venous drainage on the dorsal side of the fingers and toes. Closing the wound without tension is much more important than covering the implant. In difficult situations the wound should be left open and only closed later. In the hand, skin closure by primary flaps is sometimes necessary.

The earlier practice of using provisional thin implants requiring a second stable internal fixation has been abandoned. In peripheral areas standard procedures may be impossible for topographical reasons (approach or circulatory difficulties). The relatively unstable Kirschner wire must then be used more frequently than in other sites. The temporary arthrodesis of the distal joints by fine oblique Kirschner wires is often appropriate. After-care is then often possible without external splinting. By using these measures we have diminished the infection rate considerably.

Fig. 11 a–c. Basic technical principles: Interfragmentary compression with lag screws

a Internal fixation with cancellous screws: Simple fracture of the lateral femoral condyle. One cancellous screw is fitted with a washer in order to prevent the screw head sinking into the thin cortical bone. Principle: When using a screw with an unthreaded shank, the thread must only grip the fragment opposite the screw head (see *Manual of Internal Fixation,* 1979, Fig. 12)

b Fixation with cortex screws: The hole in the cortex nearest the screw head (gliding hole) must be as wide as the outer diameter of the screw thread. The hole in the far cortex is tapped (threaded hole). Tightening the screw produces interfragmentary compression (see *Manual of Internal Fixation,* 1979, Fig. 17)

c Correct application of the screws: Long spiral fracture of the shaft. Interfragmentary compression must exert an even effect upon the entire length of the fracture. At least one screw must be inserted at right angles to the axis of the shaft. In cross-section the screws must be placed perpendicular to the fracture plane (see *Manual of Internal Fixation,* 1979, Fig. 21)

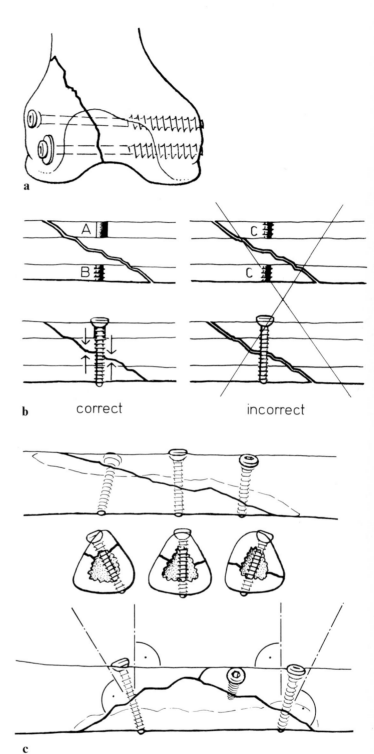

33

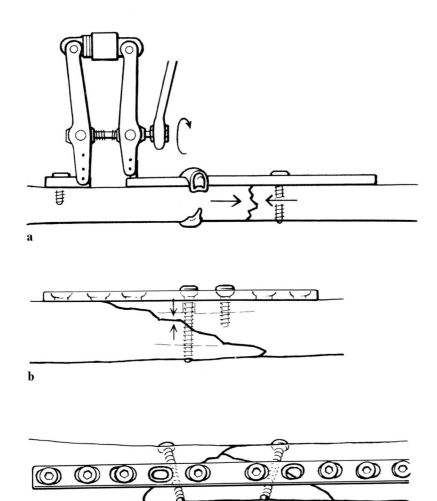

a

b

c

Fig. 12a–c. Basic technical principles: Axial compression by the tension device, lag screw through the plate, neutralization

a Axial compression by a plate: The fracture is reduced and a first screw is inserted through the plate near the fracture line. Then the articulated tension device is applied to the opposite fragment. By closing the tension device with the wrench, precise reduction and axial compression is achieved

b Lag screw through a plate: In an oblique fracture, interfragmentary compression may be produced by a lag screw through the plate, if the near cortex is provided with a gliding hole. By this screw the posterior fragment is pulled up to the plate, or the anterior fragment is compressed

between the plate and the posterior fragment (see *Manual of Internal Fixation*, 1971, Fig. 38)

c Neutralization plate in a fracture with a butterfly fragment: Interfragmentary compression between the two main fragments and the butterfly fragment is achieved by two individual lag screws. The plate, which connects the main fragments neutralizes the shearing and bending forces at the fracture lines (see *Manual of Internal Fixation*, 1979, Fig. 37). If possible this plate should be placed under tension by the DCP principle or the tension device

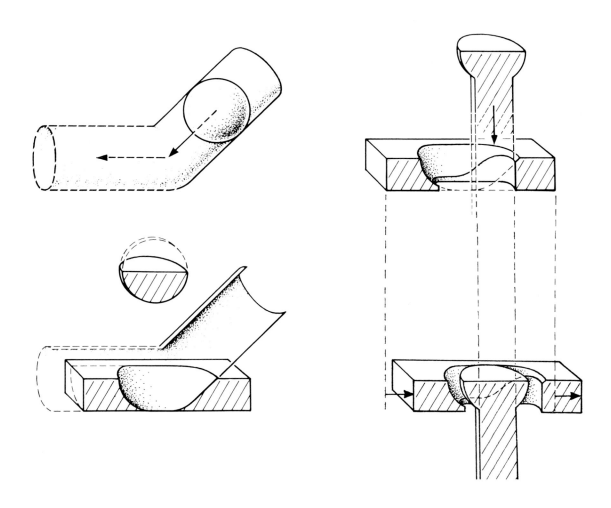

Fig. 13. Basic technical principles: Dynamic axial compression (DCP principle)

By the appropriate configuration of the oval plate-hole and using an eccentric drill-hole, a tension force is applied to the plate by driving home the screw. This principle is used for axial compression with the dynamic compression plate (DCP). This may in many cases make the use of the tension device unnecessary

35

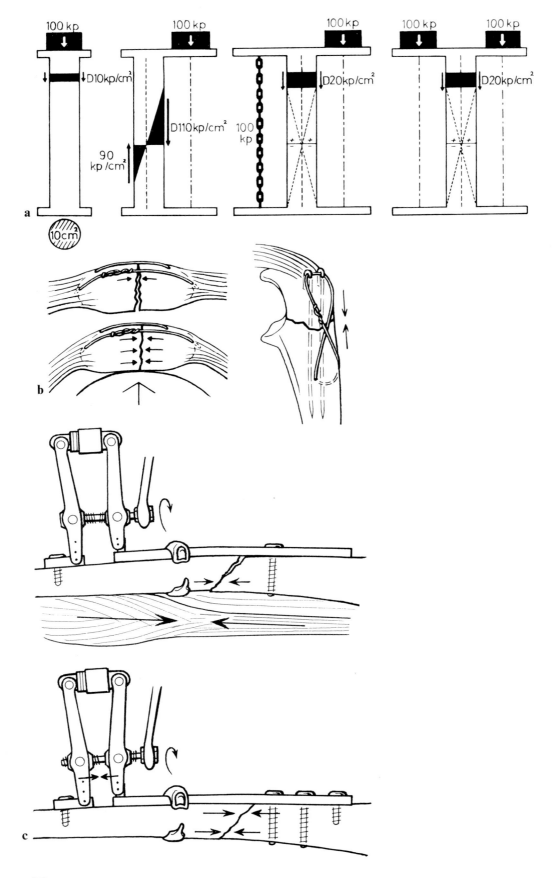

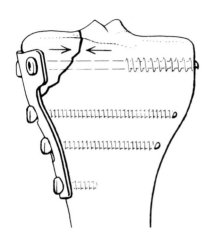

Fig. 15. Basic technical principles: Support (buttress)

The buttress plate prevents secondary depression of the epi-metaphyseal fracture. Typical example of support by a T-plate at the tibial plateau (see *Manual of Internal Fixation*, 1979, Fig. 54)

◁ **Fig. 14a–c. Basic technical principles: Tension-band principle**

a Model of the loaded T-beam after Pauwels: where the weight is placed eccentrically, it creates equal and opposite tensile and compression stresses in the interior of the column. These can be neutralized by a chain or a weight applied to the opposite side and converted into symmetrical axial compressive forces (see *Manual of Internal Fixation*, 1979, Fig. 23)

b Tension-wiring of olecranon and patella: The wire loop must overcome the tensile forces of muscles acting at the fracture line. Flexion of the joint produces compression of the fracture plane. Parallel Kirschner wires neutralize the shearing forces (see *Manual of Internal Fixation*, 1979, Figs. 25 and 26)

c A plate may also act biomechanically as a tension band. The plate is applied on the opposite side to that on which the main tensile forces fall. Interfragmentary compression on the cortex near the plate is augmented by the tension applied to the plate

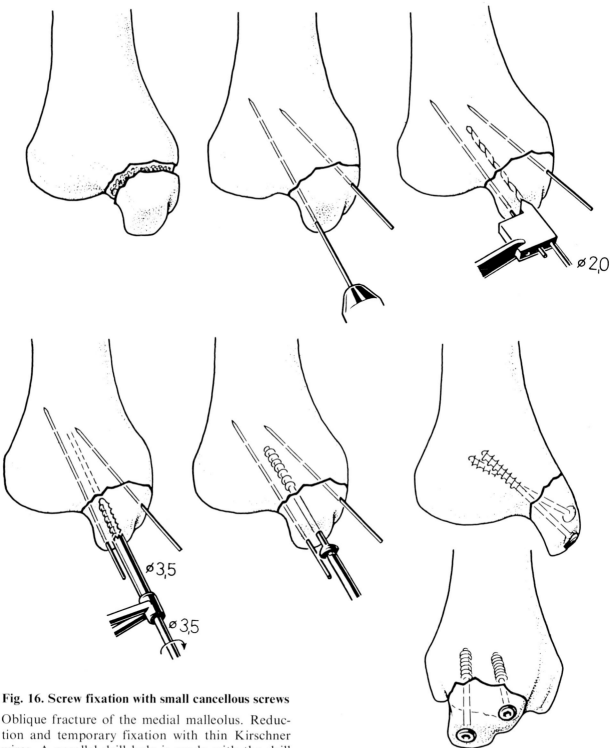

Fig. 16. Screw fixation with small cancellous screws

Oblique fracture of the medial malleolus. Reduction and temporary fixation with thin Kirschner wires. A parallel drill hole is made with the drill guide and 2.0-mm drill bit. The thread is cut with the 3.5-mm tap and tap sleeve. The first screw is inserted. The identical procedure is carried out with the second, posterior Kirschner wire. The Kirschner wires are then removed and the screws tightened

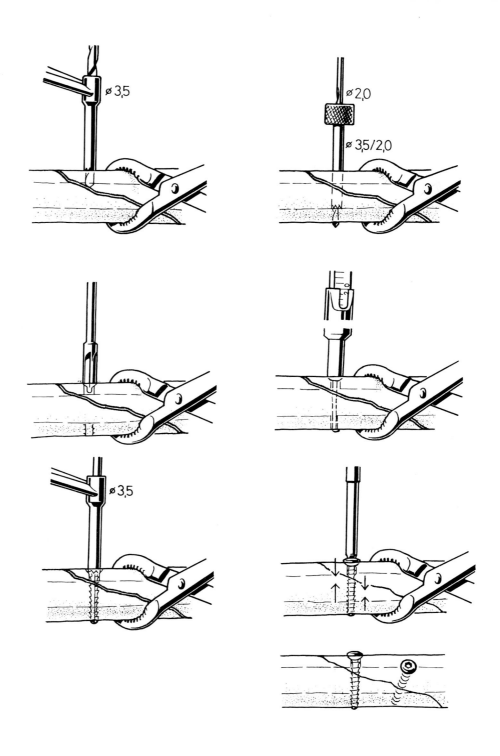

Fig. 17. Screw fixation with small cortex screws in large cylindrical bones

A spiral fracture of the shaft. Reduction and temporary fixation with reduction forceps. A gliding hole is first made in the near cortex with the 3.5-mm drill bit. The drill sleeve is inserted. The threaded hole in the far cortex is drilled with the 2.0-mm drill bit. The hole is countersunk for the screw head. The depth gauge is used to measure the required screw length. The hole is tapped with the 3.5-mm tap and the tap sleeve. After insertion of the first screw, the reduction forceps is replaced by a second screw

39

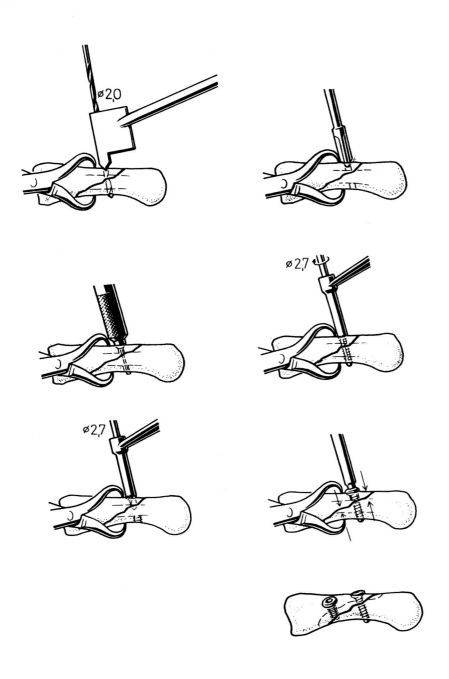

Fig. 18. Fixation with small cortex screws in a narrow tubular bone

Long oblique diaphyseal fracture. Reduction and temporary fixation with reduction forceps. Both cortices drilled with 2.0-mm drill bit and drill guide, countersinking the hole for the screw head. Depth gauge used to measure the required screw length. Both cortices tapped with the 2.7-mm tap (occasionally 3.5 mm) and tap sleeve. Over-drilling the hole in the near cortex with the 2.7-mm drill bit and tap sleeve (sometimes 3.5 mm). Insertion of the first screw. Replacement of the reduction forceps by a second screw with the same technique

40

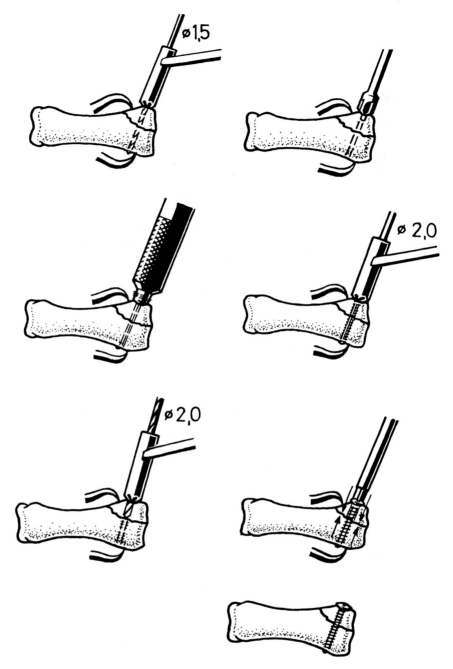

Fig. 19. Fixation of an avulsion fracture with a 2.0-mm screw

Both fragments drilled with the 1.5-mm drill bit after reduction and temporary fixation with reduction forceps. Countersinking the hole for the head of the screw with the mini countersink tool (optional). Measuring the required screw length with the mini depth gauge. Tapping the hole within both fragments with the 2.0-mm tap using the 2.0-mm drill guide as a tap sleeve. Overdrilling the hole in the near fragment with the 2.0-mm drill bit and drill guide. Driving home the screw produces interfragmentary compression.

The same technique is used for the 1.5-mm screw. The thread hole is drilled with the 1.1-mm drill bit, the gliding hole with the 1.5-mm drill bit. Measuring the screw length is not possible with the mini depth gauge in this narrow drill hole. A 0.8-mm Kirschner wire is used for this. Usually the countersink tool is not used. Because of the good grip of the screw, one may omit tapping the thread in some cases of cancellous bone

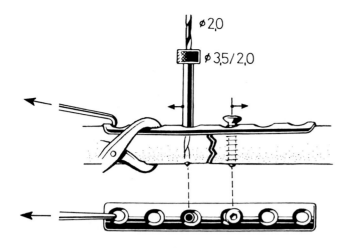

Fig. 20. Axial compression with the one-third tubular plate in a transverse fracture

The plate is loosely fixed to one fragment with a screw near the fracture. Then the plate is pulled to the opposite fragment with the help of a hook, so that the screw lies furthest from the fracture in the oval hole of the plate. An eccentric hole is drilled within the opposite fragment. In tightening the screws, their necks distract the plate, compress the fracture and put the plate under tension. This corresponds to the DCP principle. Since the plate is thin, the push and the compression are less marked

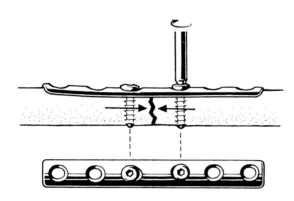

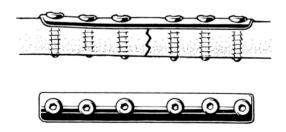

Fig. 21 a–d. Axial compression with the 3.5-mm dynamic compression plate

a The fracture is reduced and the plate fixed with reduction forceps. Drilling of the first hole near the fracture with the green end of the double drill guide: central drilling with the 2.0-mm drill bit. Cutting the thread in both cortices and inserting of the first screw

b In the opposite fragment an eccentric drill hole is made with the yellow end of the special drill guide. The arrow points to the fracture. The eccentric position of the drill bit may be checked by looking at the lower part of the drill guide, which is inserted in the screw hole of the plate. The drill hole is tapped and the screw inserted. Tightening the screw moves it a little way towards the fracture, which compresses the fragments

c Insertion of the remaining screws in the neutral position (green end of the drill guide). The drill hole is in a central position

d Angling of the screws in the plate holes in the axial and transverse plane. In the longitudinal axis of the plate, screws may be tilted up to 30°, in the transverse direction up to 15°. This prevents the possibility of hitting a lag screw which has already been inserted and provides an optimal position of the screws in the far cortex

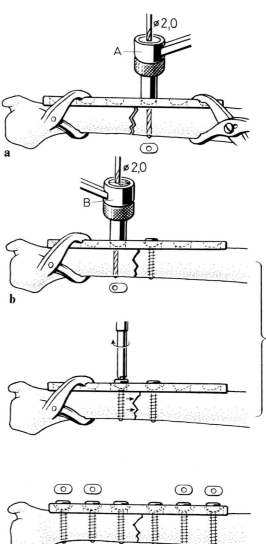

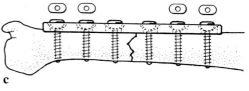

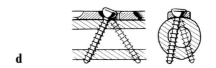

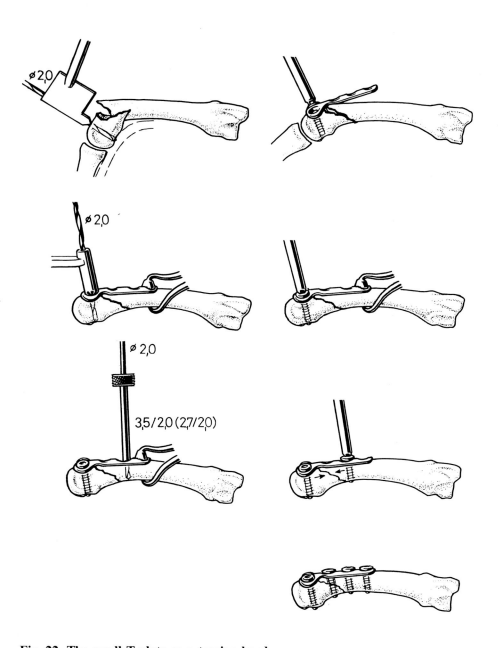

Fig. 22. The small T-plate as a tension band

Oblique metaphyseal fracture: After checking of the bone axes, the plate is fixed to the distal fragment with one screw. For reduction of the fracture, the plate is used as a lever. Temporary fixation of the plate with the holding forceps for small plates. The rotation is checked, and the second screw inserted in the peripheral fragment. Axis and rotation are checked a second time. Eccentric drilling away from the fracture in the proximal fragment (drill guide/drill sleeve or insert drill sleeve). The drill hole is tapped. Axial compression is achieved by tightening the screw. Additional stability is provided by an interfragmentary lag screw through the plate

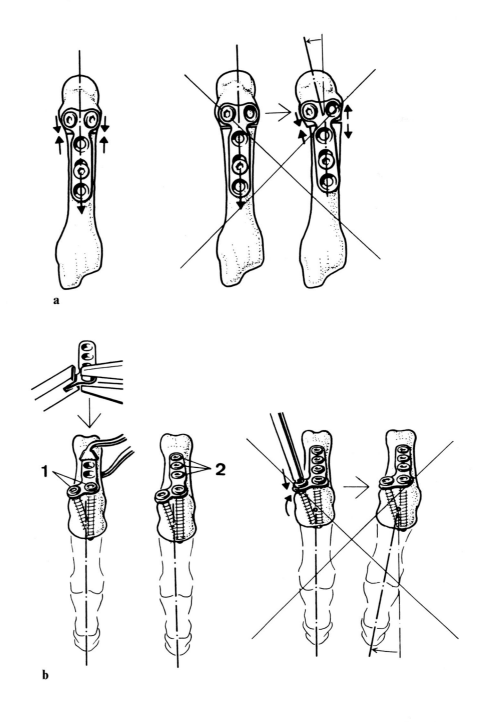

Fig. 23a, b. Two faults in applying the small plates for the hand and foot

a Small T-plate: Both screws must be fixed to the peripheral fragment before axial compression is applied. Otherwise the eccentric tensile effect produces malalignment

b Oblique L-plate: The plate must be accurately contoured to the surface of the bone using the bending pliers and the bending iron. Both distal screws must be inserted (1) before the final reduction, after which the proximal screws are driven in (2). If the procedure is reversed, the lateral distal screw produces an eccentric tensile effect which twists the fracture

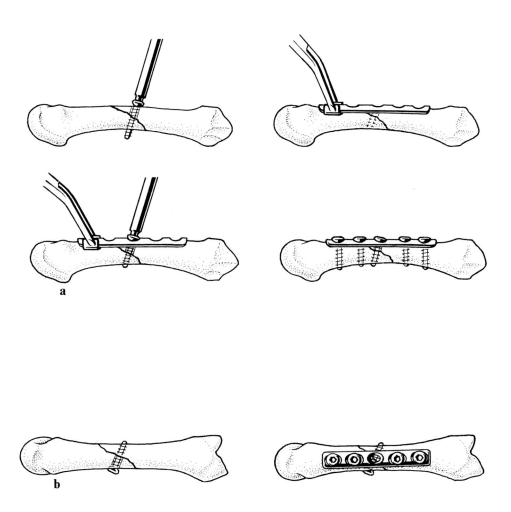

Fig. 24 a, b. The combination of an interfragmentary lag screw and a neutralization plate in a narrow bone

In an oblique fracture the plate may hide the fracture line. If the plate is screwed to the bone a displacement may remain undiscovered. Two techniques may be used to avoid this failure:

a When the tip of a fragment is in the plane of the plate, a lag screw which is a little too long is first inserted. Check the reduction and the interfragmentary compression. The plate is contoured to the bone surface, holding it with the holding forceps. Removal of the screw and reinsertion through the centre of the plate. Then the remaining screws are inserted in the neutral position

b If the tips of the fragments are not in the plane of the plate, interfragmentary compression is achieved as usual with a single lag screw. The neutralization plate is placed independently on the dorsal aspect of the bone

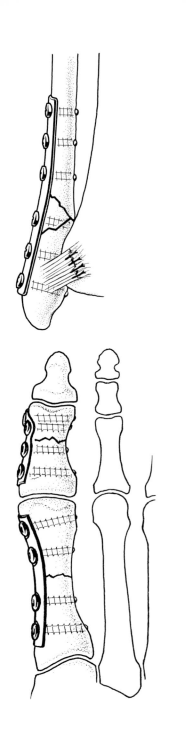

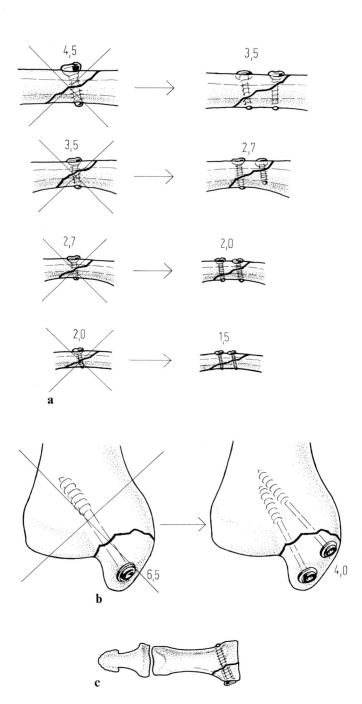

Fig. 25. Small fragment plates used as neutralization plates

The classic examples are type C malleolar fractures and transverse fractures of the first metatarsal bone or the proximal phalanx of the hallux. In the latter, the plate is applied to the lateral, not the dorsal aspect, which augments stability according to the tension-band principle

Fig. 26a–c. Stabilization rule 1: The screw fixation rule

a, b To provide stability two smaller screws are inserted near the end of the fracture line in different planes rather than a single large central screw. The gauge of the two small screws is determined by the size of the fragment. This rule applies to (a) cortical and (b) cancellous fractures

c Exception: An indented articular fragment can be fixed with a single lag screw

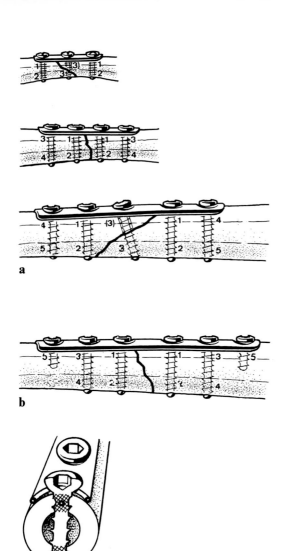

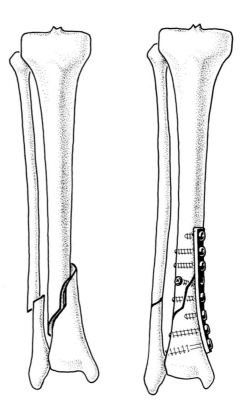

Fig. 27a–c. Stabilization rule 2: The number of threads for internal fixation with plates

a In phalanges, three cortices must be held in each fragment, in metacarpals and metatarsals four cortices. This number increases proximally to five or six, according to the type of fracture. The numbers in the drawing show the sequence of tapping and of placing the screws

Exceptions:

b In a long plate the ends of the plate have only to neutralize bending stresses. Therefore the screws at the end of the plate can be short and need only grip one cortex

c The fragments are splinted by the edges of a tubular plate. If this plate is long enough, less screws are required because of a three-point fixation mechanism

Fig. 28. Typical example of a vassal fracture in the larger skeleton

In a spiral fracture of the lower leg, the fracture of the fibula represents the vassal. Reduction of the tibia usually results in spontaneous reduction of the fibula which therefore does not require any further treatment

Fig. 29. Stabilization rule 3: Vassal rule

Mechanical interdependance of multiple fractures: The dominant fracture (metatarsal V) is being stabilized by an oblique L-plate, while the vassal fracture (metatarsal IV) reduces spontaneously. It is either left alone or fixed with an axial Kirschner wire or a single screw

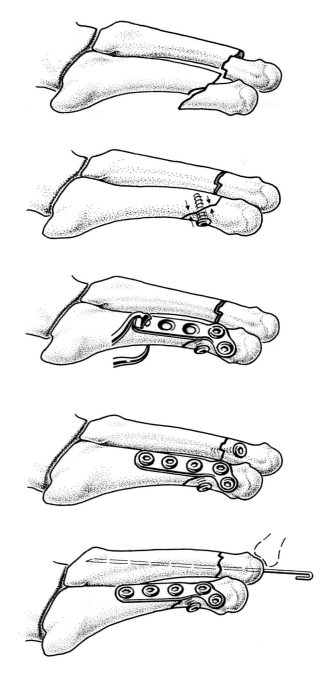

IV. Pre-operative, Operative and Postoperative Guidelines

There is a high tendency towards *post-traumatic swelling* of the hand and foot, which must be considered in the timing of the operation. Operation must either be carried out immediately, or after swelling has decreased, which means a delay of some days. Where operation is postponed, the skin of the operation site should be *disinfected* on the eve of surgery with a sterile alcohol dressing; one must, however, ensure that no moist enclosure results. Close attention must be paid to asepsis; the shapes of the hand and foot render disinfection difficult and unreliable. The use of a pressure device which forces disinfectant into the skin has proved to be suitable for these parts (Herold and Heim). This is especially important as adhesive plastic drapes cannot be used on the hand. The movement of fingers, especially in flexion, must be constantly checked during the operation to prevent any *rotational deformity*. A bloodless field is provided by a *pneumatic tourniquet* which should not be left in place longer than 2 h in younger patients.

The peripheral skeleton is surrounded by a thin delicate soft tissue layer which does not stretch easily. Careful protection of these soft tissues is even more important than in proximal areas, and the skin too must be protected from damage due to pressure or stretching. To obtain such protection can be difficult, as approaches are often limited and it may be impossible to extend incisions.

Problems of scarring are also significant. Scars on the outside of the upper limb are so conspicuous that cosmetic considerations may substantially influence indications. On the other hand, badly placed skin incisions can produce hypertrophic scars or even scar contractures. Incisions on the foot must be placed to allow comfortable walking and the use of shoes. Details are given in the special section.

Reduction and temporary holding of a fracture can be complicated. Here we use special clamps or very fine Kirschner wires, especially in the apophyses. Cerclage wires should mostly be avoided as they can produce nerve or tendon injuries. Sometimes none of these devices are suitable and we then have to perform "free-hand" reductions with the help of an able assistant. Sometimes a contoured plate may be fixed provisionally to one main fragment and used as a lever to secure reduction.

Skin is closed with Donati's sutures of Allgöwer's modification thereof, when one side of the suture is subcuticular. This helps in maintaining the vascularity of a precarious flap. Donati's sutures are, however, unsuitable for the thick skin on the flexor surface of the hand or the foot. Here it is better so secure accurate adaptation of the skin edges with fine interrupted sutures using such material as monofilament nylon. These sutures should be left until the 12th–14th day.

Suction drainage prevents postoperative haematoma formation but it cannot be used unless the wound has been made completely watertight by sutures. Air aspiration through the dressing jeopardizes asepsis. A large compression bandage with a short conventional drain, left in for 24 h, is often used in the hand and the foot. In this case a drain is better made of folded plastic sheet than rubber tubing.

Postoperative elevation of the injured limb is most important, and should be maintained as long as there is any swelling. A Braun's frame is satisfactory for the lower limb, and the arm can be conveniently suspended in a pillowcase (Fig. 30). Passive elevation should,

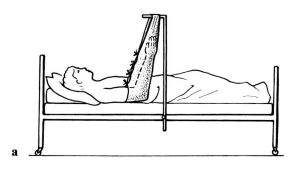

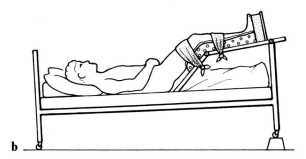

Fig. 30 a, b. Postoperative elevation

a Upper limb: In a fracture of the hand or the forearm, a reversed pillowcase is suspended on a pole. This provides elevation without pressure and gives free access to the finger tips which are free of the compression bandage

b The classic postoperative elevation of the lower limb with a sponge rubber splint on a Braun fracture frame, the leg being fixed with large non-compressing bandages

however, be interrupted every hour by active elevation for at least one minute and by extension and flexion exercise of the fingers to allow the venous pump to act. When the patient is walking, the arm should never hang down and a perfect compression bandage is then important. The sling may be used for postoperative treatment of the upper limb provided that active elbow and shoulder exercises

are executed as mentioned before. In the lower limb a well fitted elastic bandage is mandatory when the patient gets out of bed. After the first attempt at walking, the wound must be checked for swelling and haematoma formation.

Active mobilization of the joints is begun immediately after operation, as much as the bandage and the fixation will allow. The distal joints must also be moved, if necessary by assisted exercises. The shoulder especially must be moved since it easily becomes stiff by reflex action.

After operation patients should learn to walk with limited weight bearing, depending on the degree of stability achieved. They should bear 10–15 kg weight, never exceeding 20 kg. The injured limb must never be overloaded. The load applied to a leg can be tested on a weighing machine. In the upper limb all applied movement, e.g. shaking hands or rising up in the bed, are associated with stresses on the fracture. The danger of secondary displacement in internal fixation of the hand and the arm is considerable. Some psychological conditions, such as lack of judgement, obstinacy or laziness, may have undesirable consequences, and therefore individual management of each patient is necessary. Sometimes patients must be held back rather than encouraged but in other cases the reverse is true.

The time to begin actual weight bearing is estimated by the surgeon. It depends on the success of the operation but is more definitely decided by the monthly X-ray check. Bony consolidation of shaft fractures usually occurs between the 6th and 12th weeks. Full weight bearing means walking without crutches but in the upper limb it usually means the beginning of manual work.

V. Removal of Implants

It is agreed that all metal implants should be removed when their function has been overtaken by healed and remodelled bone. There are, however, several controversial questions which cannot be definitely answered by scientific proof. Removal of implants must therefore be considered individually in each case.

Metal foreign bodies implanted in the human body pose three different problems.

The Volume Factor. In the periphery implants are sometimes rather large and may limit movement and displace surrounding soft tissues. If they have to be placed directly below moving structures such as tendons, or near joint capsules or ligaments, they may produce relative shortening of these structures. They may promote adhesion between gliding layers, and by irritation produce bursae. They may sometimes hinder functional rehabilitation. The implant should be removed as soon as it is dispensable, both to provide more space and length and to enable tenolysis and capsulotomy to be performed at the same time, should they be necessary.

Implant Tolerance: Intolerance is due to corrosion or allergy.

Corrosion is produced by any metallic foreign body in contact with tissue liquid. In individual screws of the metal used in surgery, corrosion is minimal. It is increased as soon as there is contact between different metallic components, especially if they have different physicochemical properties, and in particular in the contact zone between screw and plate. Another factor which adds to corrosion is friction between implants, which must be reckoned with in any internal fixation involving screws and plates. The contact surface between screw and plate is very small in the SFS and clinical experience has shown that there is very little manifest corrosion. In the

Table 1. The average time interval between internal fixation and removal of implants in months for the different implants and sites. S, screws; P, plates; KW, Kirschner wires; TBW, tension-band wires. This only applies to typical fractures with uncomplicated healing

Clavicle	P	12–14
Non-union of the clavicle	P	16–18
Scapula	S	4–6
	P	8–12
Tuberosity of the humerus	TBW	4–6
	S	4–6
Head of Humerus	P	12–14
Distal Humerus	S	8–12
	P	12–16
Shaft of Forearm	P	24–28
Distal radius	KW	1–2
	S	6–8
	P	8–12
Scaphoid	S	12–14
Metacarpals and phalanges	KW	1–2
	S	4–6
	P	4–6
Tibial tubercle	S	6–8
	P	6–8
Intercondylar eminence	S	6–8
Insertion of ligaments	S	3–5
Malleolar fracture type C (cortical)	P	12
Malleolar fractures A and B (metaphysis)	S	6–8
	P	6–8
Talus and calcaneum, including avulsion	S	6–8
	P	6–12
Metatarsals and big toe	KW	1–2
	S	4–6
	P	8–12

larger DCP, however, some corrosion has to be expected, and has been observed in the larger bones.

Allergy had until recently been thought to be clinically irrelevant. Recent observations, however, seem to show that clinical or subclinical allergy to some components of the alloys may exist. Relation betwen allergy and resistance to infection is now being investigated scientifically. It seems that subclinical allergy may be an important indication for removal of the implant.

Alteration in the structure of the bone. This varies with different implants. The medullary nail and the medullary wire (chiefly used in the peripheral skeleton) are not very stable and may therefore produce callus. Simple screw fixation does not greatly alter the bone; changes in bone structure chiefly occur in plate fixation. The plate has been regarded for some time as an external splint and produces rarefication of the underlying cortex. Recent investigation (Matter) has demonstrated that active remodelling of the bone under the plate is partly due to vascular disturbances. In the peripheral skeleton these changes are fortunately minimal and must not be considered as serious as in the larger bones. Individual screws may therefore be left in place as they do not produce irritation of the soft tissues. This is also true for deeply inserted implants, especially if their removal is expensive or risky. In older patients, especially if they have a short life expectancy, implants may be left in place without hesitation. In younger patients, plates should normally be removed if at all possible, but cosmetic implications must always be considered.

When removing an implant it is not always necessary to re-open the whole of the original incision, but this may be better in difficult parts of the anatomy to ensure that the structures are properly identified.

The identification and removal of screws with the hexagonal socket is much easier than with the previous Phillips screws. This is also true for the mini screws with cross-slots and a central hole. Pulling cancellous screws out backwards may be best done slowly and in steps. The core of the screw may only be 1.8 mm in diameter, while the shaft may be 2.2 mm, and rough handling may thus produce a break at the junction between the thread and the shaft of the screw. The cancellous screw has therefore been modified recently so that the upper part of the thread is stronger. It is for this reason that removal of the 4.0-mm cancellous screw is advocated at 5–6 months. At this time the bone along the smooth shank has not yet become too hard and can be cut into by the thread when the screw is being withdrawn.

The optimal time for removal of implants is shorter than that for larger bones and is shorter for cancellous bone than for the cortex. In the hand it is shorter than for other sites as eventual tenolysis may be required.

Table 1 provides a guide to selection of optimal time for removal of implants.

VI. Autogenous Bone Graft Combined with the Use of the SFS

The use of cancellous or corticocancellous grafts is often indicated in treating injuries of the peripheral skeleton. With increasing experience, accepted indications for their use have increased in recent years: Besides the classic indications – to fill up bony defects and to give support in comminuted areas, especially in open fractures in the distal tibia and lower radius etc. – attention has been directed to their use in small defects of biomechanical importance, e.g. the end of the radius, the base of the first metacarpal, the talus and the metatarsals. The cancellous bone graft considerably accelerates bone healing and helps to prevent displacement and loosening of implants. Using bone grafts together with metal implants increases the biological potency of the operation and its stabilizing effect considerably by buttressing a fracture area when filling up a defect and by increasing the hold of screws in the grafted bone.

Where there are large defects of the skeleton but satisfactorily preserved soft tissue elements, as in a dorsal defect of the thumb and fingers, primary insertion of bridging corticocancellous grafts has proved to be very useful (Segmüller). Such grafts may be fixed by screws or fine tension-band wires. The details of this technique are given in the special section.

When internal fixation is employed for delayed union or non-union, or an osteotomy for malignment, the biological condition of the fragments must be considered. If there is strong callus present in a hypertrophic or reactive non-union, bone grafting is not required. It is only necessary to provide stabilization to secure rapid bone healing.

If there is osteoporosis, however, or if the fragments are non-reactive, fixation with metallic implants is inadequate. In these cases autogenous cancellous grafting is required together with shingling of the bone, if possible. In very bad osteoporosis a corticocancellous graft may be required to give a better grip for the screws.

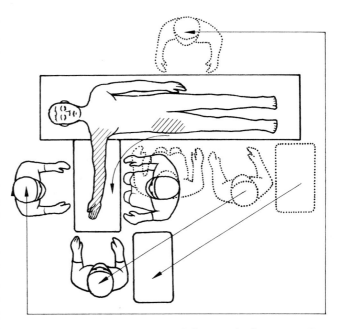

Fig. 31a, b. Arrangement of the surgical team and preparation for taking a cancellous bone graft from the iliac crest in internal fixation of the upper limb

a Removal of the bone graft (dotted line): The surgeon sitting, assistant on the opposite side, sister at the right of the surgeon

b Change of position for the internal fixation (drawn out): The surgeon turns around 90°. The assistant moves to the opposite side of the limb. The sister is between the assistant and the surgeon, the table with the instruments between the surgeon and the instrument sister

For operation on the lateral side of the arm or the dorsum of the hand the surgeon and the assistant may change positions

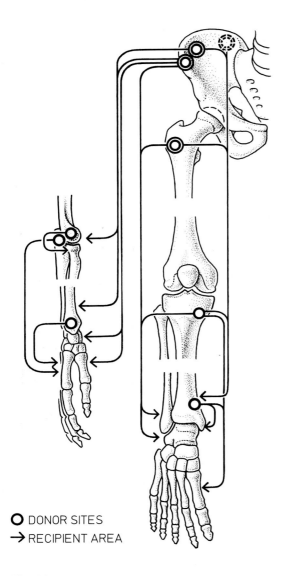

O DONOR SITES
→ RECIPIENT AREA

Fig. 32. Autogenous bone grafting

Donor sites and recipient areas in peripheral internal fixation:

Main donor sites: iliac crest, iliac fossa, posterior iliac spine, greater trochanter.

Occasional donor sites: lateral epicondyle of the humerus, olecranon, distal metaphysis of the radius, tibial head, distal metaphysis of the tibia

The surgeon must ensure that proper preparations are made for taking a bone graft before the operation. The donor site must be decided on and the patient placed in a suitable position so that this area can be properly disinfected and covered by drapes. It is as well to prepare a donor site, even if it turns out that the graft is not necessary. This means additional work for operating theatre staff, so it is important to discuss the possibilities with them (Fig. 31).

It is biologically best to obtain pure cancellous bone from the iliac crest and corticocancellous bone from the inner aspect of the anterior, and external aspect of the posterior part of the iliac bone. Even in elderly patients these sites contain haemopoietic bone marrow with the best trabecular structure.

There are other considerations, however, in the choice of a donor site: The volume of cancellous bone required varies and waste must be avoided. Tourniquet time will limit the length of the operation, and to reduce the chance of sepsis it is better to remove bone from a single site. Small grafts are therefore better removed from the neighbourhood of the recipient area but proximal to it, where there is a good independent blood supply.

Donor sites are thus often not the same as those used for obtaining grafts for larger bones. Besides the classic sites of the pelvis and the greater trochanter, grafts may be obtained from the epicondylus of the humerus for defects in the radial head, from the olecranon and the lower epiphysis of the radius for use in the hand and from the upper or lower end of the tibia for fracture of the lower end of the tibia or the foot. Suitable combinations of donor site and recipient areas are shown in Fig. 32. When epiphyseal lines are still open in young people, the choice must be limited.

VII. Use of the SFS for Reconstructive Operations

There are many indications for secondary operations on the peripheral skeleton. Peripheral fractures are less conspicuous and may be primarily overlooked, or their functional significance underestimated. The approved methods of conservative treatment, especially in the hand, seem to have met with too little recognition, or have actually been forgotten. Deformities of rotation, angulation or shortening call more frequently for operation than do pseudarthroses. Painful post-traumatic arthrosis, as well as rheumatic affections of joints, can be either corrected or made pain-free by arthrodesis. Here fixation with small implants has proved to be very useful and has largely replaced the application of unstable Kirschner wires, which often interfere with joint fusion. Good internal fixation often makes external fixation in plaster unnecessary. Intensive, active mobilization of the neighbouring joints and immediate partial weight bearing give surprisingly good functional results. However, this cannot be expected if there has been a previous long period of immobilization or if much osteoporosis or dystrophy is present.

In our experience, autogenous bone grafting combined with metal fixation is the safest procedure. In many cases, however, secure arthrodesis can be achieved without any grafting. The requirements are good vascularity, a broad contact surface on each fragment and faultless compression. From the different available methods, the most suitable can be chosen for each individual case.

1. Bone Pegging Combined with a Plate

This method is especially indicated for osteotomy and for the treatment of a displaced mobile pseudarthrosis, but less often for arthrodesis. The fragments must be mobilized and the medullary canal reamed in each and drilled through. The resulting holes are filled with a spindle-shaped corticocancellous bone peg which holds the fragments together, maintaining the longitudinal axis while still allowing rotation to be corrected if necessary. The osteotomy is then stabilized by a plate, longer than the graft, and fixed on both sides by screws (Fig. 33a). Shortening of bone may to some degree be corrected by pegging (Fig. 33b).

2. Graft Interposition Combined with a Plate

At a primary or secondary operation, a defect can be filled in with corticocancellous graft to occupy the whole width of a long bone, which is fixed and compressed by a posterior tension-band plate (Fig. 34). This method is indicated for bridging larger defects in primary or secondary operations. To achieve distraction in a lengthening osteotomy, the articulated tension device may be applied in the opposite direction (e.g. in the lateral malleolus). An external fixator can also be used for this purpose.

3. Compressed Bridging Graft Combined with a Plate

This technique is used in a pseudarthrosis or an osteotomy when pegging cannot be carried out because of restricted mobility of the fragments, or in an arthrodesis where there is defective blood supply. The dorsal cortex is opened and a deep bed made in both fragments, or, in an arthrodesis, in the metaphysis bordering the joint. This is done with a fine chisel or a reamer. Alignment and rotation must be checked first, as they cannot be corrected later. The prepared corticocancellous graft is embedded in the groove which should be slightly smaller than the graft. The tension-band plate is then fixed with screws, compressing the graft, which organizes quickly (Fig. 35).

A compressed bridging graft may be combined with bone pegging (Fig. 35c).

4. Excision of Joint and Subsequent Arthrodesis Using a Tension-Band Plate

This is indicated for arthrodesis in a slightly flexed position when a little shortening is not detrimental, as in the metacarpophalangeal joint of the thumb. A standard excision of the joint is carried out, the position is corrected, and fixation is obtained with a dorsally applied tension-band plate (Fig. 36). The thumb may be used immediately after the operation.

5. Excision of a Joint Followed by Screw Fixation from Proximal Distally

This technique is indicated for arthrodesis in mild flexion of 20° or more, as in the proximal interphalangeal joint of a finger (Fig. 37). The joint is approached by a dorsolateral incision and longitudinal splitting of the extensor tendon. The joint is excised with correction of the deformity. A Kirschner wire is passed pro-

ximally from the plane of resection and the hole made by the wire is then widened by the drill bit used for making a gliding hole. A place can be made for the screw head by drilling the dorsal cortex transversely, after which the gliding hole in the proximal fragment can be made obliquely to the plane of resection of the joint. The thread hole is then drilled in the distal phalanx in the appropriate direction, after which it is tapped. The seat for the screw head must now be countersunk and the screw itself must be long enough to grip the distal fragment and to compress the two phalanges lag-wise. The danger of displacement when the screw is tightened is only present if the bed for the screw head has not been properly prepared.

6. Excision of a Joint Followed by Screw Fixation from Distal Proximally

This technique is indicated for arthrodesis of the distal interphalangeal joints in a straight position (Fig. 38). A standard excision of the joint is carried out through a dorsal H-shaped incision with correction of the alignment of the phalanges. A hole is drilled in the distal phalanx from the resection plane starting with a Kirschner wire and then widened to the diameter of the screw selected for fixation, thus providing a gliding hole. A transverse incision is made over the finger tip 4 mm from the nail. The thread hole is then drilled in a retrograde direction in the middle phalanx, which can be done in a slightly flexed position. The thread is tapped and then the hole in the distal phalanx is widened to make it a gliding hole. A long screw is then inserted from the finger tip and tightened to compress the arthrodesis lag-wise.

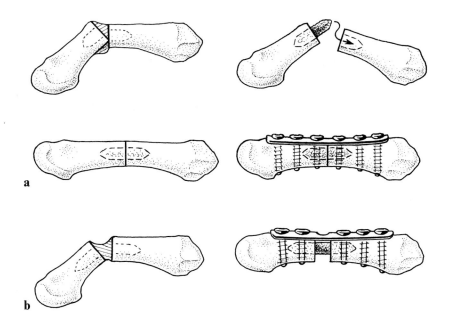

Fig. 33a, b. Bone pegging combined with a plate

a In osteotomy and mobile pseudarthrosis: Mobilization of the pseudarthrosis, drilling through both medullary canals, insertion of a corticocancellous bone peg. Screw fixation of a tension-band plate, which must be anchored beyond both ends of the graft

b In pseudarthrosis with a bone defect: bone pegging with an elongation effect

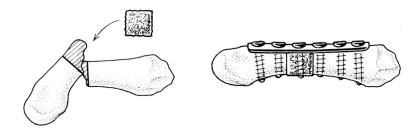

Fig. 34. Graft interposition

In a short pseudarthrosis, the defect is filled with a cancellous bone block, replacing the entire width of the bone. Two screws on each side guarantee plate fixation of the main fragments. The plate also stabilizes the interposed cancellous graft

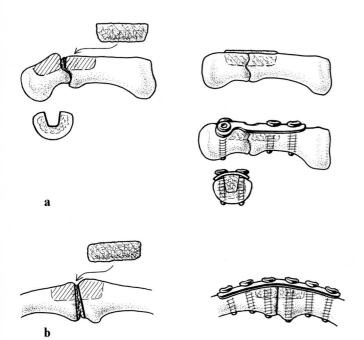

Fig. 35 a–c. Compressed bridging graft

a In pseudarthrosis: Opening of the dorsal cortex and drilling a bed in both fragments. Insertion of the graft which is slightly longer than the bed. Screw fixation of a plate, which must be longer than the graft. The graft is thus compressed in its bed

b In arthrodesis: Similar procedure to a. A dorsal bed is chiselled in both metaphyses. In most cases excision of the joint is unnecessary

c Combination of bone pegging and compressed bridging graft:
A distal hole is drilled to accommodate the peg, while proximally a bed is chiselled in the dorsal cortex. Compression is obtained with a plate which is longer than the graft at both ends

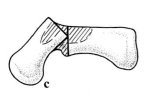
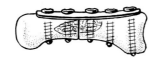
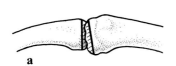
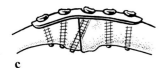
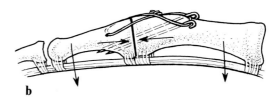

Fig. 36 a–c. Arthrodesis with joint resection and internal fixation with a tension-band wire or tension-band plate

a Typical limited resection of the joint to give the required angle

b Internal fixation with two parallel Kirschner wires and a tension-band wire loop

c Internal fixation with a dorsal plate. The central screw should cross the osteotomy and is inserted preferably as a lag screw

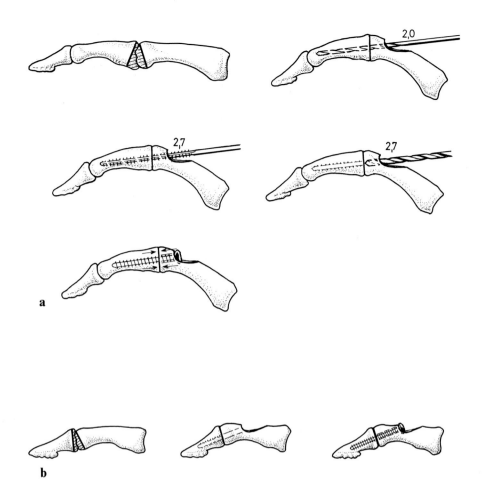

Fig. 37 a, b. Arthrodesis with screw fixation proximodistally

a PIP joint of a finger:
Resection of the joint at the required angle. Drilling of a wide dorsal groove in the proximal phalanx. Drilling through the resection line of the distal phalanx with a drill bit of 2.0 mm. Cutting the thread in both phalanges with a 2.7-mm tap. Drilling the gliding hole in the proximal phalanx with the 2.7-mm drill bit. Inserting the 2.7-mm lag screw which compresses the osteotomy. The screw head must lie within the medullary canal on the palmar cortex to prevent secondary flattening of the chosen angle

b Distal interphalangeal joint from proximal to distal. Same technique. The minimal angle of flexion is 15°. A deep groove for the screw head is of outmost importance to avoid additional flexion on tightening the screw

Fig. 38a, b. Arthrodesis with screw fixation of the DIP joint from the distal end

a Approach by an H-shaped incision. Division of the extensor tendon over the joint, division of the collateral ligaments and limited excision of the joint

b Drilling the medullary canal of the distal phalanx in a flexed position with a 1.5-mm Kirschner wire mounted in the small chuck. Perforation of the tip of the phalanx.
- Transverse incision at the finger tip, 3 mm from the nail.
- Drilling the medullary canal with the 2.0-mm drill bit (occasionally the 1.5 mm). Retrograde insertion of a Kirschner wire through the osteotomy in the proximal phalanx, watching the chosen angle of flexion. Drilling with the Kirschner wire may be carried out in the axis of the medullary canal or in a slightly flexed position. The drill bit will now follow the prepared canal.
- Tapping the thread in the proximal phalanx. Drilling the gliding hole with the appropriate drill bit. Insertion of the screw from the finger tip. Since the standard sizes are usually too short, screws of extra length may be asked for. Checking the rotation and compression of the osteotomy by tightening the screw. Suture of the extensor tendon and of the skin. Functional treatment without an external splint with immediate careful use.

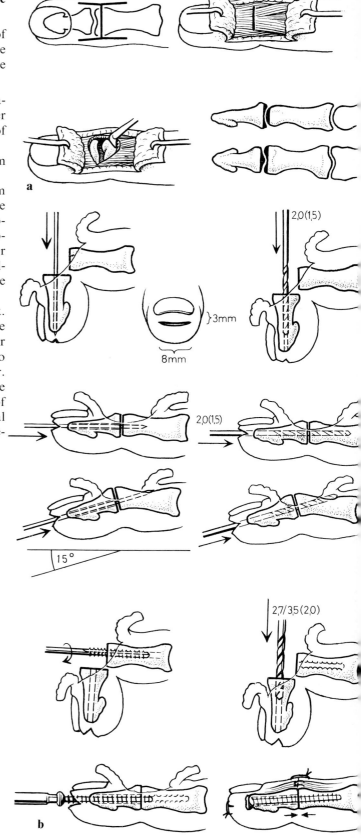

Special Section

VIII. Introduction and Overview

Fractures of the small bones of a limb and associated articular fractures are regular indications for the use of the SFS; injuries in these areas will therefore be described systematically. As small implants can also be applied to larger bones, typical examples of these will also be described.

There are, however, some internal fixations of small bones which cannot be carried out with small screws and plates. The semitubular plate is often used in places where small implants would normally be used. Tension-band fixation with wire is also used in the olecranon and the malleolus, where it achieves excellent results.

We cannot avoid repeating some material already published in the *Manual of Internal Fixation,* and figures from this work have been adapted to our purposes, but problems of positioning, approach and postoperative treatment are only dealt with in as far as they differ from those advocated with the use of standard implants.

Two types of examples are presented:

– *Technical examples* illustrate the fracture and its operative treatment, especially for malleolar fractures. There is a special need for precise descriptions of approaches and techniques, and therefore considerable space has been devoted to semi-schematic drawings of typical situations. Extensive research in this area has solved the problems of indications for internal fixation and the functional results achieved thereby.

– *Clinical examples.* It seemed imperative to illustrate actual cases and to this end a series of clinical X-rays has been added to each chapter, and described in extracts from the case histories to show the final result. These examples are intended to show variations that can occur from the standard examples illustrated. Besides our own cases, we have drawn on the extensive material in the AO/ASIF Documentation Centre.

In addition to the description of internal fixations, the indications and techniques for reconstructive operations have been considered.

IX. The Shoulder Girdle

Fractures in this region have increased as a result of larger numbers of traffic accidents and sport injuries. The scapula and head of the humerus are chiefly affected. For most of these injuries conservative treatment is undisputed, aiming chiefly at restoring good function to the shoulder joint. Immobilization should be as brief as possible and there is little place for the abduction splint or shoulder-arm spica. Besides the rare open fractures, internal fixation is indicated in avulsion fractures, unstable displaced fractures, and fracture-dislocations.

1. Clavicle

a) Fractures in the Middle Third

Of these fractures, 90%–95% are treated conservatively with a figure-of-eight bandage or clavicle rings. This fixation must be checked at frequent intervals and the function of the shoulder must be maintained. The few indications for primary internal fixation include open fractures, which are rare, a pointed fragment threatening the skin, an irreducible fragment, and finally injuries involving the subclavian artery and the brachial plexus. Internal fixation may be advocated to aid the nursing management of multiply injured patients. Fixation of the clavicle can also be very helpful if there is difficulty in respiration or if there are other fractures in the same limb.

Approach and Internal Fixation. Approach to the clavicle is always made through a sabre-cut or brace incision, giving the best cosmetic result in an area which is very susceptible to hypertrophic scar formation (Fig. 39). This gives good access to both medial and lateral fragments. It is important to protect the deep surface of the medial end of the bone as the subclavian vessels are closely related.

Reduction of a comminuted fracture may be difficult, and it is wise to fix any small butterfly fragment to the main fragment. Most fractures, however, are simple and oblique, and reduction is easy. Provisional stabilization with a reduction forceps is usually impossible. We always use the small DCP with 3.5-mm screws and the plate should have 6–8 holes. It may be difficult to contour the plate to the shape of the clavicle and the technique shown on p. 71 has proved to be very useful. The plate is bent to match one fragment only and then screwed to it and used as a lever. The first screw has usually to be removed once or even twice together with the plate until adaptation to the second fragment is completed (Fig. 39). The soft tissues must be protected by Hohmann retractors when the bone is being drilled and the threads tapped. If there is a defect or loss of blood supply, autogenous cancellous bone grafting is mandatory.

The plate may also be placed on the ventral surface of the clavicle. In this position damage to the vessels is less likely but the brachial plexus is endangered and contouring the plate to the shape of the clavicle is more difficult.

b) Fractures of the Lateral Third

If there is little or no displacement of the fragments, treatment is the same as in the middle third, with a figure-of-eight bandage. Internal fixation is indicated if there is much displacement, especially if the clavicle rides high over the shoulder due to rupture of the coracoclavicular ligament, in comminuted fractures which may lead to non-union, or if the acromioclavicular joint is involved.

Approach and internal fixation. The approach is the same as for fractures of the middle third and reduction is not very difficult. Temporary fixation can be established with Kirschner wires, drilled in through the acromion. Depending on the size of the fragment, stabilization is achieved with a small T-plate or a one-third tubular plate (Fig. 40). If the clavicle rides high, one of the screws through the plate should be driven down to get a grip in the coracoid process. The hole for this screw must be over-drilled in both cortices of the clavicle with a wider diameter than usual, to protect the screw from breaking under bending stresses when the shoulder is mobilized. If the coracoclavicular ligament is ruptured, which can easily be seen, it should be sutured before screw fixation.

Alternative technique: Instead of screw fixation it is possible to pass a cerclage wire round the coracoid process and fix it to the clavicle, or the plantaris tendon can be used instead.

The hold of a screw in the small, thin acromion is unstable and loosens very quickly. Tension-band wiring can be used for lateral fractures of the clavicle but long immobilization of the shoulder is needed.

c) Secondary Operations

These are mostly indicated for pseudarthrosis of the clavicle in its middle third or for deformity with shortening. Pain and limitation of shoulder movement are the chief indications for reconstructive operation.

Shortening of the clavicle is treated by interposing a corticocancellous bone graft and plate fixation (Fig. 34), while pseudarthrosis only needs simple internal fixation with a plate, as used in a fresh fracture. Contouring the plate may be difficult if there is a limited area of contact between the fragments. The fragments must be joined without force and malrotation must be avoided to prevent post-traumatic arthrosis in the acromioclavicular joint. The length of the clavicle should be accurately restored.

In a hypertrophic non-union the callus, which may need to be removed for reconstruction, can be used as an autogenous graft. In an atrophic non-union, additional cancellous bone must be applied. In all instances the 3.5-mm DCP is used for fixation.

2. Scapula

a) Fractures of the Articular Surface

Fractures of the anterior and inferior glenoid, which are sometimes seen as isolated fractures, may lead to subluxation of the head of the humerus. They can only be treated by open reduction in which the fragments are first stabilized with provisional Kirschner wires; fixation is then performed with small screws, sometimes supplemented with metal washers (Fig. 41).

The approach is by an incision in the deltopectoral groove, with either division of the subscapularis muscle or osteotomy of the coracoid process. Both structures are repaired at the end of the operation.

b) Fracture of the Coracoid Process

This is sometimes seen following direct trauma in traffic accidents, but repair is more often necessary following osteotomy performed to give an approach to the front of the shoulder. Because of the strong muscles taking origin from the coracoid, firm reconstruction is important. Depending on the diameter of the process a 6.5-mm cancellous screw with washer, a malleolar screw or a small cancellous screw is used, together with a tension-band wire loop alone or with Kirschner wires combined with a tension-band wire.

c) Fractures of the Acromion and the Spine of the Scapula

There is usually little displacement of these fractures but they produce considerable pain and may lead to non-union because of the pull of the deltoid and trapezius muscles. Lateral avulsions are fixed by Kirschner wires and a tension-band wire loop, but in more medial fractures a tension-band plate, usually the one-third tubular plate, is useful. Internal fixation allows active shoulder movements to begin as soon as the wound was healed (Fig. 42).

d) Fractures of the Neck of the Scapula

If the fragments are only slightly displaced or are impacted, the shoulder should be immobilized in a bandage for 1–2 weeks, after which active exercises are begun. Badly displaced or mobile fractures can only be adequately stabilized by internal fixation, and a one-third tubular plate fixed with screws to the prominent axillary margin has proved best for this purpose.

The patient is placed prone and the fracture approached through a slightly curved incision between the teres minor and infraspinatus muscles or immediately proximal to the detached infraspinatus muscle. The nerves and vessels to this muscle must be protected. Details can be seen in the *Manual of Internal Fixation* (2nd edn. 1979, p. 164).

3. Head of the Humerus

a) Avulsion of the Tuberosity

Operation is not indicated for minor displacement of the tuberosity as this heals with a few weeks of conservative treatment and may be used fully after 4–6 weeks. Open reduction is only necessary for widely displaced fragments of the tuberosity which become trapped between the humeral head and the acromion. Internal fixation is accomplished with small screws alone, small screws combined with a wire loop, or Kirschner wires combined with a wire loop (Fig. 43a). The approach is by an incision in the deltopectoral groove and the deltoid muscle may be detached to some extent from the clavicle.

b) Subcapital, Comminuted Fractures of the Head of the Humerus

Internal fixation is mandatory for an irreducible fracture-dislocation. Relative indications are gross displacement and instability, especially in younger patients. The clover-leaf plate has proved to be useful in some comminuted fractures of the head of the humerus, and with this the multiple fragments can be assembled atraumatically and given solid connection with the stem of the plate to the shaft of the bone (Fig. 43b).

The fracture is approached by a wide incision in the delto-pectoral groove. The coracoid process should usually be osteomized. If the reduction is difficult the subscapularis and the long head of biceps may be divided. For reconstruction the tendon of the long head should be sutured to the tendon of the short head. A cancellous bone graft should be applied whenever there is a defect.

4. Clinical X-ray Examples: Figs. 44–48

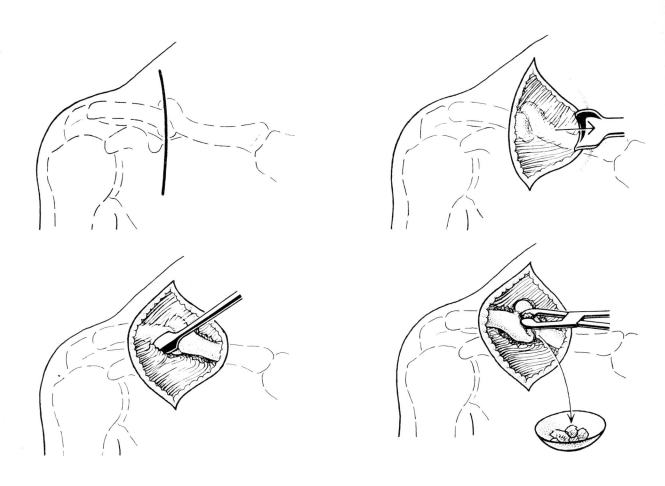

Fig. 39. Internal fixation of a hypertrophic pseudarthrosis of the clavicle

Approach is through a sagittal incision over the pseudarthrosis. Exposure of the fragments by alternate retraction of the wound edges. Detachment of the muscles with a periosteal elevator. Excision of the hypertrophic callus with a Luer forceps. Elevation of the fragments and preparation of their posterior surface.

Reduction of the fragments, checking the length and rotation. Contouring of a 3.5-mm DCP and temporary fixation with a screw to one fragment, protecting the underlying soft tissues with a Hohmann retractor. Removal of the screw and correction of the bend and twist of the plate. Fixation of the plate with screws. The previously removed pieces of callus are packed against the fracture site. Finally the insertions of the muscles and the skin are sutured

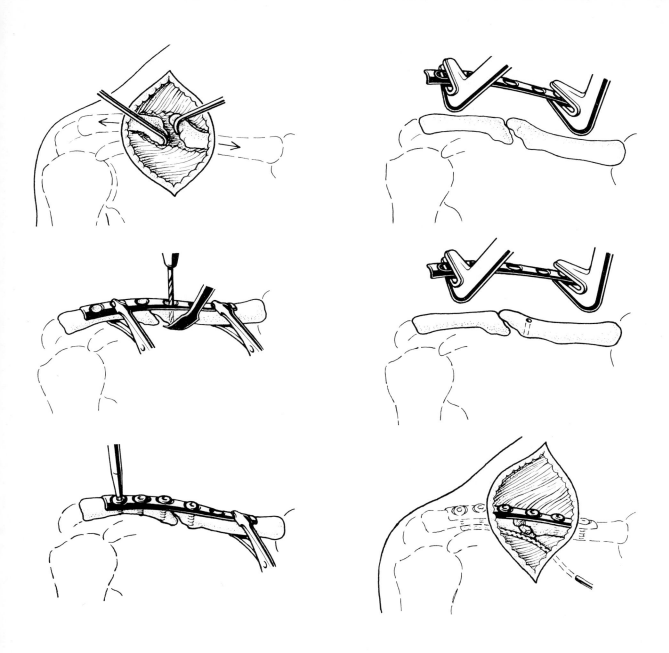

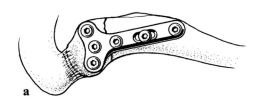

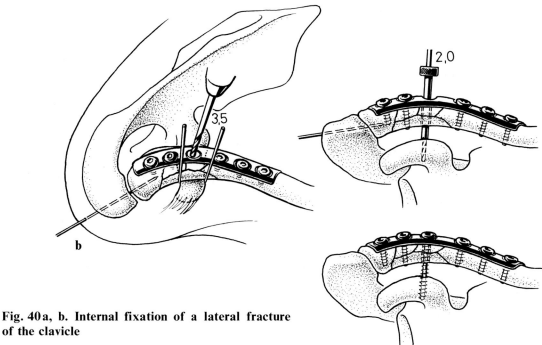

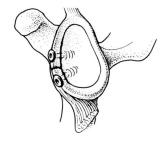

Fig. 40a, b. Internal fixation of a lateral fracture of the clavicle

a Lateral transverse fracture: Internal fixation with a transverse or oblique 3.5-mm T-plate. Three screws must be inserted in the broad, thin-walled lateral fragment

b Comminuted lateral fracture: Internal fixation is achieved with a one-third tubular plate, anchored to the coracoid process. Reduction of the fracture and, if there is instability of the acromioclavicular joint, temporary transfixion with a Kirschner wire is carried out. Contouring of a long one-third tubular plate which is temporarily fixed to the clavicle. The coracoid process is marked with two Kirschner wires, which are put in on both sides. Drilling of a 3.5-mm gliding hole through the plate over the process. Inserting the straight drill sleeve and drilling of the coracoid process with the 2.0-mm drill bit. Insertion of a cortex screw, which pulls the plate to the coracoid process. It is important to have a gliding hole in the clavicle of sufficient width to prevent the screw breaking during movements of the shoulder. If a larger screw has to be used for better stability then the drill hole in the clavicle must be correspondingly wider

Fig. 41. Screw fixation of the limbus of the scapula

Fixation of the limbus with two small cancellous screws is the operation for recurrent dislocation of the shoulder.
The same procedure is used in fractures of the anterior border of the glenoid in fracture-dislocation of the head of the humerus

72

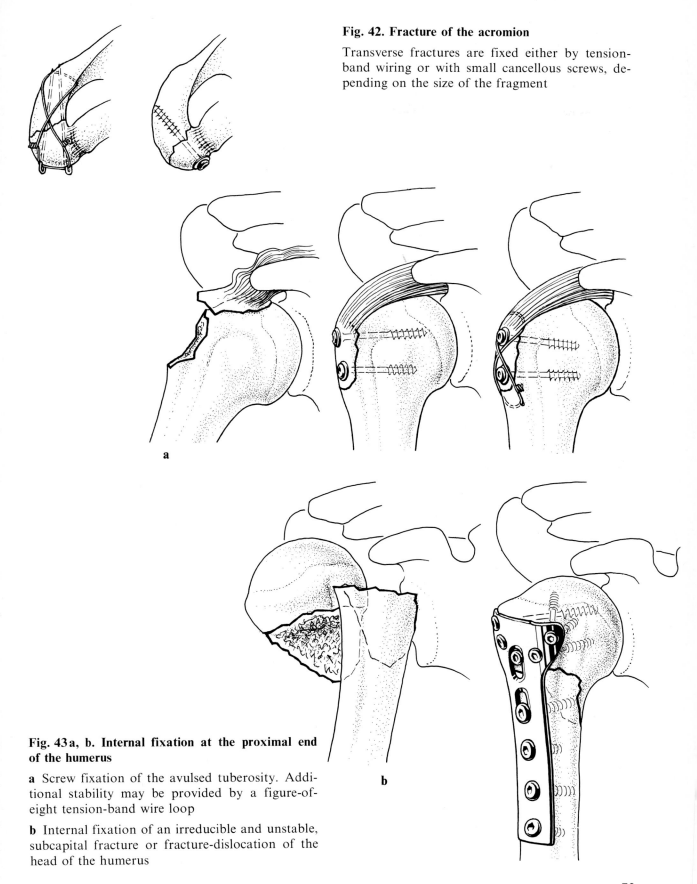

Fig. 42. Fracture of the acromion

Transverse fractures are fixed either by tension-band wiring or with small cancellous screws, depending on the size of the fragment

Fig. 43a, b. Internal fixation at the proximal end of the humerus

a Screw fixation of the avulsed tuberosity. Additional stability may be provided by a figure-of-eight tension-band wire loop

b Internal fixation of an irreducible and unstable, subcapital fracture or fracture-dislocation of the head of the humerus

73

Fig. 44a–c. Clinical example: fracture of the middle third of the clavicle

B., Karl, a 42-year-old civil servant. Fall on the shoulder in a football game

a Comminuted fracture of the middle third of the clavicle. Perforation of the skin is threatened

b Unsuccessful attempt at reduction. Internal fixation using a 3.5-mm DCP with eight holes and two separate 3.5-mm lag screws.
Uneventful course. Functional postoperative treatment. Back at work as a civil servant after 2 weeks. Unrestricted mobility of the shoulder achieved after 8 weeks

c Final review after 9 months: No pain. Inconspicuous scar. Full mobility of the shoulder. Primary fracture healing. Removal of the metal arranged

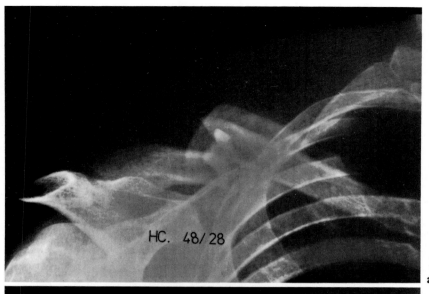

a

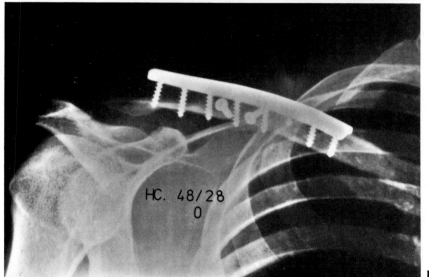

b

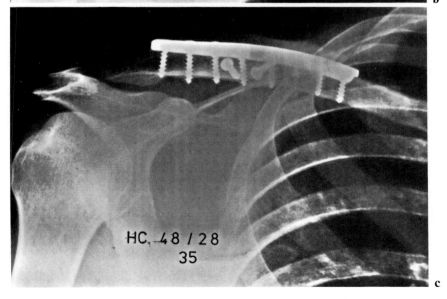

c

75

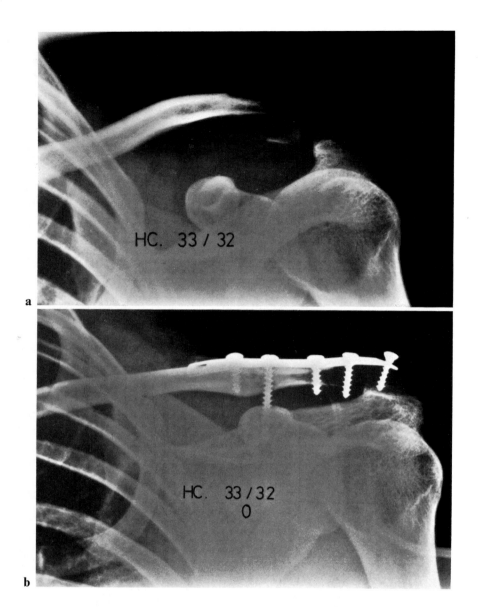

Fig. 45a–e. Clinical example: Lateral fracture of the clavicle with damage to the acromioclavicular joint

M.P., Anita, 26-year-old needlework teacher. Fall on the shoulder in gymnastics. Concussion

a Lateral fracture of the clavicle with upward displacement due to rupture of the coracoclavicular ligament

b Internal fixation after 2 days: Open reduction and stabilization with a contoured one-third tubular plate. Anchoring of a screw passed through the plate into the coracoid process.
Uneventful course. Relative fixation with a sling on discharge from hospital

c 2 weeks after operation, the screw in the acromion is loose and is removed through a small incision

d Full working capacity and mobility of the joint. Removal of the implants after 5 months

e Final review at $3^{1}/_{2}$ years. Unlimited mobility of the shoulder. Inconspicuous scar. Full activity in gymnastics. A little subclavicular calcification of the soft tissues is seen on X-ray

76

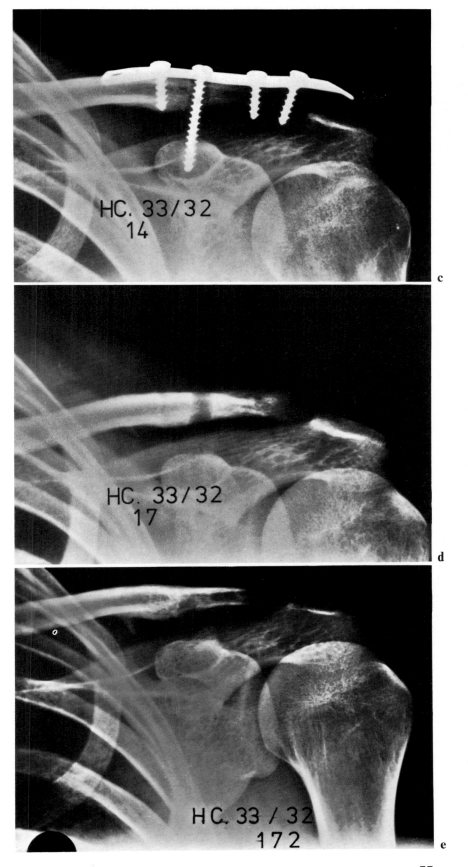

c

d

e

77

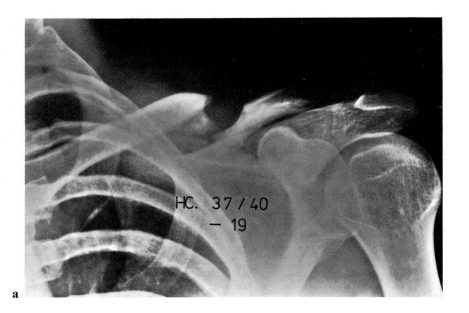

a

Fig. 46 a–d. Clinical example: Pseudarthrosis of the clavicle with bone defect

B., Pius, 28-year-old policeman. Motorcycle accident. Concussion, fracture of the clavicle, which has not been treated. Pain in the shoulder and limited strength of the left arm. Almost 2 years later the diagnosis of pseudarthrosis is made

a Pseudarthrosis of the left clavicle with bone defect

b Two years after the injury internal fixation with a 3.5-mm DCP with eight holes. Six cortices are drilled in each fragment. The defect is filled with an autogenous cancellous bone graft from the iliac crest. Uneventful course. Full capacity for work and full lifting power after 8 weeks

c Review and removal of the implants after 1 year: Full and painless mobility, linear scar, the pseudarthrosis is healed

d Review after 3 years: The structure of the bone has become normal. The patient has participated in two ski marathon competitions

78

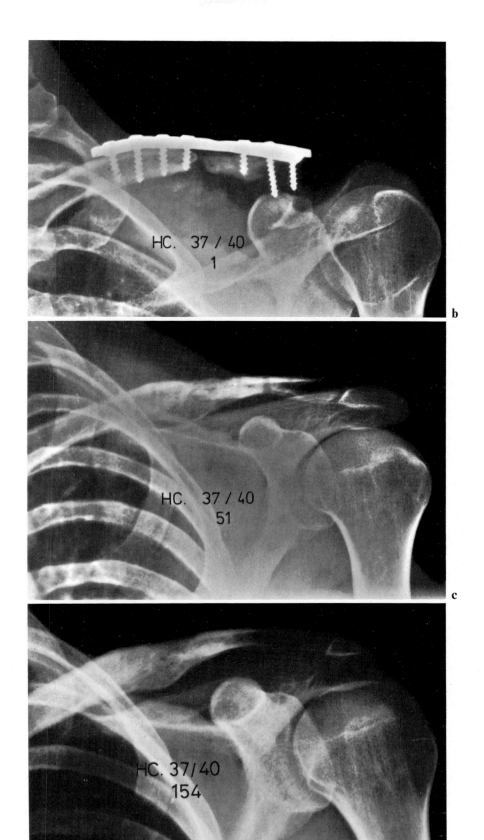

b

c

d

79

Fig. 47 a–c. Clinical example: Fracture of the anterior edge of the glenoid

N., Liselotte, 43-year-old secretary. Fall on the right shoulder while skating. Two days later was first seen by a doctor, who referred her to hospital

a Fracture of the anterior edge of the glenoid

b Internal fixation 3 days after injury. The displaced and mobile fragment is reduced and fixed with three small cancellous screws. Osteotomy of the coracoid process for the approach, and reconstruction with a malleolar screw and a washer.
Uncomplicated course. Pendulum exercises of the arm after one week, active mobilization from the 3rd week

c Review and removal of the metal after 6 months. Some limitation of elevation of the arm and of rotation. Small linear scar. Removal of the screw from the coracoid process. No removal of the deep screws is proposed

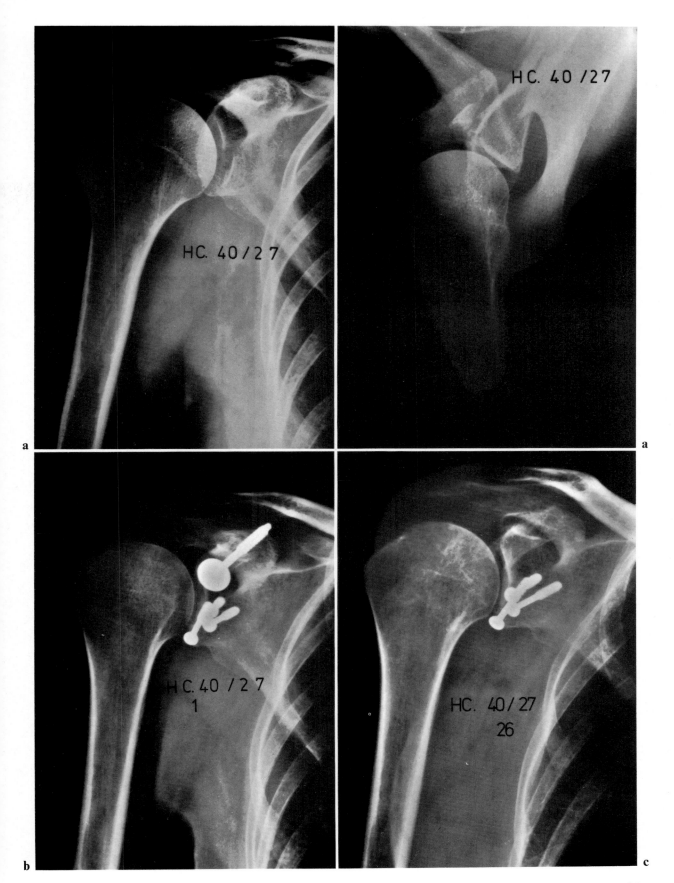

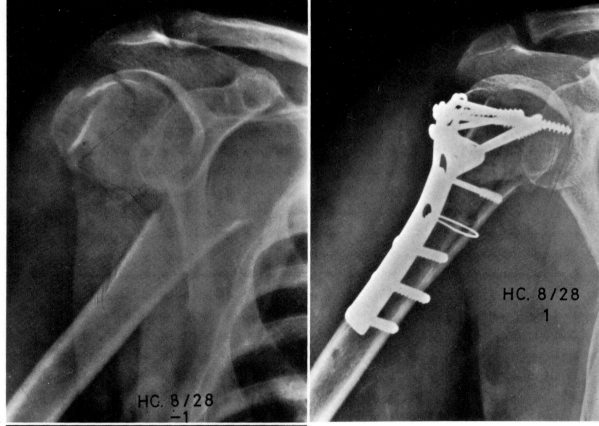

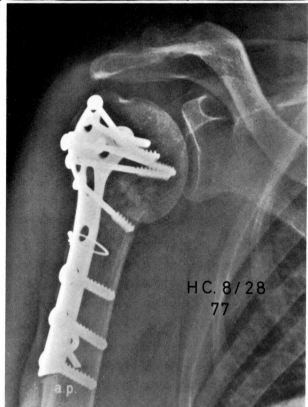

Fig. 48 a–c. Clinical example: Internal fixation of a subcapital fracture of the humerus with the clover leaf plate

W., Rosa, 58-year-old housewife. Fall on icy steps

a Grossly displaced and very mobile subcapital fracture of the humerus. In the same limb a Colles fracture of the radius is not yet healed, movements are limited and there is some circulatory disturbance

b Internal fixation with a clover leaf plate at 4 days. Uneventful course, functional postoperative treatment

c X-ray after $1^1/_2$ years shows a healed fracture in slight varus. The patient refuses the removal of the implants

At 8 years the patient claims to have painless full function of the shoulder. She refuses a review examination and an X-ray, which she considers unnecessary in view of her condition

X. The Elbow

The elbow consists of three joints: the hinge between olecranon and trochlea, which allows flexion and extension; the proximal radio-ulnar joint, which has some of the functions of a ball bearing joint and allows pronation and supination; and the radiohumeral joint, which takes part in both movements and transfers stress from the radius to the humerus via the discoid articular surface and which is largely responsible for the stability of the hinge joint.

Limitation of extension and flexion of the elbow can be compensated for by the patient but limitation of pronation and supination is very disabling. The small steps in the articular surface, and especially instability of the joint, can give rise to bad post-traumatic arthrosis, especially in the radial head.

Fractures of the elbow are mostly unstable and in adults can seldom be accurately reduced by conservative means. SFS implants have an important place in the stabilization of these slender bony structures. Operative treatment has proved to be effective and the technical details are therefore described. Figure 49 shows two typical positions for internal fixation of the elbow.

1. Distal Humerus

a) Fractures of the Condyles and Avulsion Fractures of the Epicondyles

These fractures, which often occur in adolescents and children, must be accurately reduced to prevent later malalignment. The strong muscular attachments to bony fragments in adults may also cause considerable displacement. Bony fragments can be displaced and

enter the joint. The indications for operative treatment are therefore absolutely clear.

Access is obtained by a medial or lateral incision. In the medial approach the first step is to isolate and protect the ulnar nerve. Fixation is with small cancellous screws or in adults with 3.5-mm cortex screws, sometimes with a washer (Fig. 50).

b) Intra-articular Fractures of the Lower End of the Humerus

Internal fixation is indisputably indicated for these fractures which are of two different types.

The Simple "Y" Fracture with Slight Displacement

A bilateral approach is used and the fracture stabilized with lag screws alone and this is often enough in this fracture. The best method is to use small cancellous screws for the trochlea and long malleolar screws to fix the articular fragment to the humeral shaft (Fig. 51).

The Complex Comminuted Fracture with Displacement of Fragments of the Trochlea

Reduction of these fractures may be extremely difficult. As a rule reduction can be accurately achieved, provided that a systematic operative procedure is followed.

Anaesthesia. A general anaesthetic with an endotracheal tube is necessary. The patient should lie prone with the forearm hanging at the side of the table with the elbow over an accurately adjusted and well-padded roller. It must be possible to flex and extend the joint during the operation (Fig. 49b). A high pneumatic tourniquet is used and the posterior part of the iliac crest is prepared so that a cancellous bone graft can be taken from it.

Incision. A slightly curved incision measuring 25–30 cm is made, preferably on the radial side so as to avoid the olecranon itself. The exposure must allow a full view of the back of the elbow joint (Fig. 52a). The ulnar nerve is first identified and protected by retraction with a tape (Fig. 52b).

Osteotomy of the Olecranon. This is recommended to give perfect exposure of the trochlea. Our experience is that it heals rapidly in the well vascularized bone of the elbow. First a hole is drilled from the tip of the olecranon into the medullary canal of the ulna tapped to take the large 6.5-mm cancellous screw (Fig. 53a). The olecranon is then osteotomized at a right-angle to the axis of the trochlea, using a narrow osteotome or an oscillating saw. The olecranon with its attached triceps can now be turned up proximally (Fig. 53b), providing a complete exposure of the lower end of the humerus and the comminuted trochlea.

The replacement of the osteotomized olecranon is carried out using a long 8–9 cm cancellous screw and a washer. A tension-band wire should also be used as the screw itself cannot grip well in the medullary canal of the ulna. The triceps can pull on the olecranon and loosen the screw, but the addition of the tension wire makes everything secure. Alternatively the osteotomy can be fixed by passing two Kirschner wires down and using a tension-band wire as for a fracture of the olecranon (Fig. 53c).

Reconstruction of the Trochlea. The most important step of the internal fixation is precise reconstruction of the trochlea. Fragments of the humerus are often considerably displaced, but even devitalized or completely detached fragments should be accurately replaced, not removed. Major defects are rare in these fractures but when they do occur they must be grafted with autogenous cancellous bone.

We use Kirschner wires for provisional reduction and fixation of the fracture complex.

The first wire serves as a guide and its accurate placement is decisive. It should penetrate the radial fragment from the side of the fracture, which means the ulnar side. We apply it as a lever to help in the reduction and drill it through the central trochlear fragment or fragments, then back into the ulnar fragment (Fig. 54a, b). After reduction, a hole is made parallel to the guide wire using the drill sleeve as a guide (Fig. 54c). A small cancellous screw of sufficient length is inserted into this hole to provide interfragmentary compression. If necessary the Kirschner wire may be left in place or removed and replaced by a second cancellous screw to maintain rotational stability (Fig. 54d).

Joining the Trochlea to the Shaft of the Humerus. Having stabilized the trochlea, the joint complex must be connected to the metaphysis of the humerus. For this two one-third tubular plates with five–seven holes are indicated, one on each side; each must be accurately fitted by being appropriately bent. The plates and screws must be kept clear of the olecranon fossa and the coronoid notch. Moreover, the plates should have no immediate contact with the ulnar nerve, and on the radial side must not limit extension of the elbow. It may be difficult to contour the plate accurately. Holding the proximal end of both plates with a single screw improves the stability but it is then much more difficult to bend and twist the plates accurately. We therefore prefer to apply each plate on the side of the humerus with independent screws. This makes the internal fixation easier as well as the subsequent removal of the plates. Plates are fixed with 3.5-mm cortex screws or occasionally 4.0-mm small cancellous screws (Fig. 55).

In simpler fractures, the second plate can be replaced by a long screw of the small cancellous or malleolar type (Fig. 55d). Special Y-shaped plates have been developed for internal fixation of such complex elbow fractures, and the contouring of these plates is easier.

Internal Fixation of the Olecranon. The olecranon is replaced as described above (Fig. 53c).

Closure. A Redon suction drain is inserted and the wound is simply closed with skin sutures and the arm elevated. In most cases a protective, padded plaster splint is applied.

Postoperative treatment depends on the stability achieved. A removable plaster splint, with the elbow flexed to about 80°, is often advisable for several weeks. Consolidation of comminuted fractures may take 12 weeks or more. Recovery of flexion is always quicker than that of extension.

Only after firm consolidation can the metal be removed and this should usually be done in two steps. The first is a thorough clinical and possibly electromyographical check of the ulnar nerve. If there is evidence of irritation or paresis, the removal of the plate can then be combined with anterior transposition of the ulnar nerve. The nerve must always be re-identified and isolated when an implant is removed from the ulnar side.

c) Secondary Operation

Non-union of the lower end of the humerus is uncommon. Instability must be suspected if there is pain and this is an indication for reoperation. The deformities that occur are mostly complex, since the radial and ulnar pillars are not equally involved. Careful planning of the operation is mandatory. In every case autogenous bone is used to provide a graft and for internal fixation the 3.5-mm DCP has proved to be better than the one-third tubular plate because it is stronger.

2. Radial Head

Displacement of a fracture of the radial head is nowadays often considered an indication for internal fixation. The following points must be kept in mind.

Associated lesions are not rare. Ligaments may be ruptured, or there may be small avulsion fractures on the ulnar side which interfere with the stability of the elbow and must be considered in postoperative treatment. These injuries can be caused by a real dislocation of the joint. If ruptured ligaments are left unsutured, limitation of extension and flexion may result or ectopic calcification may occur. In the presence of joint instability, therefore, suture of the ligaments is recommended. Rupture of the interosseous membrane, which is most important for stability of the forearm, cannot be clinically diagnosed, but may be suspected if the radial head is found to be very easily exposed during internal fixation. There is no specific treatment available. It is believed that some ruptures heal more easily with functional treatment, which is possible when internal fixation is firm, than with an external cast. Full restoration of pronation and supination can always be achieved after internal fixation of the radial head.

Fracture of the radial head may also occur in fracture-dislocations. In the Monteggia fracture-dislocation the radial head dislocates to the ventral surface and remains intact. This dislocation usually reduces spontaneously when the ulna is firmly fixed and surgical treatment is not then necessary. When posterior dislocation occurs, the ulna is usually fractured in its proximal third, and a sheared or comminuted fracture of the head of the radius is frequent. In such cases a dorsal approach is used, giving simultaneous access to the ulna. As with fractures of the lower humerus, the patient is placed in the prone position and the forearm hangs down over the padded roller (Fig. 49b). Stabilization is then achieved using the techniques described below.

Removal of fractured parts of the radial head has been found to give rise to severe arthrosis and has been abandoned. Excision of the whole radial head is only exceptionally carried out.

There are three different types of fractures to be considered when planning internal fixation:

a) Comminuted Fractures

Fractures which preclude any type of reconstructive operation are rare. By the use of a wide exposure, reduction is almost always possible if connecting bridges of periosteum are preserved between the shaft and the articular fragments. The fragments are fixed by using multiple very small screws. Any defects are grafted with cancellous bone. In exceptional cases small T-plates may be used to stabilize the fragments but they have to be removed early, as they limit pronation and supination considerably. From a biological standpoint this procedure is to be preferred to primary excision of the whole radial head. In the rare case when this is necessary, the head should be replaced by a prosthesis to avoid secondary valgus deformity. In our experience Swanson's silastic prosthesis, with a specially long shaft, has proved very useful. There are also metal prostheses available which can be cemented in the bone or fixed by a bolt mechanism (Fig. 56c).

b) Fissure Fractures

In this fracture the head remains intact while a sharp edged fragment is split off and displaced to a greater or lesser degree (Fig. 56a). On X-ray film the displacement and instability are not fully evident, but there is often an indication for internal fixation. The fragments are fixed by screws.

c) The Cap-Over-Ear Depressed Fracture

Cap-like depressions of the circumference as well as central depressions of the articular surface are frequent, but they are often scarcely visible on X-ray films (Fig. 56b). The interposition of shorn-off fragments of the articular cartilage of the humerus between the fragments of the radial head is often seen and interferes with reduction of the fracture. Bony defects in the centre of the articular surface or in the periphery should be filled in with cancellous bone graft to encourage rapid revascularization. The metaphysis of the distal end of the humerus can be conveniently used as a donor site. It is easily reached by enlarging the exposure a little.

d) Approach and Internal Fixation

Standard exposure. A lateral longitudinal incision is made, beginning at the lateral epicondyle (Fig. 57a). The extensor muscles are split, avoiding the radial nerve which lies more anteriorly. The incision must therefore be kept dorsal, opening the joint capsule over the radial head, which can be felt. The annular ligament is only a reinforcement of the capsule and is rarely felt as a separate ligament. The radial head is then exposed by rotating the forearm. It is not advisable to insert Hohmann retractors on the ventral aspect of the head, as they may compress the radial nerve (Fig. 57b), and the assistant must be instructed accordingly. The radial head may be elevated to some degree by a retractor resting on the lateral epicondyle. Interposed fragments are removed from the articular surface with a small hook (Fig. 58a) and any depressed or avulsed fragments can be reduced, while preserving the periosteum. Provisional stabilization is maintained with pointed reduction forceps or fine Kirschner wires (Fig. 58b). Internal fixation is achieved by using at least two screws, but three to five screws may occasionally be necessary. In recent years we have almost always used 1.5-mm screws, which can be introduced without any harm into the articular surface.

The screw heads are countersunk and do not disturb the proximal radio-ulnar joint. All defects are grafted with cancellous bone before the final reconstruction (Fig. 58c).

The joint is closed with sutures which unite the capsule and the fibrous layer. Suture of the usually unidentifiable annular ligament is not necessary. A Redon suction drain is introduced in every case.

Extended Approach. In an occasional complex fracture or when the first exposure has been insufficient the incision may be extended in the dorsoproximal direction. The enlargement is made with an angled incision (Fig. 57a). A drill hole is made in the exposed epicondyle, which is then tapped to take the small cancellous screw which can be provided with a metal or spiked polyacetal resin washer. A screw of 24–28 mm in length is introduced, making sure that it obtains a good grip and is well seated. The screw is then withdrawn and the epicondyle osteotomized with a narrow osteotome. The fragment can then be reflected together with the lateral capsule. This gives a very good exposure of the whole radial head. Good cancellous bone from the osteotomized surface of the humerus can be obtained with a small spoon without jeopardizing the reconstruction. The osteotomy is closed with a prepared screw after internal fixation of the radial head. The joint is closed as in the standard method.

Dorsal Approach. Operation on a dorsal fracture-dislocation of the elbow is performed with the patient in the prone position. Preparations are the same as for fractures of the distal humerus (Fig. 49b). The incision to reveal the olecranon or fracture of the ulna first exposes the dislocated prominent radial head. The fracture of the radial head is first reduced and reconstructed with screws as described above. Reduction of the fracture of the ulna then follows and leads to spontaneous reduction of the dislocation of the radial head. Because of the difficulties of approach, removal of the screws from the radial head is usually omitted.

e) Postoperative Treatment

The arm is immobilized in a removable dorsal plaster splint and is kept elevated. Exercises are started after the wound has healed, including flexion and extension and pronation and supination. Depending on the type of fracture, the elbow is protected by the removable splint for 3–6 weeks. Full function is not allowed in depressed or comminuted fractures before 10–12 weeks. The implants should be removed early in fractures of the cancellous area.

f) Secondary Operation

Indications for secondary operation are posttraumatic arthrosis after conservative treatment, or painful deformity caused by rheumatoid arthritis. Reconstructive procedures are then impossible and the radial head has to be removed. It should be replaced by a prosthesis to maintain the length of the radius and the stability of the elbow. Swanson's silastic prosthesis can be used here, as in primary replacement.

3. Olecranon

Most fractures of the olecranon can be primarily fixed with a tension-band wire, followed by functional postoperative treatment. This is well described in the *Manual of Internal Fixation* (Muller et al. 2nd edn., 1979, p. 188). The use of the SFS is restricted to the following special conditions.

a) Oblique Fracture

In the standard method of tension-band wiring, the parallel Kirschner wires act as a splint and the tension-band wire resists the pull of the triceps muscle. In an oblique fracture this produces asymmetrical compression, so an additional screw is recommended to apply interfragmentary compression (Fig. 59a). Simple screw fixation may also be justified in a long oblique fracture or a simple undisplaced fissure, especially in children.

b) Fractures of the Coronoid Process

Small fragments of bone may be shorn off during spontaneous or manipulative reduction of an elbow dislocation. They do not need internal fixation but can be treated with a plaster splint. Larger fragments may interfere with the congruity of the hinge joint. The fragment is held under tension by the brachialis muscle, and if it is not fixed, instability and arthrosis may follow. Internal fixation is best achieved by a screw (Fig. 59b), usually a small cancellous screw if there is only a single fracture. The approach is from the ulnar side, carefully protecting the ulnar nerve.

c) Comminuted Fractures

Simple tension-band wiring may be inadequate for holding such a fracture. Internal fixation with the one-third tubular plate has been successful in this type of fracture. The plate should have six to eight holes and be exactly contoured to the shape of the bone. The first screw is placed in the tip of the olecranon. The plate is then put under tension by drilling the screw hole eccentrically or by using the articulated tension device (Fig. 59c). Additional screws are needed in different planes. Bony defects must be filled in with autogenous cancellous bone.

d) Approach and Operative Procedure

An inhalation anaesthetic or a brachial plexus block should be used. The patient lies on his back and a tourniquet is applied. The forearm is placed over the chest and the hand held with a towel, to be controlled by an assistant, fixed with a towel clip to the drapes, or provided with a weight hanging down on the opposite side of the table (Fig. 49a). A slightly curved incision is made on the radial side of the olecranon. In complex fractures it is mandatory to identify and protect the ulnar nerve. The fracture is then reduced and temporarily fixed by forceps, hooks or fine Kirschner wires.

e) Fracture-Dislocations

In a posterior fracture-dislocation, which is often combined with a fracture of the radial head (p. 87), the operation is done with the patient lying prone with the arm hanging down on the side of the table (Fig. 49b). The incision is the same as used in the approach to the badly fractured lower end of the humerus (p. 84). After reducing the ulna the radial head usually falls back into place without difficulty. The fracture of the olecranon or the shaft of the ulna is fixed by the technique described for comminuted fractures. If the fracture is more distal in the diaphysis, the use of the stronger DCP with 3.5-mm screws is recommended rather than the one-third tubular plate.

f) Secondary Operations

In the unusual non-union of the olecranon, fixation and compression can be obtained with a tension-band plate of either the one-third tubular or the 3.5-mm DCP type. In an atrophic non-union an additional cancellous bone graft is needed, sometimes helped by shingling of the bone.

4. Clinical X-ray Examples: Figs. 60–68

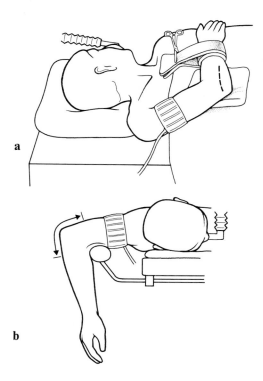

Fig. 49 a, b. Typical positions for internal fixation of the elbow

a Internal fixation of the olecranon: supine position. Anaesthesia is by inhalation or plexus block. A pneumatic tourniquet is used. The limb is placed across the chest with the elbow flexed. The hand is fixed to the drapes, which are not illustrated, by a sling and a towel clip. The incision is curved and on the radial side of the olecranon

b For complex articular fractures and fracture dislocations, the prone position with the arm hanging down is used. The patient is intubated, and a pneumatic tourniquet used. The arm hangs at the side of the operating table, the elbow is supported by a well-padded roller. Passive flexion of the elbow must be free

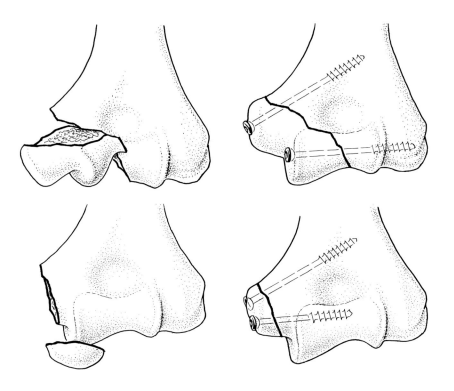

Fig. 50. Fractures of condyles and epicondyles in adults

Internal fixation with small cancellous screws by
a lateral approach. On the ulnar side the ulnar
nerve must be exposed and protected

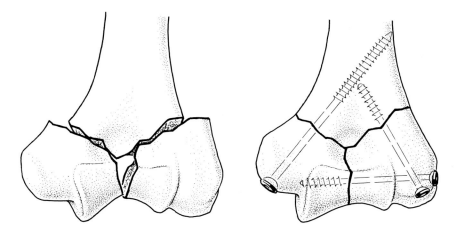

**Fig. 51. Articular Y-fracture of the distal humerus
with slight displacement**

Bilateral approach. The trochlea is stabilized by
a small cancellous screw. The pillars are fixed by
small cancellous or malleolar screws

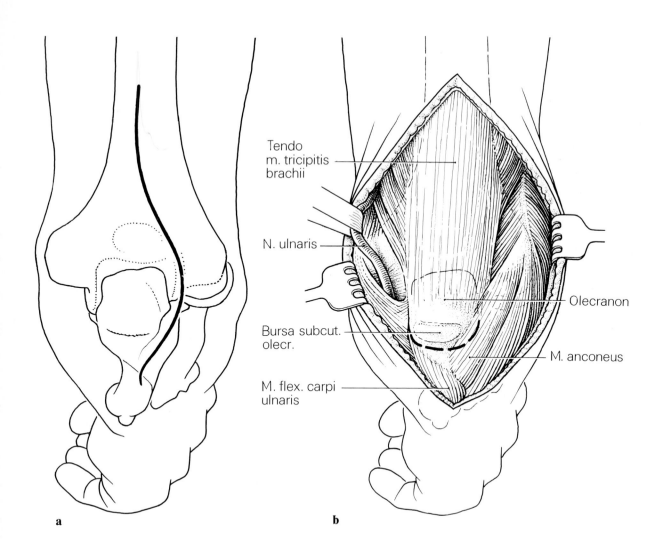

a

b

Tendo
m. tricipitis
brachii

N. ulnaris

Bursa subcut.
olecr.

M. flex. carpi
ulnaris

Olecranon

M. anconeus

Fig. 52 a, b. Comminuted intra-articular fracture of the lower humerus

a Incision: The olecranon is bypassed on the radial side

b Approach to the olecranon, retraction of the ulnar nerve

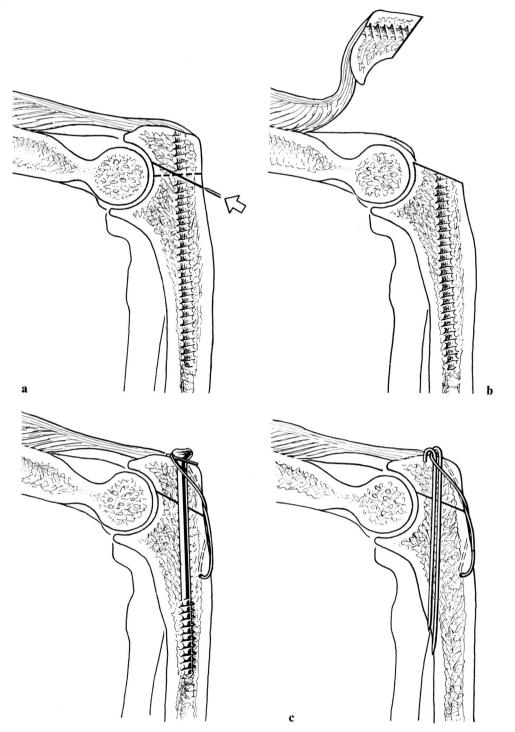

Fig. 53a–c. Osteotomy of the olecranon for access to a comminuted intra-articular fracture of the lower humerus

a Drilling and tapping of the olecranon for a long large cancellous screw (6.5 mm). Oblique or perpendicular osteotomy of the olecranon with the oscillating saw, depending on the articular involvement of the fracture

b Turning up the osteotomized olecranon together with the triceps muscle and tendon

c Replacement of the olecranon with the 6.5-mm cancellous screw, a washer, and additional figure-of-eight tension-band wire loop, or with two parallel Kirschner wires and additional tension-band wire loop

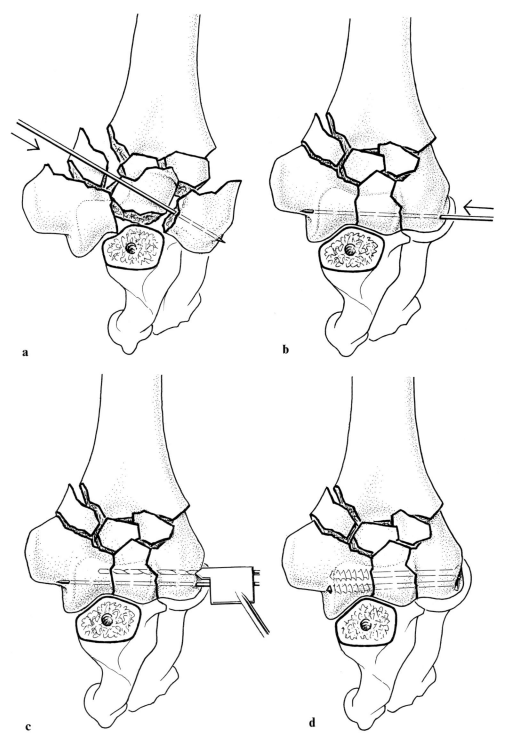

Fig. 54a–d. Internal fixation of an intra-articular fracture of the lower humerus: reconstruction of the trochlea

a Insertion of a guide wire (1.8 mm) into the lateral fragment from the medial side

b Drilling back of the guide wire into the medial fragments. The wire may be used as a lever for reduction of the fragments

c Drilling of a hole parallel to the guide wire with the drill sleeve. Insertion of the first small cancellous screw

d Replacement of the guide wire by a second small cancellous screw

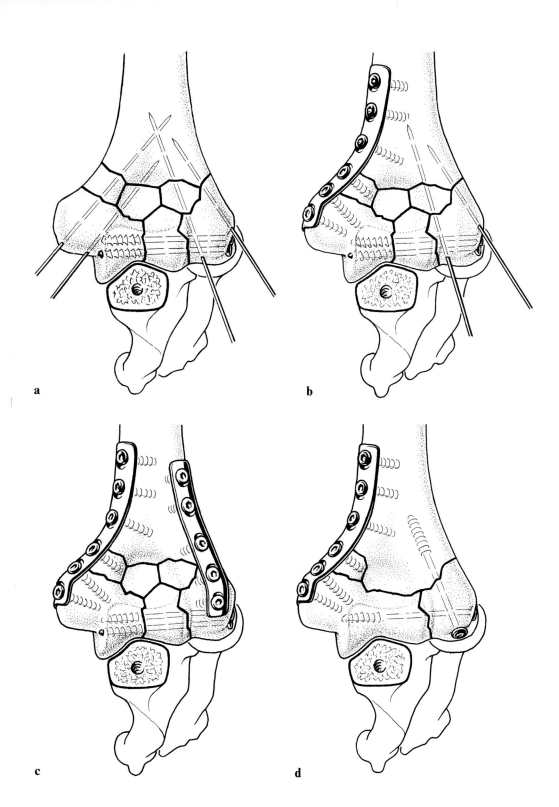

Fig. 56a–c. Typical fractures of the radial head

a Fissure fracture in the lateral view. The periosteal connection to the shaft is intact. Sheared off small fragments from the capitellum humeri are frequently interposed within the fracture. Frontal view from above with the triangular fragment and the articular step

b Impacted fracture. The cancellous bone defect is seen in longitudinal cross-section. A central defect of the cancellous bone before and after reduction

c Irreducible comminuted fracture

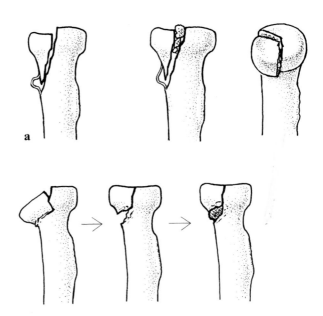

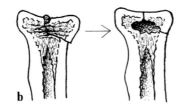

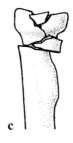

◁ **Fig. 55a–d. Internal fixation of an intra-articular, comminuted fracture of the lower humerus: The trochlea joined to the humeral metaphysis**

a Reduction and temporary fixation with Kirschner wires

b Placing a one-third tubular plate on the medial pillar

c Internal fixation with two plates

d One small cancellous screw on the radial side is sufficient for simpler fractures

95

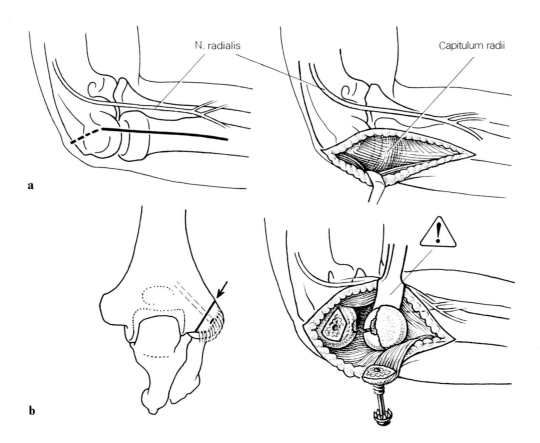

Fig. 57a, b. Approach for the internal fixation of the radial head

a Straight incision at the radial side of the joint from the capitellum distally. Division of the muscle fibres and the joint capsule, protecting the deep branch of the radial nerve. If necessary an angled extension at the proximal end of the incision

b If exposure is not sufficient, the lateral epicondyle is osteotomized. First a drill hole is made and tapped for a small cancellous screw which is fitted with a spiked polyacetal resin washer. The lateral collateral ligament can now be reflected and the whole circumference of the radial head may be inspected. Beware of pressure damage to the radial nerve by the Hohmann retractor. Small fragments which have been sheared off from the capitellum humeri are interposed with the fracture

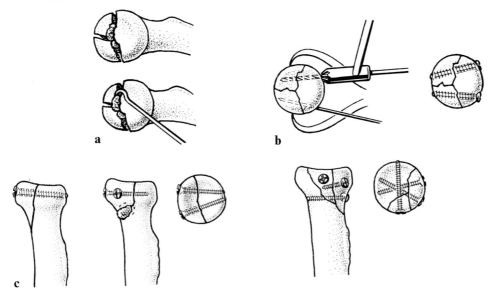

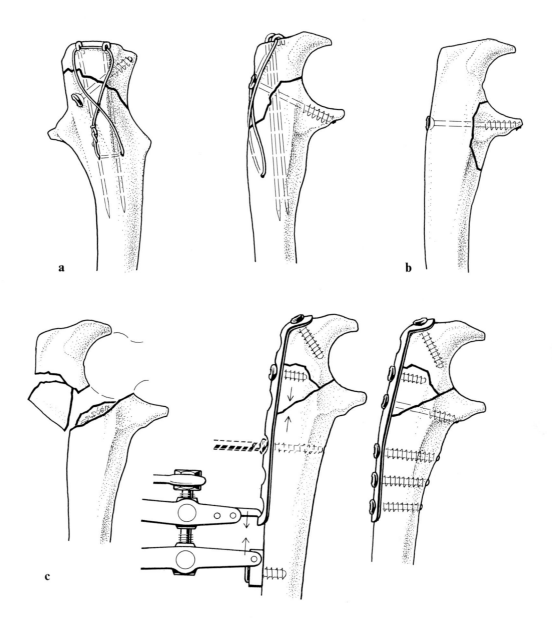

◁ **Fig. 58 a–c. Screw fixation of fractures of the radial head**

a Removal of small, interposed fragments with a small hook

b Reduction and temporary fixation with a reduction forceps and fine Kirschner wires. Drilling with a 1.1- or 1.5-mm drill bit depending on the size of the fragments

c Position of the screws and the cancellous bone graft, frontal and lateral view. Screws in different planes in a comminuted fracture

△
Fig. 59 a–c. Internal fixation of the olecranon with the SFS

a Combined fixation of an oblique fracture with a screw, Kirschner wires and a tension-band wire

b Screw fixation of a fracture of the coronoid process

c Internal fixation of a comminuted fracture with a long one-third tubular plate as a tension band. For optimal axial compression the articulated tension device is suitable. The third and fourth screws are only inserted after interfragmentary compression has been applied

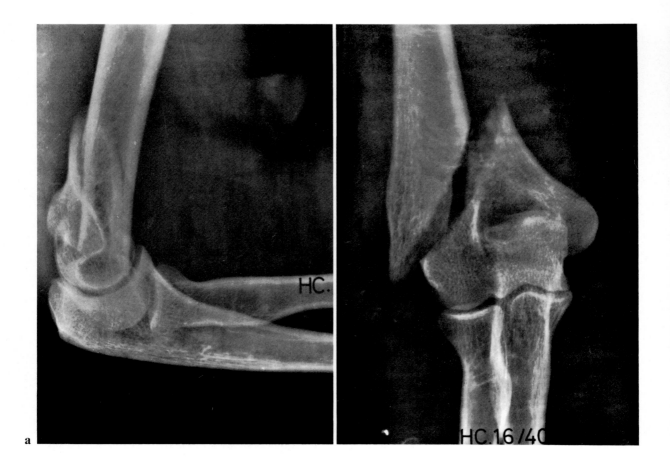

a

HC.

HC.16/40

Fig. 60 a–c. Clinical example: Supracondylar fracture of the elbow

W., Lilly, a 50-year-old housewife. Household accident

a Displaced oblique supracondylar fracture of the humerus

b Internal fixation as an emergency: By a radial approach the fracture is fixed with a one-third tubular plate. The screws avoid the olecranon fossa and the coronoid fossa.
Uneventful postoperative course. Dorsal plaster slab for 4 weeks. Then the patient was lost and did not have the implants removed

c Review after 7 years. No complaints. Flexion deficit of 10°. Full extension, pronation and supination. The metal can be felt through the soft parts. Some of the screws have loosened as shown by X-rays. Removal of implants is refused by the patient

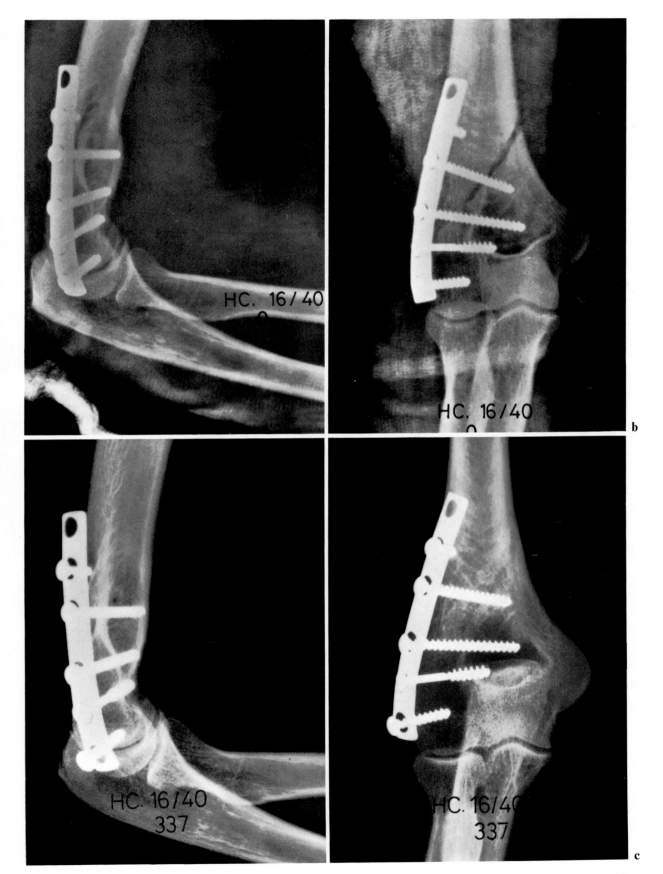

HC. 16 / 40

HC. 16 / 40

b

HC. 16/40
337

HC. 16/40
337

c

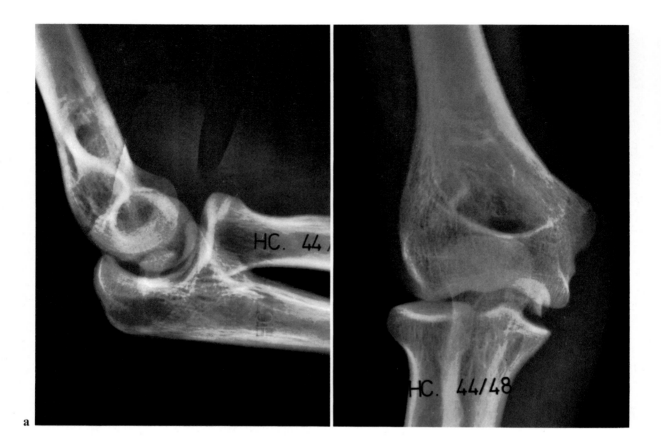

a

Fig. 61 a–c. Clinical example: Avulsion fracture of the medial epicondyle and interposition into the joint

B., Rene, a 15-year-old school boy. Skiing accident

a Avulsion fracture of the medial epicondyle. The fragment is displaced into the medial compartment of the joint. Paraesthesia of the ulnar nerve

b Immediate internal fixation on the day of injury. Exposure of the ulnar nerve. Reduction and fixation of the fragment with a small cancellous screw and additional Kirschner wire to prevent rotation. Uneventful course. Dorsal plaster slab for 3 weeks. Functional treatment thereafter. Removal of implants elsewhere

c Review after 16 months. No complaints. Full function, normal radiological appearances

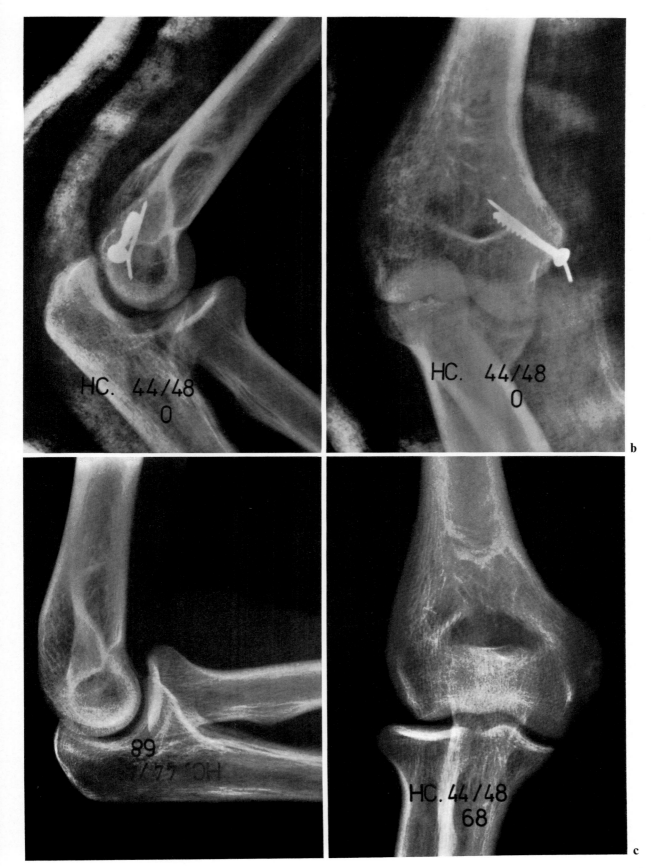

HC. 44/48
0

b

HC. 44/48
0

89

HC. 44/48
68

c

101

Fig. 62 a, b. Clinical example: Shearing fracture of condyle

Sch., Ursula, 69-year-old farmer's wife. Household accident. Diagnosis only established in this pain-resistant woman after 2 weeks

a Shearing fracture of the lateral condyle with anterior displacement.
Screw fixation by a radial approach at 2 weeks.
Uneventful course. Dorsal plaster splint for 6 weeks. Unlimited lifting and farming work after 4 months

b Review at 14 months: No complaints, full working capacity and full range of motion. No arthrosis, implants without reaction. The patient refuses removal of implants

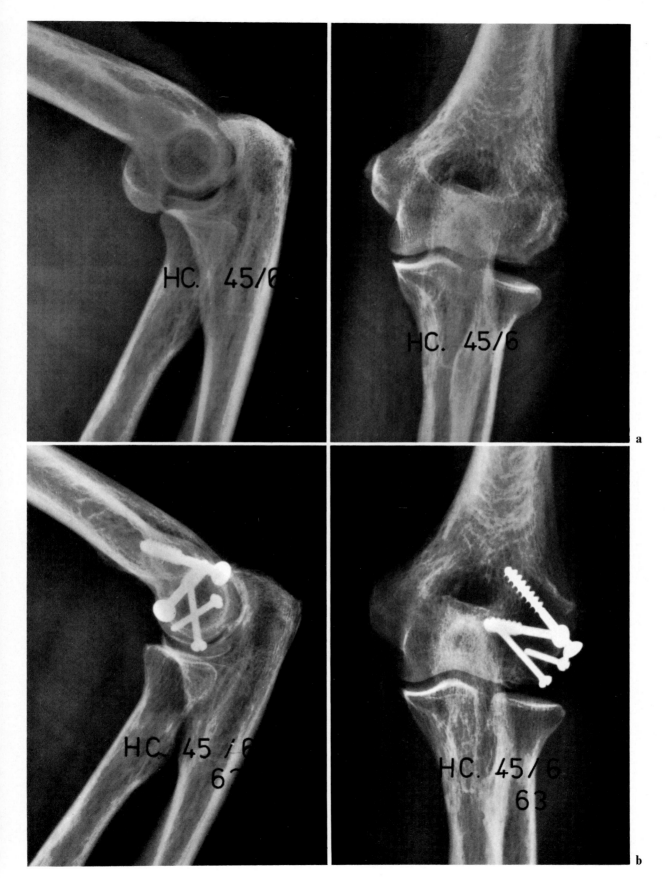

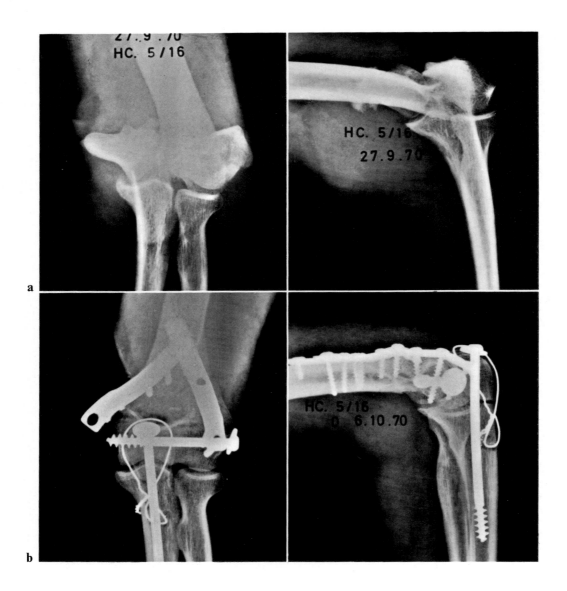

Fig. 63a–d. Clinical example, Comminuted intra-articular fracture of the humerus

H., Rene, 30-year-old director of a sports resort. Fall while playing football

a Distal intra-articular comminuted fracture of the humerus

b Internal fixation as an emergency: Osteotomy of the olecranon. Stabilization of the trochlea with a large cancellous screw, lateral one-third tubular plates between the condyles and the shaft.
Postoperative course without complications. Dorsal plaster splint for 6 weeks. Removal of the implants and anterior transposition of the ulnar nerve after 9 months

c Review after 17 months: Slight limitation of extension and flexion, pronation and supination equal on both sides. No arthrosis. Slight discomfort at times

d After 10 years: No complaints. The strength of the arm is somewhat limited and there is some atrophy of the muscles. Lack of extension 20°, of flexion 5°, pronation and supination are full. There is no arthrosis seen on X-ray

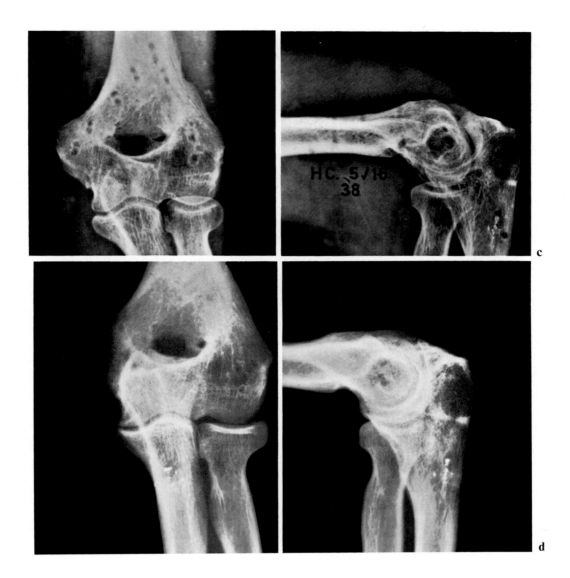

c

d

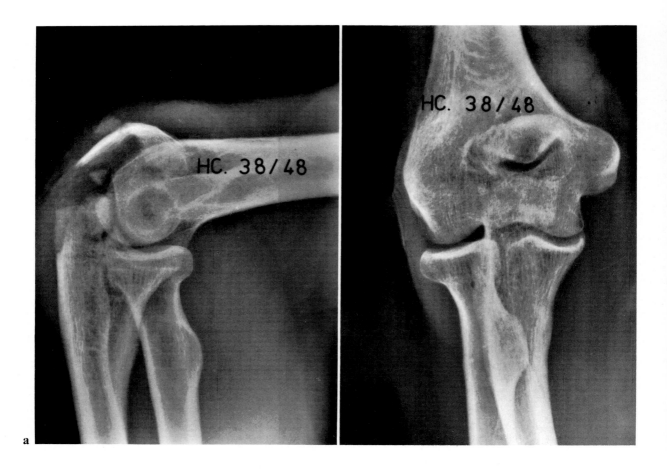

a

Fig. 64a–c. Clinical example: Comminuted fracture of the olecranon

L., Anton, 46-year-old commercial employee. He was struck by a car while riding a motorcycle and fell on his arm

a Comminuted fracture of the right olecranon

b Emergency operation: Two parallel Kirschner wires combined with figure-of-eight tension-band wire loop with two twists. The oblique fractures and the additional fragments are fixed by small cancellous screws.
Uneventful course. Removable dorsal splint for 4 weeks. Full weight lifting after 8 weeks. Full working capacity after 9 weeks

c Review and removal of implants after 8 months. No complaints, full range of motion, primary fracture healing, no arthrosis

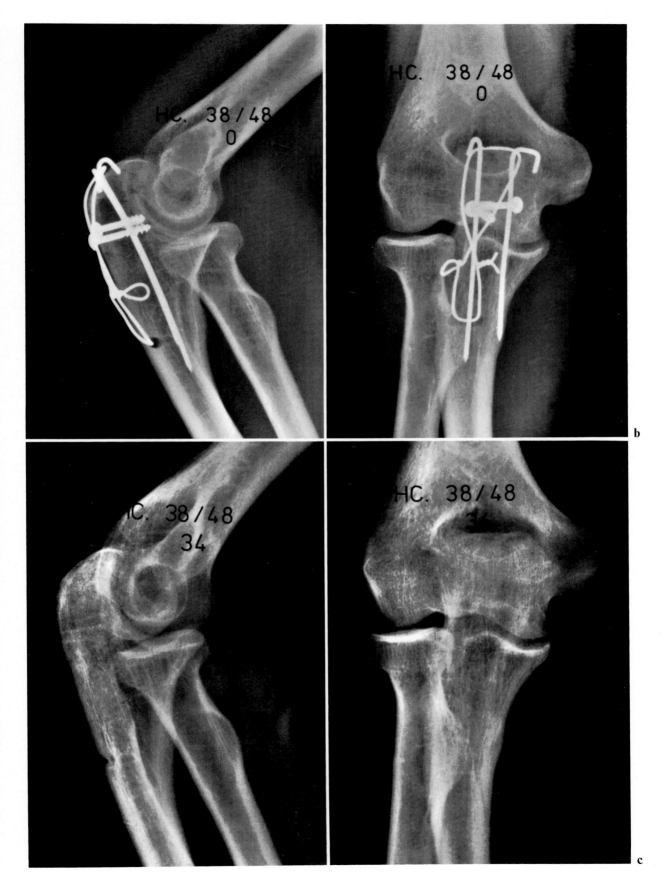

Fig. 65 a–d. Clinical example: Fissure fracture of the radial head

C., Maria, 61-year-old woman, working as a florist. Fall on a rock

a Fissure fracture of the radial head of the right arm with considerable displacement. Primary plaster cast fixation. Admission to hospital after on week

b Internal fixation at 11 days. Reduction after removal of interposed cartilagineous fragments of the humeral articular surface. Fixation by three 1.5-mm screws.
Uneventful course. Removable plaster splint for 4 weeks. Full weight lifting after 10 weeks. Full working capacity after 12 weeks. Removal of the implants at 5 months

c, d see page 110 f.

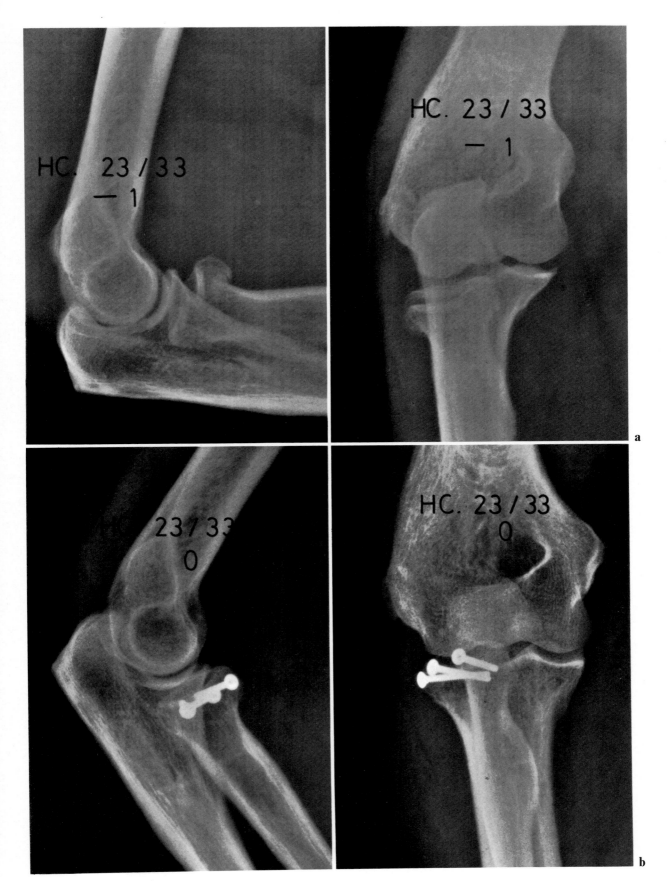

Fig. 65 c, d

c Review at 10 months: Pain-free full function of the joint, primary bone healing, no arthrosis

d After $5^1/_2$ years: No change in clinical and radiological findings

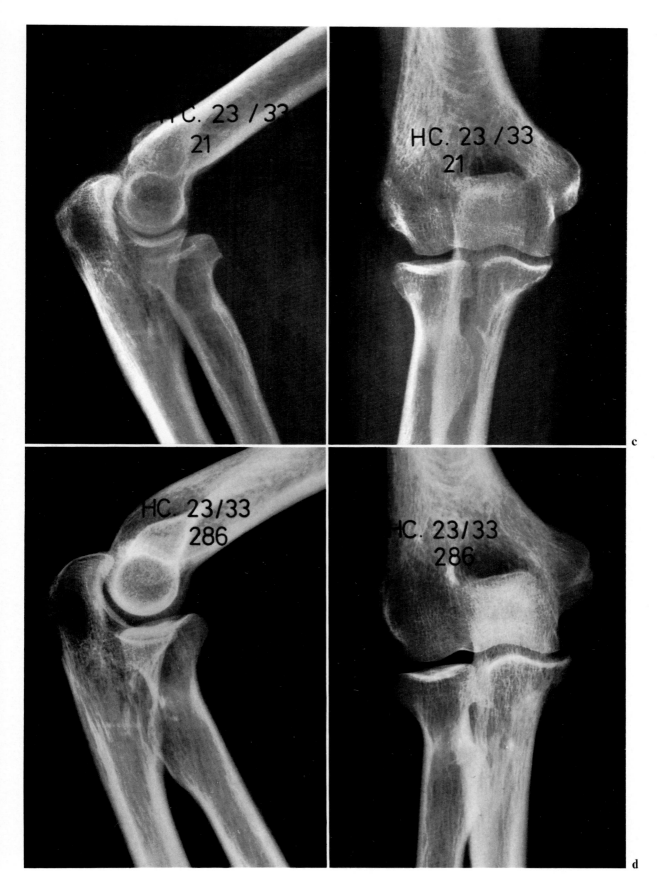

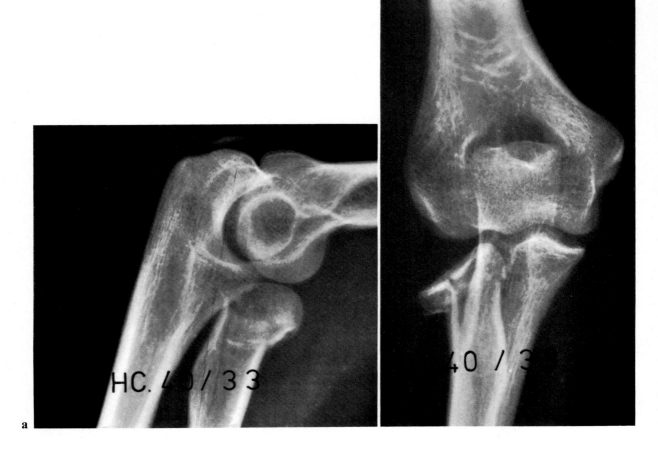

a

Fig. 66a–c. Clinical example: Depressed fracture of the radial head

St., Pia, 23-year-old commercial employee. Fall on an icy street

a Cap-over-ear depressed fracture of the radial head with impaction of the metaphysis

b Immediate internal fixation through a wide extended approach (osteotomy of the epicondyle): Fixation by two 1.5-mm screws, cancellous bone graft from the lateral epicondyle.

No complications postoperatively. Dorsal plaster splint for 8 weeks. Full use of the arm after 10 weeks

c Review and removal of the screws at 10 months: No complaints, full range of movements, primary fracture healing, no arthrosis. A further review was impossible, since the patient left the country

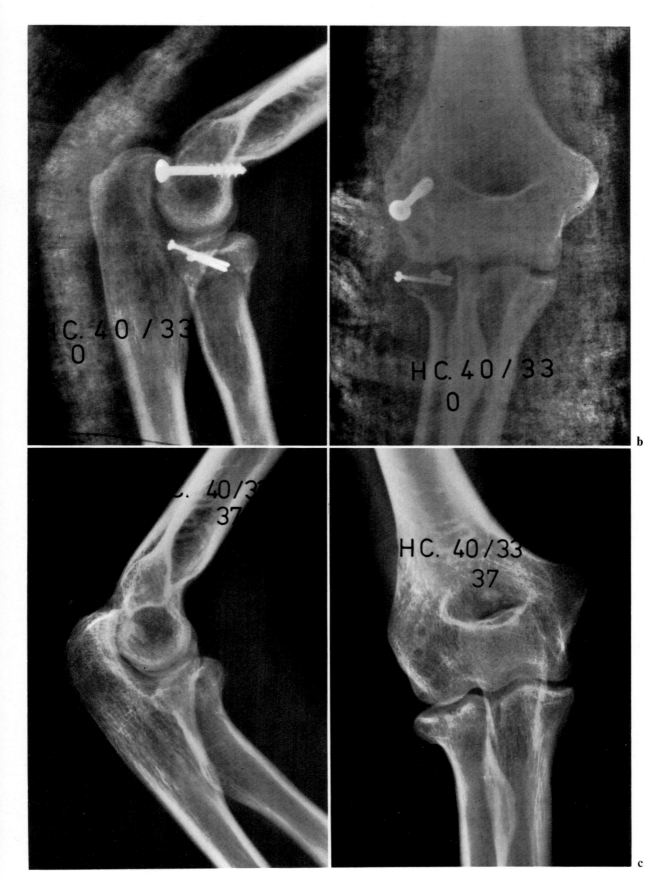

C. 40 / 33
0

HC. 40 / 33
0

b

C. 40/33
37

HC. 40 / 33
37

c

113

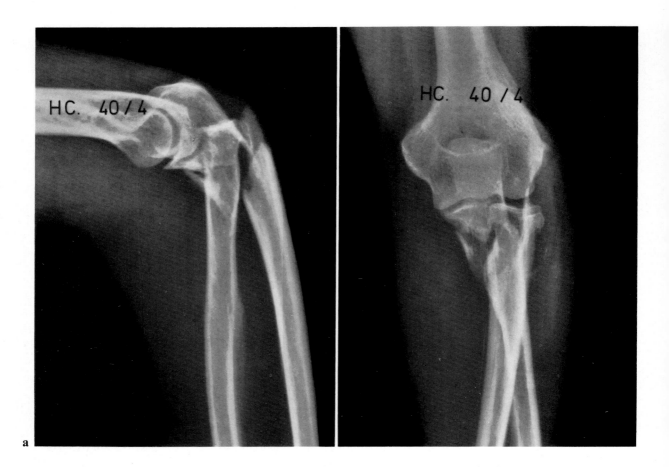

a

Fig. 67 a–c. Clinical example: Reversed Monteggia fracture, comminuted fracture of the olecranon, fracture-dislocation of the radial head

C., Elisabeth, 60-year-old housekeeper. Fall on a staircase

a Comminuted fracture of the left olecranon combined with a fracture-dislocation of the radial head and dorsal displacement

b Internal fixation as an emergency: Prone position of the patient and dorsal approach. First the internal fixation of the radial head was done with three 1.5-mm screws, then the head was reduced and the ulna fixed with two lag screws and a one-third tubular plate of six holes.
Uneventful course. After wound healing a plaster cast was applied for 6 weeks, followed by active mobilization of the joint

c Review and removal of the implants at 15 months: No complaints, full function of the joint, the fracture has healed primarily, no signs of arthrosis are seen. One screw was left behind at removal of the metal from the dorsum

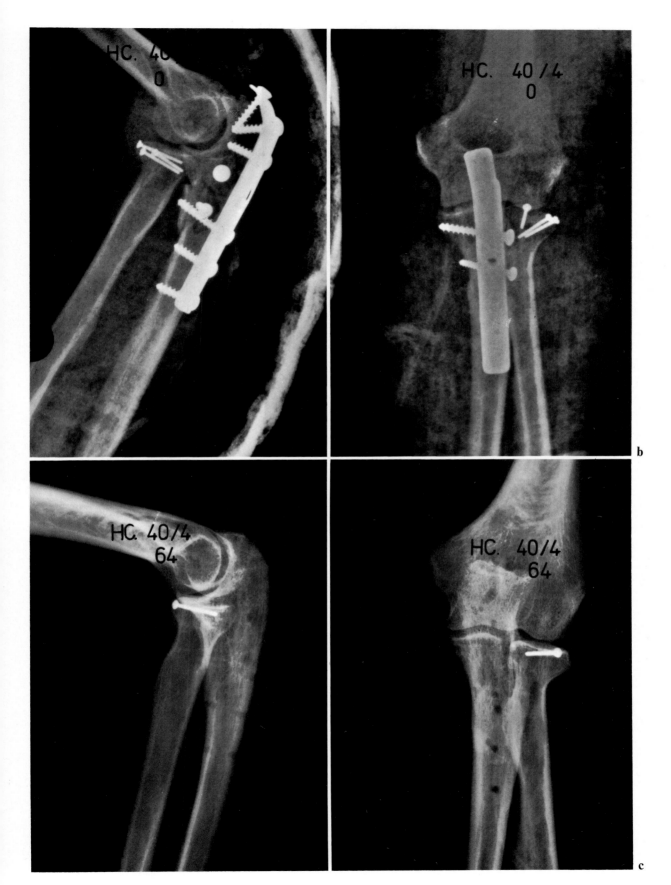

b

c

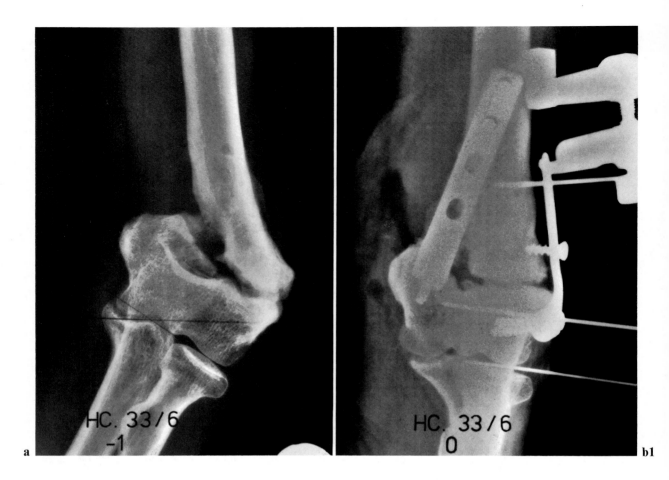

HC. 33/6 -1

a

HC. 33/6 0

b1

Fig. 68 a–c. Clinical example: Non-union of the distal humerus

G., Ilse, 36-year-old woman physician. Accident in horse riding: open supracondylar fracture of the left humerus. The patient was left handed. Primary treatment with unstable internal fixation followed by chronic osteitis and prolonged plaster cast fixation. Since then a painful, mobile non-union has been present

a At 3 years supracondylar non-union of the humerus with malposition in varus and internal malrotation

b1 Internal fixation: Support of the medial pillar with interposition of a corticocancellous bone graft and a 3.5-mm DCP. On the radial side compression is achieved by a small T-plate. The operation X-ray shows the application of the compression device

b2 The postoperative X-ray demonstrates the restoration of the axis.

Postoperative course was uncomplicated. A removable splint of synthetic material was applied for 3 months. Thereafter weight lifting was allowed progressively. Full working capacity was achieved at 5 months. The implants have been removed elsewhere after 1 year

c Review after 2 years: The patient is pain-free and fully able to work as a physician. There is a loss of 10° of extension and 35° of flexion. Pronation and supination are full. The pseudarthrosis is united and there is no arthrosis

116

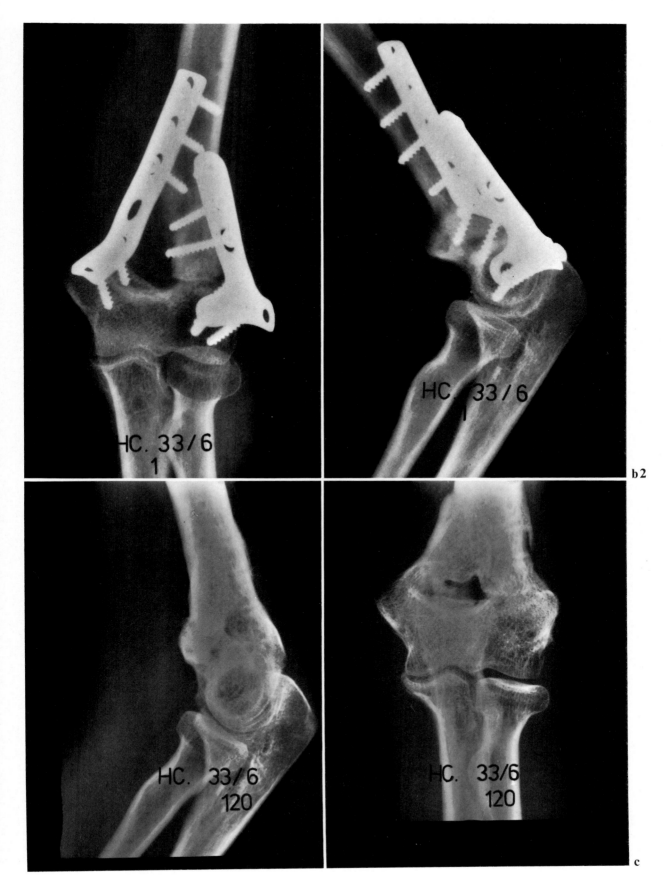

HC. 33/6
1

HC. 33/6
1

b2

HC. 33/6
120

HC. 33/6
120

c

117

XI. The Shafts of the Forearm Bones

1. Internal Fixation

It is agreed that there is a definite indication for internal fixation in fractures of the shafts of the forearm bones and also for fracture of one bone in isolation as in the Monteggia or Galeazzi type. Only with stable internal fixation is early mobilization possible, and this is necessary to guarantee recovery of pronation and supination.

The necessary techniques, approach, details of internal fixation and post operative treatment are described in the *Manual of Internal Fixation* (Muller et al. 2nd edn., Springer 1979 pp. 186–192).

It has been found that the larger straight plates with round holes and 4.5-mm screws are too bulky for use in the radius, especially in women where the bone may be very slender. Sometimes driving these large screws home can produce additional fissure fractures and the width of the plate can often prevent one seeing the accuracy of the reduction on X-ray.

Since the introduction of the 3.5-mm DCP, the SFS is often used to overcome these problems. The DCP's thickness of 3 mm gives enough strength and occupies little space. It is easier to mould it to the curved shape of the radius. The 3.5-mm screws are the right size and do not cause further trouble.

It is important to use plates of sufficient length (seven or eight holes). In a pure transverse fracture the articulated tension device can be used to obtain accurate reduction and precise axial compression. In oblique fractures either an additional lag screw is inserted in a different plane or an interfragmentary lag screw is used through the plate itself (Fig. 14c). This ensures perfect stability. If there are defects or avascular areas, cancellous bone should be grafted.

In secondary operations for refracture or non-union the DCP with 3.5-mm screws has proved to be as satisfactory as in primary cases.

2. Clinical X-ray Examples
Figs. 69–72

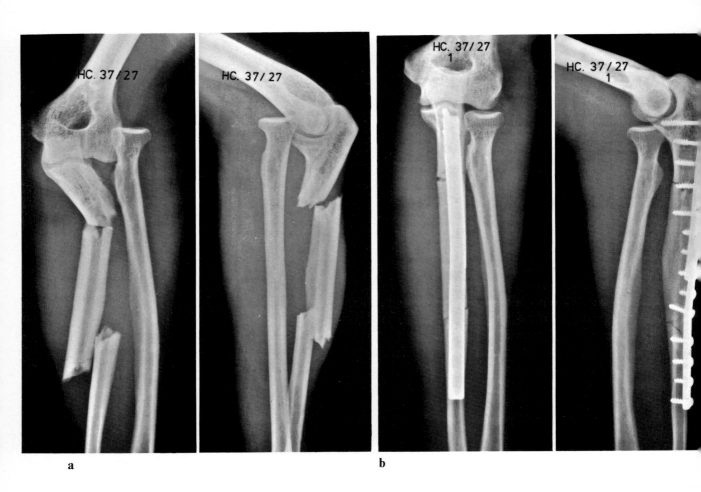

a   b

Fig. 69a–e. Clinical example: Non-union of the ulna after a Monteggia fracture-dislocation

M., Luigi, 50-year-old factory worker. His left arm was hit by a machine

a Monteggia fracture-dislocation with dislocation of the radial head and two level fracture of the ulna

b Immediate internal fixation of the ulna by two superimposed one-third tubular plates with eight holes. The radial head reduced spontaneously. The annular ligament was not sutured. A dorsal plaster splint was applied.
Uneventful course. Functional postoperative treatment was started after 3 weeks

c The proximal fracture remained painful and only partial working capacity could be achieved. Five months after the initial treatment a tight fibrous pseudarthrosis of the proximal fracture was diagnosed, caused by incorrect positioning of the screws in the proximal plate

d Second operation after 5 months: Removal of the proximal one-third tubular plate and application of a 3.5-mm DCP. A cancellous bone graft was not done. The non-union was healed after 3 months. The implants were removed 16 months after the second operation

e Review 3 years after the accident. The patient is pain-free and has a full range of movement. Full working capacity. The scar is slightly adherent to the periosteum

120

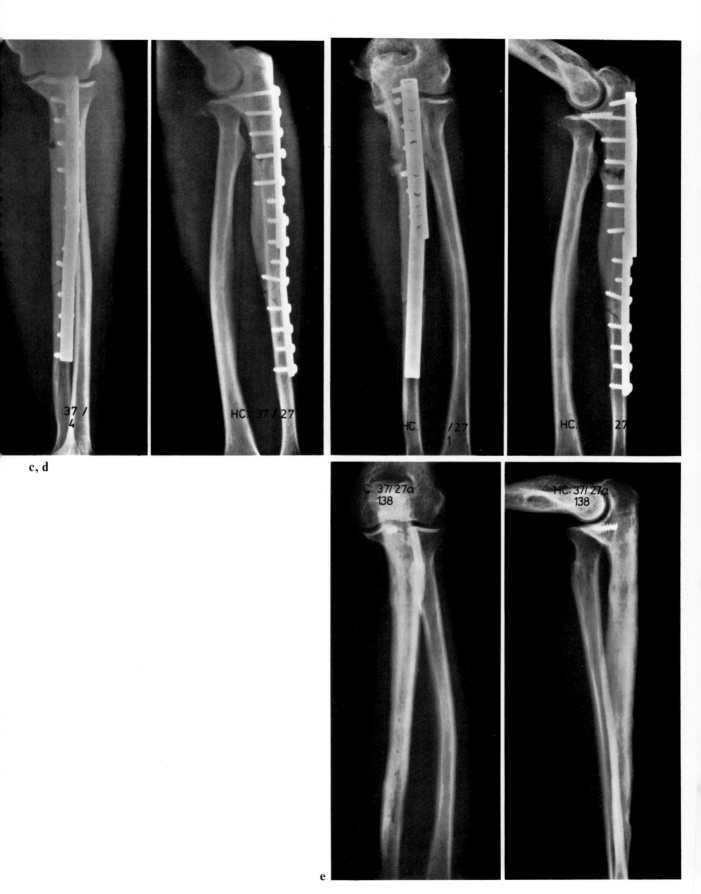

c, d

37 /
4

HC. 37 / 27

HC. / 27
1

HC. 27

C 37/ 27a
138

HC. 37/ 27a
138

e

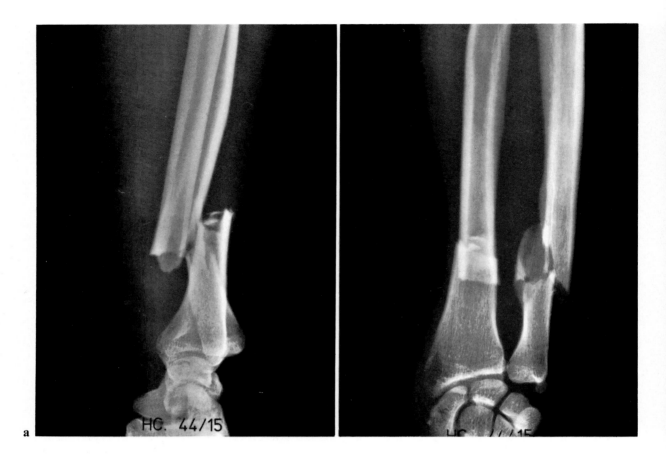

a

Fig. 70a–c. Clinical example: Forearm shaft fracture

D., Tibor, 42-year-old turner. His left forearm was squeezed in his machine

a Forearm shaft fracture with a butterfly fragment of the ulna

b Internal fixation the same day by two longitudinal incisions. Both fractures have been fixed by a 3.5-mm DCP and the separate fragment of the ulna stabilized by an additional lag screw. Because of considerable oedema, a fasciotomy was also performed.
Postoperative course was uneventful. For 6 weeks a removable posterior plaster splint was applied, after which functional treatment was started. Full working capacity was achieved after 26 weeks

c After 14 months the patient is pain-free and presents full function of the joints and primary healing of both fractures. The implants have been removed

122

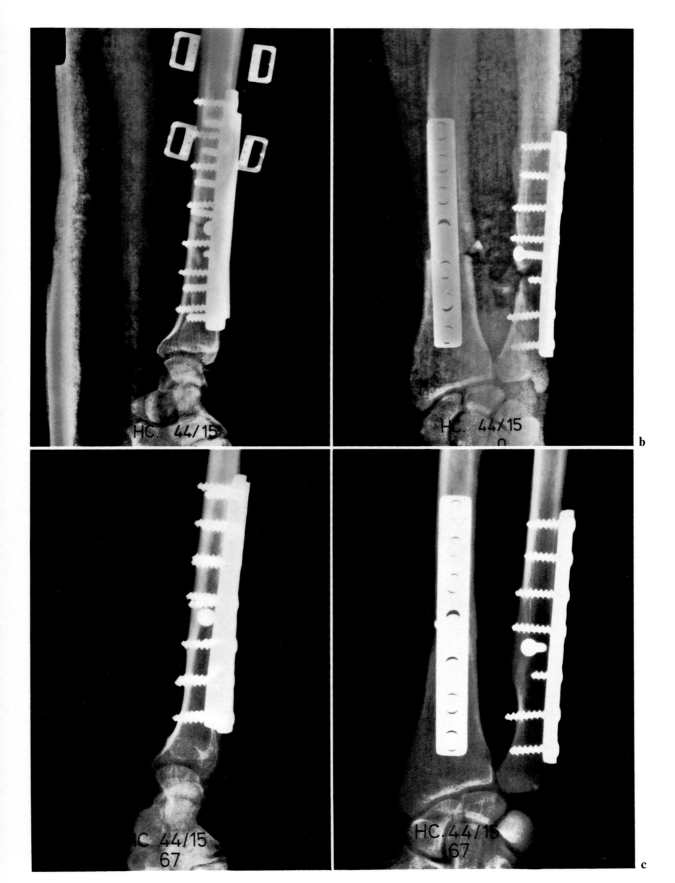

HC. 44/15

HC. 44X15
0

IC 44/15
67

HC.44/15
67

b

c

123

Fig. 71 a–c. Clinical example: Open fracture of the forearm

E., Rosa, 46-year-old farmer's wife. Fall while skiing

a First degree open fracture of the left forearm with butterfly fragment of the radius and an incomplete wedge fracture of the ulna

b Internal fixation as an emergency operation: By two incisions both fractures have been stabilized using a 3.5-mm DCP with seven holes and an additional separate lag screw applied to the radius.
No complications after operation. A removable splint was applied for 3 weeks, followed by functional treatment. Full working capacity at farming at 4 months

c Review at 5 months: Full range of motion, no atrophy of the muscles, slight intermittent hypoaesthesia of the long finger and swelling of the hand after work. The fractures are healed. Removal of the metal is planned for $1^1/_2$ to 2 years after the accident

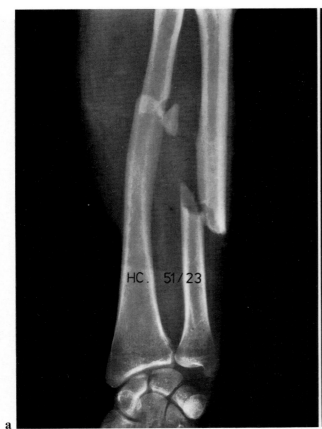

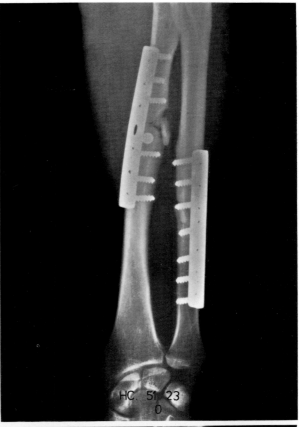

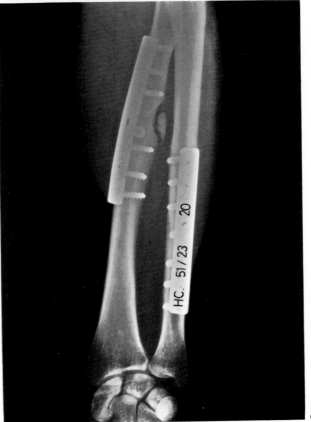

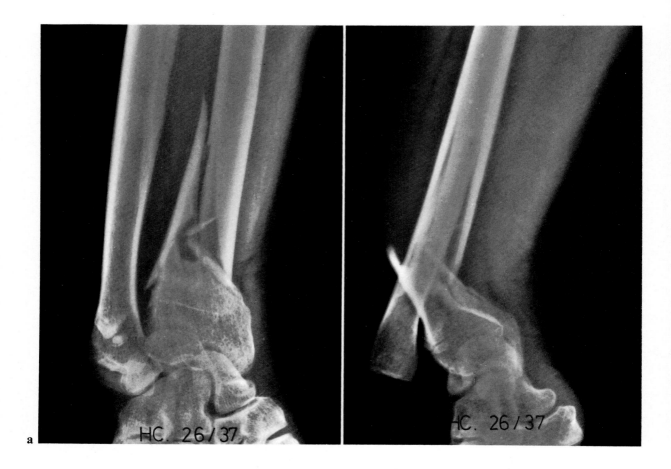

Fig. 72a–c. Clinical example: Galeazzi fracture-dislocation

V., Hans, 52-year-old civil servant. Skiing accident

a Galeazzi fracture-dislocation with a comminuted fracture of the distal shaft of the radius and posterior dislocation of the ulna. Avulsion of the styloid process of the ulna

b Immediate internal fixation of the radius with a long T-plate and additional lag screw. The ulna reduced spontaneously.
Uncomplicated postoperative course. A removable plaster splint was given for 9 weeks. Full weight lifting and working capacity after 12 weeks

c Removal of the implants one year later. The patient is free of pain and has a full range of movement. No muscular atrophy and good skin scar. The X-ray shows persistent pseudarthrosis of the ulnar styloid process but no arthrosis of the distal radio-ulnar joint

126

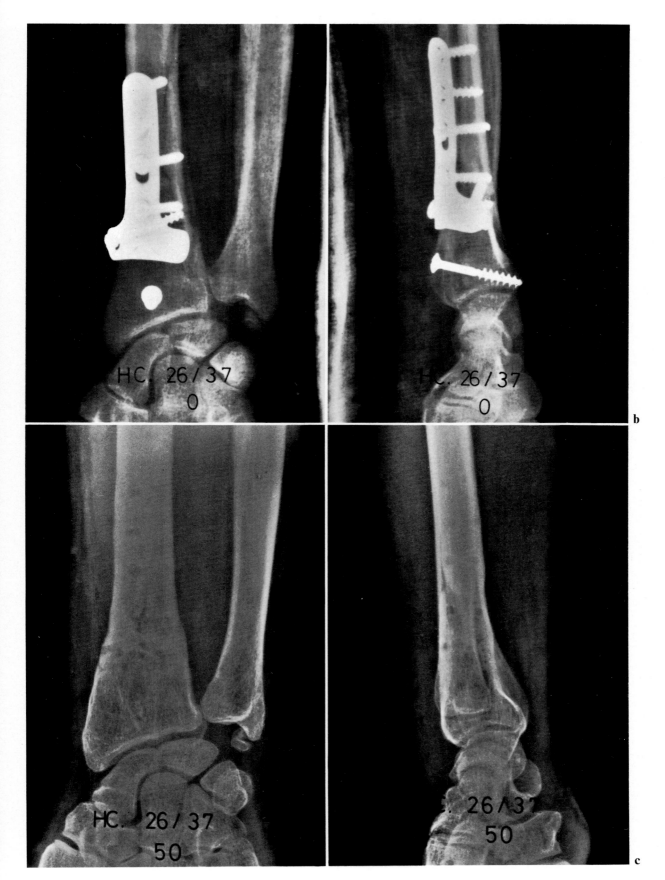

HC. 26/37
0

HC. 26/37
0

b

HC. 26/37
50

26/37
50

c

127

XII. The Wrist Joint

1. Distal Radius

The most frequent fracture in this region, and perhaps the most frequent fracture in man, is the Colles fracture. In German this fracture is called "the fracture of the radius loco classico or loco typico" and in French "Pouteau-Colles fracture". It is a compression fracture of the distal end of the radius with a dorsal and/or radial tilt of the articular surface and a variable degree of shortening of the bone. Most cases are treated conservatively, but serious disability may result if the reduction is inadequate or secondary displacement occurs, which may happen in some 50% of cases. The simple insertion of Kirschner wires percutaneously can be very helpful where there is instability (Fig. 73), but it does not prevent secondary displacement in every instance. This injury should not be considered trivial just because it occurs in elderly patients whose disability need not affect their work or their earnings.

Open reduction and stable internal fixation is indicated in young people if there is a step in the articular surface.

Open reduction is commonly recommended in flexion fractures of the Smith or Barton type, which the French call the Goyrand fracture. Here all or part of the joint surface has a tilt in the palmar direction and there is some shortening of the bone. The proximal row of the carpus is subluxated. Closed reduction of these fractures is very unstable, and percutaneous Kirschner wires do not hold the reduction well enough. In most cases open reduction and rigid internal fixation is needed.

Fractures with an extension as well as a flexion component, which are clear on the lateral X-ray as a Y-shape, are borderline cases, as are comminuted fractures. Each case has

to be treated individually and the indications are limited, but excellent results can be obtained from internal fixation by a well trained surgeon.

Internal fixation can only be stable when screws can obtain a firm grip on the distal fragment, especially in the large fragment of the radial styloid or on the palmar edge of the radius. French and Belgium surgeons often use what they call "bipolar traction", inserting Kirschner wires transversely through the first metacarpal and the radial shaft and incorporating them in a plaster cast. Recently the use of the external fixator has been recommended for such comminuted fractures. The typical and well proven internal fixations with the SFS implants are now described:

a) Isolated Fracture of the Radial Styloid

In only some of these fractures is there an important displacement, but they are always unstable. In some cases they are the visible sign of a trans-scaphoid-perilunar fracture-dislocation, which has spontaneously reduced. An additional scaphoid fracture must therefore be excluded in every case. Internal fixation is better than the uncertain immobilization in plaster. It is achieved by simple screw fixation using two 3.5- or 4.0-mm screws if possible (Fig. 74). In very small fragments a preliminary Kirschner wire may be left in place to prevent rotation deformity.

b) Comminuted Articular Fractures

This type of fracture, which is chiefly seen in road accidents and in athletic injuries to young people, is often characterized by impacted fragments which cannot be reduced by closed manipulation. They are mostly of the extension type and may have steps in the articular surface. Stabilization is usually carried out from the dorsal surface with a small T-plate and 3.5-mm screws, or with the new oblique T-plate using the same screws (Fig. 75).

c) Flexion Fractures (Smith, Barton, Goyrand)

The palmar fragments are difficult to reduce by closed manipulation and are not well held in plaster casts. They press on the flexor tendons and the median nerve in the carpal tunnel. These fractures are therefore classic indications for the use of the buttress plate. The small T-plate with 3.5-mm screws has been developed especially for this and it is easily made to fit the palmar surface of the radius. There may be bony defects which have to be filled in with cancellous bone grafts. The radial styloid cannot be fixed from the palmar surface and additional oblique or transverse screws or Kirschner wires may be needed (Fig. 76).

d) Y-Fractures

These have a flexion and an extension component. A plate needs to be applied to one side of the bone and then cannot support the opposite side, which may then break off because it is not fixed. Experience has shown that the plate should be placed on the least stable side, which is the area of greatest comminution. A large shell-like fragment on the opposite side can be safely fixed by screws through the plate, while small comminuted fragments are better compressed by the plate itself. The image intensifier is helpful here in reduction. After exposure of the fracture site, reduction is achieved by continuously pulling the thumb. The invisible shell-fragments on the opposite side must be stabilized by pressing on a hard support or, with the help of a single finger or a Hohmann retractor, hooked round the radius after mobilization of the tendons of

the extensor pollicis brevis and abductor pollicis longus. This pressure must be maintained while the plate is applied and the screws inserted. Screws in the transverse part of the plate must be long enough (usually cancellous screws of 22–28 mm) to obtain a firm grip on the opposite cortex. The best grip, even in osteoporotic bone is on the palmar articular margin of the radius. In some instances it may be advisable to set the first screw through the oval hole in the shaft of the plate, thus giving support to the comminuted area. Distal fragments are then fixed by inserting screws in the transverse part of the plate and, if possible, by an interfragmentary lag screw through the end hole of the plate. Again any defects must be filled in with cancellous bone graft.

e) Approaches and Technique for Internal Fixation

Experience has shown that surgeons avoid operations of the wrist joint because of the complex anatomy. Especially on the dorsal surface, the many layers of intersecting tendons and nerves make a direct approach to the bone difficult if all the soft tissues are to be left intact. The approaches that have proved successful for the osteosyntheses mentioned are therefore described in detail below.

Approach to the Radial Styloid Process

The guide point for this incision is the tip of the styloid or the radial border of the anatomical snuff box. A slightly curved incision is made in the skin over the dorsoradial aspect of the wrist. Branches of the superficial radial nerve are identified and retracted in an ulnar direction. The styloid process of the radius is exposed between the tendons of extensor pollicis brevis and extensor carpi radialis. The extensor retinaculum must be divided and the fibrous tendon sheaths incised in a longitudinal direction. The tendons of the abductor longus and extensor brevis to the thumb can now be retracted to the radiopalmar side and the fracture exposed, as well as the dorsoradial surface of the wrist joint.

Approach to the Back of the Distal Radius

A lazy S incision begins distally over the base of the second metacarpal (Fig. 77). The superficial branches of the radial nerve are retracted radially. The extensor retinaculum is divided over the tendon of the abductor pollicis longus and reflected to the ulnar side by dissecting its insertion into the dorsal radial crest. This is more effectively performed with a scalpel than a periosteal elevator. The back of the radius can now be exposed by retracting radially the tendons of the extensor pollicis longus, the extensor carpi radialis brevis and longus, the extensor pollicis brevis and the abductor pollicis longus. The tendons of extensor indicis and extensor digitorum communis are retracted to the ulnar side. If necessary the fascia on the radio-palmar edge of the radius may be divided, giving access to the pronator quadratus muscle and the palmar aspect of the radius for a surgeon's finger or a Hohmann retractor (Fig. 77a).

The oblique T-plate, using 3.5-mm screws, is appropriate for this area; the screw holes are such that the plate can be used for either hand. The oblique part of the plate covers the dorsal surface of the styloid process (Fig. 75).

After fixing the plate, the retinaculum may be reconstructed over it and the extensor tendons, but as we know from the surgery of rheumatic disease, this is not mandatory and the retinaculum may be passed between the plate and the extensor tendons, which now lie in the subcutaneous tissue (Fig. 77c). The rounded shape of the screw heads preclude any danger of tendon injuries, and active movement after the operation prevents adhesions of the tendons, especially of extensor pollicis longus.

Approach to the Distal Radius from the Palmar Surface

The guide point here is the tendon of flexor carpi radialis. A wide exposure is important to allow decompression of the median nerve in the carpal tunnel at the same time as the internal fixation of the distal radius. The flexor retinaculum must therefore be divided in its whole length to give satisfactorry decompression of the tendons, nerves, and vessels.

The S-shaped incision begins in the thenar crease and crosses the wrist joint towards the ulnar side (Fig. 78a). The median nerve is identified on the ulnar side of the tendon of flexor carpi radialis and is followed through the carpal tunnel. Its sensory branch to the thenar skin must be protected. It arises some distance above the wrist from the median nerve and runs parallel to the main branch distally, crossing the flexor carpi radialis tendon on its way to the skin of the thumb.

After dividing the ulnar side of the flexor retinaculum the median nerve and its branch are held radially, together with the flexor carpi radialis (Fig. 78b), and the flexor tendons within their tendon sheaths are retracted to the ulnar side. Occasionally the median nerve may be retracted to the ulnar side, together with the digital flexors. The palmar edge of the radius and the pronator quadratus muscle are now exposed. The muscle is incised at its radial insertion and reflected to the ulnar side with a periosteal dissector (Fig. 79). The fracture is exposed and the wrist joint identified by inserting a needle or Kirschner wire or the capsule may be incised transversely for reduction. It is difficult to expose the radial styloid using this approach.

Second Approach

Where the distal radio-ulnar joint must be exposed, the approach is made from the ulnar side and the flexor tendons, together with the median nerve, are retracted laterally (Fig. 79). The flexor carpi ulnaris tendon together with the ulnar vessels and the nerve is retracted medially.

Closure of the Wound

Only the skin is closed in either approach but a suction drain is always inserted. A well-padded posterior plaster slab is applied until wound healing is complete. This allows elevation of the limb and mobilization of the fingers with the wrist in a functional position. If stability is doubtful the slab may be left in place for several weeks, but movements of the fingers may be started immediately after operation.

Removal of the Implants

Incisions are made in the line of the original wounds but because of subcutaneous fibrous tissue formation it may be difficult to protect the branches of the radial nerve posteriorly. It is easier therefore to remove palmar plates than those on the dorsum, though the sensory branch of the median nerve must be protected.

f) Secondary Operation

Secondary Internal Fixation

The best results are obtained when redisplacement of a reduced extension fracture is discovered before consolidation is complete. There must be no atrophy or impairment of circulation if a secondary operation is to be successful. Using a dorsal approach, the dorsal impaction of the articular surface, the radial impaction, and the shortening of the radius are corrected. This leads to a defect in the metaphysis which must be filled in with cancellous bone graft. In cases of severe osteoporosis a corticocancellous graft may be required. For stabilization the small T-plate or the small oblique plate is used, and must be accurately contoured.

Pseudarthrosis of the Distal Radius

In the rare instances when this occurs, it is fixed by a dorsal T-plate or a 3.5-mm DCP, depending on the shape of the non-union. Bony defects are again filled with cancellous bone.

Osteotomy

This is most often indicated for correction of malunion after conservative treatment of a Colles fracture involving dorsal and radial impaction of the articular surface and shortening of the bone. X-ray evidence of malposition is not in itself an indication for osteotomy; the deciding factors are the functional limitation of the hand and wrist and the associated pain. Carpal tunnel compression may also be present and the median nerve must therefore be checked by neurography before secondary operation. If there is median nerve entrap-

ment, decompression of the nerve must be performed at the same time as the correction osteotomy, using the same technique and implants as for secondary internal fixation.

As a rule articular steps cannot be corrected by secondary operation. An osteotomy does not relieve the post-traumatic arthrosis here.

If, in elderly patients, there is marked limitation of pronation and supination caused by the relative elongation of the ulna, the operation on the radius must be combined with resection of the head of the ulna.

Osteotomy for lengthening or shortening is very rarely needed in the distal radius. When necessary, fixation can be achieved by the small T-plate or straight plate of the SFS.

2. Distal Ulna

In the narrow part of the distal ulna transverse or short oblique fractures occasionally occur, either in isolation or in combination with fractures of the lower end or shaft of the radius. These fractures are placed under stress in pronation and supination and are therefore unstable and need to be fixed by internal means. This is best done using the one-third tubular plate or the small DCP with 3.5-mm screws. As the distal ulna is subcutaneous the approach is simple.

Secondary operation: Indications for secondary operation to the distal ulna are fairly frequent. Such operations are mostly needed for malposition of the lower radius, where there is subluxation of the distal radio-ulnar joint and relative lengthening of the ulna. Painful arthrosis of the distal radio-ulnar joint or trouble in the lower end of the ulna in rheumatoid disease are indications for resection of the head of the ulna. Stability of the wrist joint is little affected by this procedure.

In corrective procedures for malunion of the radius in young patients, osteotomy to shorten the ulna may be necessary. This sometimes restores pronation and supination.

3. Scaphoid

a) Indications

Undisplaced fractures of the scaphoid treated conservatively usually heal after 8–12 weeks in a suitable plaster cast, while solitary fracture of the tubercle will settle down after 3–4 weeks. From long experience it is clear that indications for primary internal fixation of the scaphoid are limited.

Internal fixation is justified in displaced fractures of the middle third which cannot be easily reduced by closed methods. This is especially true for the perilunate trans-scaphoid fracture-dislocation described by De Quervain, 50% of which end in pseudarthrosis. Internal fixation is also indicated for the uncommon vertical oblique fracture which, like Pauwels type III fracture of the neck of femur, is especially exposed to strong shearing forces, so that development of pseudarthrosis is six times as common as in any other type of fracture. The established method is fixation with a small cancellous screw if the proximal fragment is large enough to accommodate the whole thread, but otherwise one uses a 3.5- or 2.7-mm cortex screw inserted lag-wise.

b) Approach and Internal Fixation

A curved dorsoradial incision is made in the anatomical snuffbox (Fig. 80a). The superficial branches of the radial nerve and the tendon of extensor pollicis longus are retracted together posteriorly. The tendons of extensor pollicis brevis and abductor pollicis longus are retracted together with the radial artery in a radial direction (Fig. 80b). The wrist joint is opened at the dorsal edge of the radial styloid process. The hand is held in strong palmar and ulnar flexion. The fracture is exposed and reduced with the help of a fine elevator or hook (Fig. 80c). The articular cartilage must be carefully protected. Provisional transfixion with a fine Kirschner wire inserted from the tubercle is the next step. The position and length of the wire can be verified by X-ray. Using the triple drill guide and a 2.0-mm bit,

an axial hole is drilled parallel to the wire. After tapping the thread, a small cancellous screw is inserted into this hole. In order to prevent rotation of the proximal fragment, the guide wire should only be removed after the screw has been tightened (Fig. 81).

The primary partial excision of the radial styloid to give improved exposure of the fracture is disputed, because it may disturb the blood supply.

c) Secondary Operation

Delayed union of a fracture after conservative treatment is an excellent indication for screw fixation. The bony fragments must be alive if success is to be achieved, and subsequent immobilization in plaster is indispensable.

A real pseudarthrosis with sclerosis and poor vascularity of the fracture surfaces resembles the atrophic pseudarthrosis in other bones. This cannot be treated by a screw alone; cancellous bone grafting, as described by Matti and Russe, is the most reliable method.

4. Other Parts of the Carpus

Fractures of other bones of the carpus are rare, but when they occur internal fixation is indicated as long as large and easily approached fragments are present. Small screws can be used.

5. Fusion of the Wrist Joint

Arthrodesis is indicated in severe comminution of the carpus, in painful post-traumatic arthrosis, in destruction of the joint by chronic inflammatory disease like rheumatic fever or tuberculosis, or in cases of instability or subluxation. After removal of any remaining articular cartilage, internal fixation is carried out with a plate to fix the distal radius across the carpus to the second or third metacarpal. The DCP is suitable for this purpose. The

3.5-mm screw version can be used where the skeleton is slender, but if the bones are heavier the normal 4.5-mm screw DCP is more suitable. Bony defects are filled in with cancellous bone graft and the carpus is bridged from the radius to the capitate with corticocancellous bone taken from the pelvis. Before the plate is screwed to the carpus a lag screw is inserted through the radial styloid process to the capitate, pulling the carpus to the radial side and thus preserving the distal radio-ulnar joint (Fig. 82).

6. Clinical X-ray Examples
(Figs. 83–91)

Fig. 73. Displaced, articular T-fracture of the distal radius

Stabilization by Kirschner wires which are introduced percutaneously

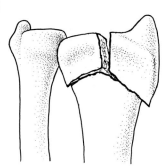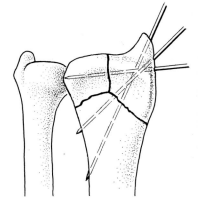

Fig. 74. Unstable fracture of the styloid process of the radius

Screw fixation

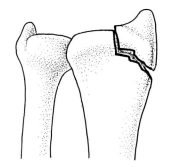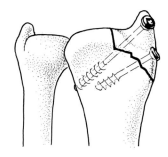

Fig. 75. Unstable fracture of the lower end of the radius with dorsal displacement (Colles-Poutteau)

Internal fixation by an oblique T-plate applied posteriorly

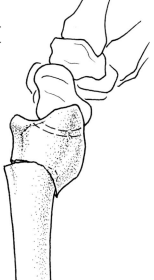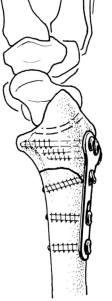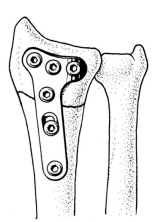

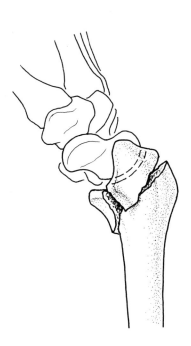
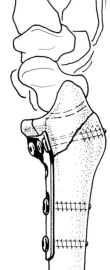

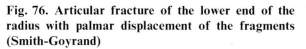

Fig. 76. Articular fracture of the lower end of the radius with palmar displacement of the fragments (Smith-Goyrand)

Internal fixation by a palmar T-plate. In a fracture of the styloid process of the radius a separate, oblique lag screw is needed

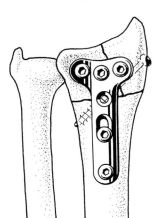

Fig. 77 a–c. Approach to the radiodorsal aspect of the lower radius

a S-shaped incision:
1) Approach to the styloid process of the radius through a small incision between the tendons of the extensor pollicis brevis and the extensor carpi radialis.

2) Approach to the distal metaphysis of the radius by division of the extensor retinaculum between the extensor carpi radialis brevis and the extensor pollicis longus tendons.

3) Combined approach for dorsal positioning of a plate and control of reduction on the palmar aspect. Division of the extensor retinaculum at the palmar border of abductor pollicis longus tendon sheath and reflection of the retinaculum to the dorso-ulnar side. With one finger the surgeon may now control the reduction of the palmar cortex below the pronator quadratus muscle

b The approaches in cross-section:
1) Between the tendons of extensor pollicis brevis and extensor carpi radialis longus.

2) Between the extensor carpi radialis brevis and ▷ the extensor pollicis longus tendon with reflection of the tendon sheaths.

3) At the palmar edge of the abductor pollicis longus tendon with reflection of the extensor retinaculum to the dorso-ulnar side

c At the end of the internal fixation, the extensor retinaculum may be sutured back below the tendons for protection of the latter, which is not possible in all instances

EI Tendon of Extensor indicis
EDC Tendon of Extensor digitorum communis
EDQ Tendon of Extensor digiti quinti
ECU Tendon of Extensor carpi ulnaris
FCR Tendon of Flexor carpi radialis
PL Tendon of Palmaris longus
FDS Tendon of Flexor digitorum superficialis
FDP Tendon of Flexor digitorum profundus
FCU Tendon of Flexor carpi ulnaris

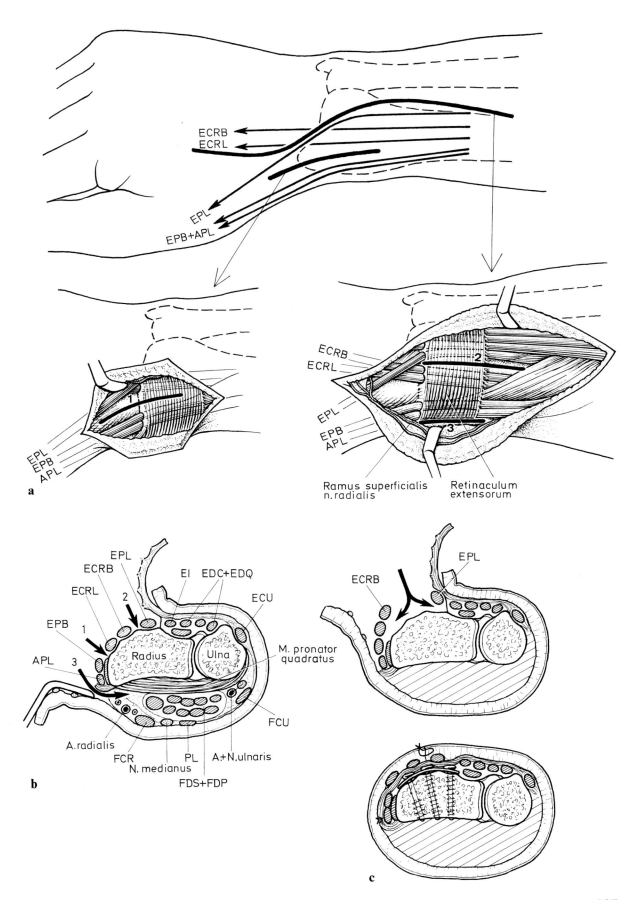

a

ECRB
ECRL

EPL

EPB+APL

EPL
EPB
APL

ECRB
ECRL

EPL
EPB
APL

Ramus superficialis   Retinaculum
n. radialis   extensorum

b

EPL
ECRB
ECRL

EPB

APL

EI   EDC+EDQ

ECU

Radius   Ulna   M. pronator
quadratus

FCU

A. radialis

FCR   PL   A.+N. ulnaris
N. medianus
FDS+FDP

ECRB   EPL

EPL

c

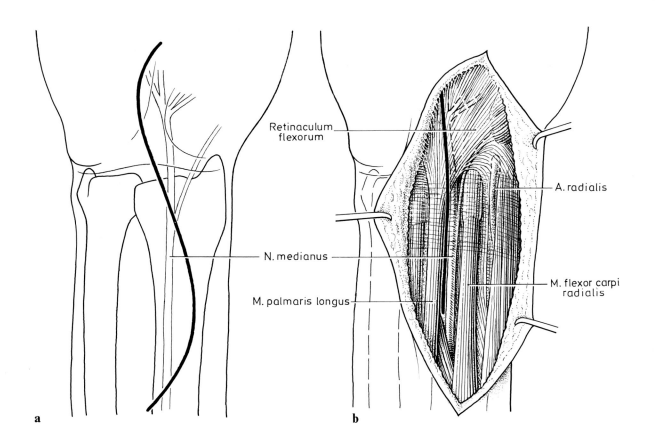

a

b

Retinaculum
flexorum

A. radialis

N. medianus

M. flexor carpi
radialis

M. palmaris longus

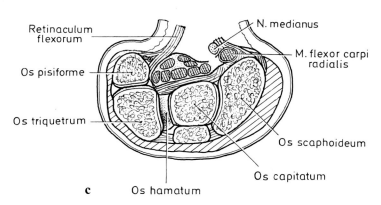

Retinaculum
flexorum

N. medianus

M. flexor carpi
radialis

Os pisiforme

Os triquetrum

Os scaphoideum

Os capitatum

c   Os hamatum

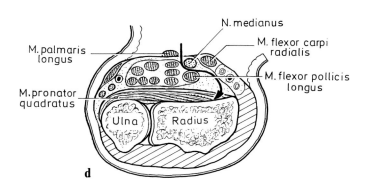

M. palmaris
longus

N. medianus

M. flexor carpi
radialis

M. flexor pollicis
longus

M. pronator
quadratus

Ulna   Radius

d

**Fig. 78 a–d. Approach to the palmar aspect
of the lower end of the radius**

a Long, S-shaped skin incision

b Division of the flexor retinaculum and
approach medial to the flexor carpi radialis tendon. For protection of the palmar
branch, which leaves the median nerve
just above the wrist joint, the median
nerve is drawn to the radial side together
with the palmar branch

c Distal cross-section at the level of the
flexor retinaculum. The median nerve is
retracted to the radial side

d Proximal cross-section at the level of
the distal end of the radius

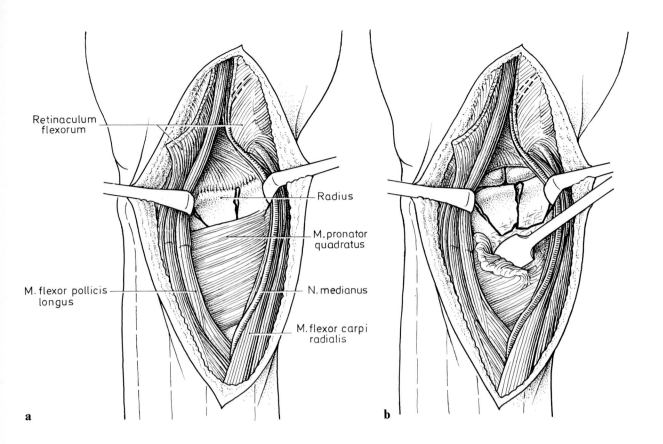

Retinaculum flexorum

M. flexor pollicis longus

Radius

M. pronator quadratus

N. medianus

M. flexor carpi radialis

a

b

Fig. 79 a–c. Approach to the lower end of the radius from the palmar aspect, deep layer

a The median nerve and the flexor carpi radialis tendon are retracted laterally. Exposure of the fracture and the pronator quadratus muscle

b Division of the pronator quadratus muscle at its radial insertion and reflection to the ulnar side. If necessary for reduction, the radiocarpal joint may be opened and inspected

c Second approach: The tendons are retracted laterally to expose the distal radioulnar joint

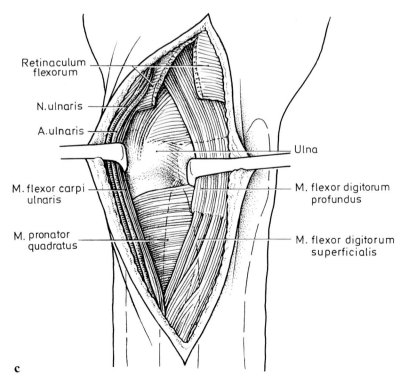

Retinaculum flexorum

N. ulnaris

A. ulnaris

M. flexor carpi ulnaris

M. pronator quadratus

Ulna

M. flexor digitorum profundus

M. flexor digitorum superficialis

c

139

Fig. 80a–c. Fracture of the scaphoid: incision and exposure

a Incision of the skin

b Topography: The tendons of the extensor pollicis longus and the extensor carpi radialis longus are retracted dorsally together with the branches of the superficial radial nerve. Some other branches of the radial nerve and the radial artery are retracted to the palmar side

c The wrist joint is opened at the dorsal margin of the styloid process of the radius. The fracture is reduced with the help of a fine hook

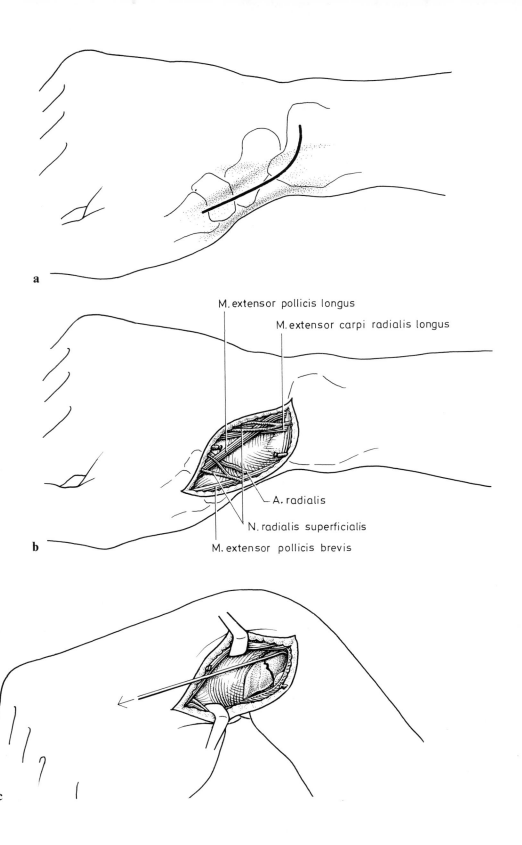

a

M. extensor pollicis longus

M. extensor carpi radialis longus

A. radialis

N. radialis superficialis

M. extensor pollicis brevis

b

c

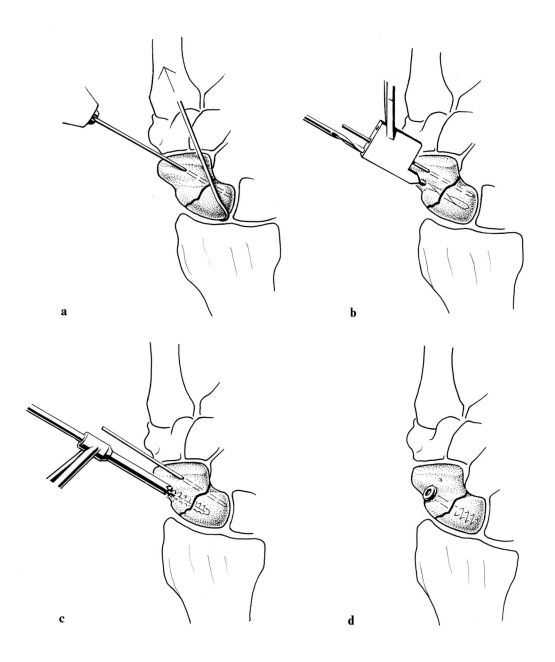

Fig. 81 a–d. Internal fixation of a fracture of the scaphoid

a Transfixion of the reduced fracture with a fine Kirschner wire in the distal part of the bone. X-ray control

b Using the drill guide to place the drill hole parallel to the guide wire

c Tapping the thread

d Insertion of the screw and removal of the Kirschner wire

142

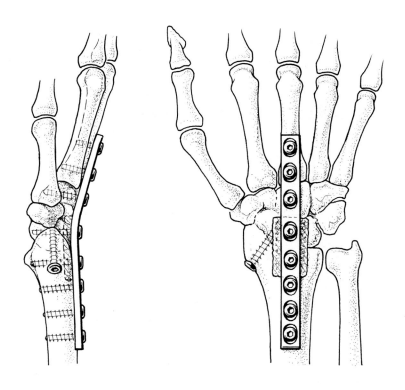

Fig. 82. Arthrodesis of the wrist joint with the 3.5-mm dynamic compression plate

The cartilage is removed from the radiocarpal and the intercarpal joint surfaces. Defects are filled in with cancellous bone. A 3.5-mm lag screw is introduced through the styloid process of the radius into the capitate bone. It fixes the carpus to the radial styloid and keeps clear of the distal radioulnar joint.

A flat, rectangular, corticocancellous bone graft from the iliac fossa is inserted in a prepared bed between the carpus and the distal radius.

Internal fixation is achieved by a 3.5-mm DCP with eight holes. Compression of the radiocarpal joint is exerted with one screw in the capitate bone and one screw in the radius, proximal to the bone graft. The graft is compressed in the transverse plane by cortical or cancellous lag screws. The plate must be fixed to the third (exceptionally to the second) metacarpal bone by two or three screws and to the radius by four screws.

In the large skeleton of heavy workers arthrodesis of the wrist joint is preferred with the 4.5-mm DCP

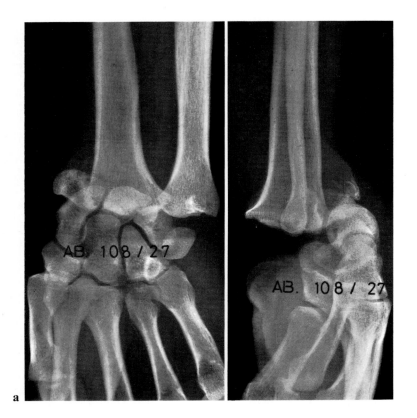

a

Fig. 83a–c. Clinical example: Screw fixation of a radiocarpal fracture-dislocation

R., M., 33-year-old construction draughtsman

a Fracture dislocation of the wrist joint with avulsion of the radial styloid process caused by a fall while playing football

b Primary reduction and internal fixation with one 4.0-mm cancellous screw and a 3.5-mm cortex lag screw. Removable splint for the wrist joint for 4 weeks. Working capacity of 50% after $2^1/_2$ weeks, of 100% after $2^1/_2$ months. Removal of the screws at $5^1/_2$ months

c Review after $13^1/_2$ months: Small defect within the articular surface of the radius, no arthrosis. The patient was pain-free and had full strength of the hand. Flexion was limited by 15°, the range of motion being otherwise the same in both wrists

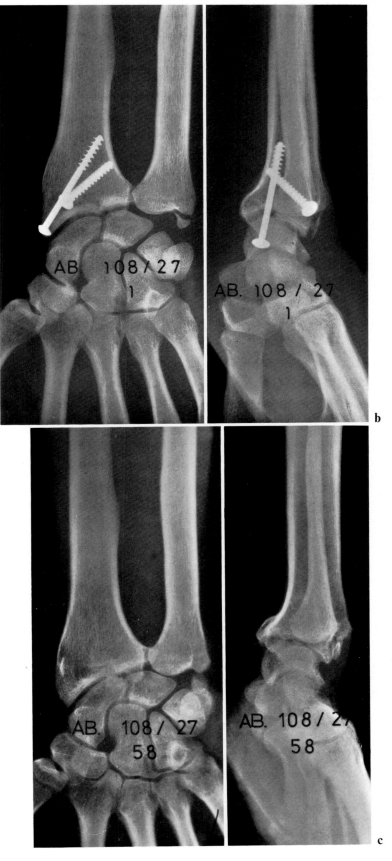

b

c

145

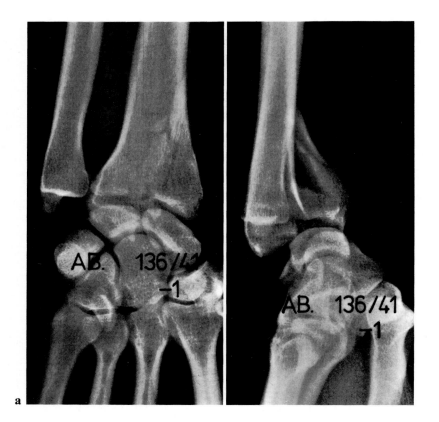

a

Fig. 84a–c. Clinical example: Internal fixation with a palmar plate of a fracture of the lower radius with palmar displacement (Smith-Goyrand)

G., J., 40-year-old worker at a chemical factory

a Fracture of the distal radius of the Smith-Goyrand type caused by a motorcycle accident. The attempted conservative treatment had failed. Therefore internal fixation was done after 10 days with a palmar T-plate. Functional treatment without stress was started immediately

b X-ray picture after 4 weeks. Working capacity was partial after 3 months and complete after 4 months

c After 13 months a slight irregularity is present at the articular surface. The patient has no pain even on hard work, the range of motion is full. Since the patient is not disturbed by the implants, these are left indefinitely

146

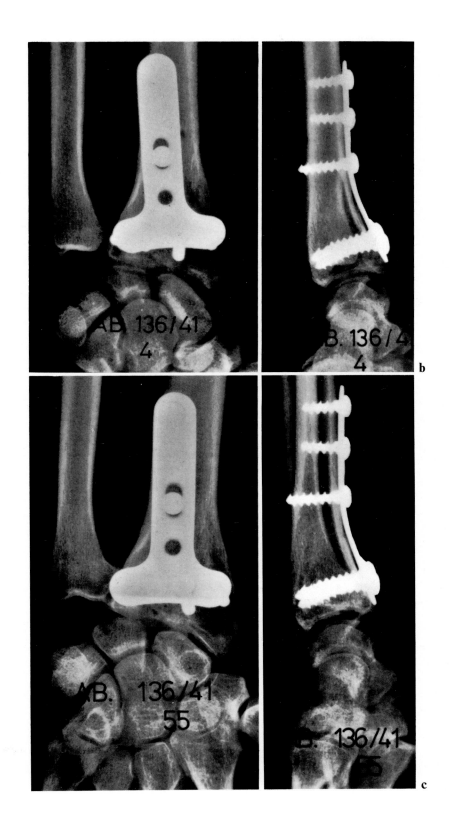

AB. 136/41
4

B. 136/4
4

b

AB. 136/41
55

B. 136/41
55

c

147

Fig. 85a–d. Clinical example: Palmar T-plate at the lower end of the radius for a comminuted fracture with median nerve compression

M., Gertrud, 44-year-old secretary. Skiing accident with fall on the outstretched left hand. Paraesthesiae in the index and long finger were present at once

a Displaced, comminuted fracture of the distal end of the radius. The X-rays do not show the full displacement on the palmar aspect

b At immediate operation the median nerve was found riding on a bone fragment, which has perforated through the flexor tendons. Internal fixation with T-plate. Bony defects were filled in with cancellous bone graft from the iliac crest. The median nerve was decompressed by division of the flexor retinaculum as far as the palmar arterial arch. Postoperative course without complications. Functional treatment protected by a removable plaster splint. Full weight lifting after 8 weeks

c, d see page 150f.

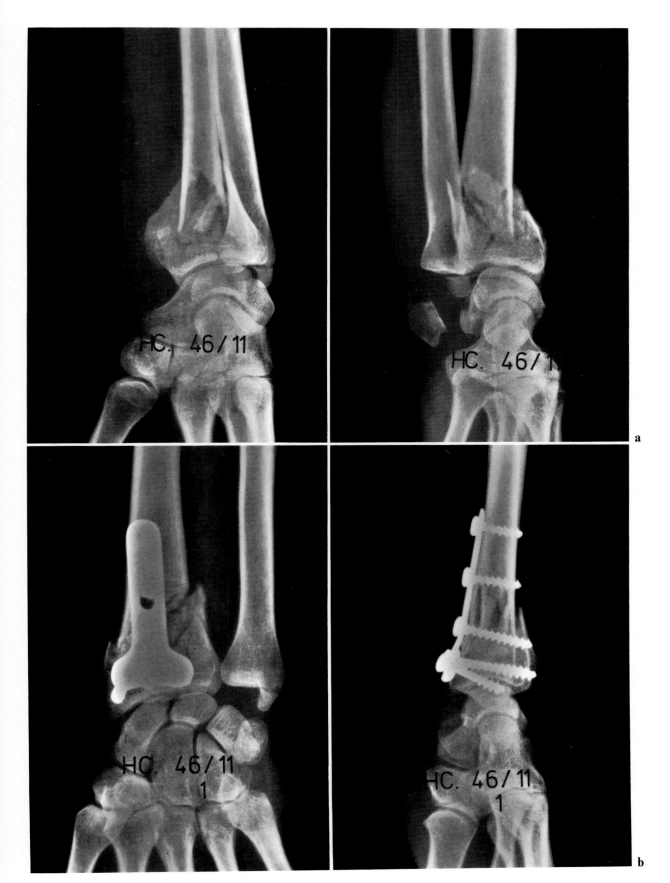

a

b

149

Fig. 85c, d

c Removal of the implants after 8 months: A loose screw caused synovitis of the flexor tendons and partial erosion of one tendon

d Review at $1^1/_2$ years: No complaints. The patients is still working as a secretary and has a full range of joint movement. There is no atrophy of the muscles and no arthrosis

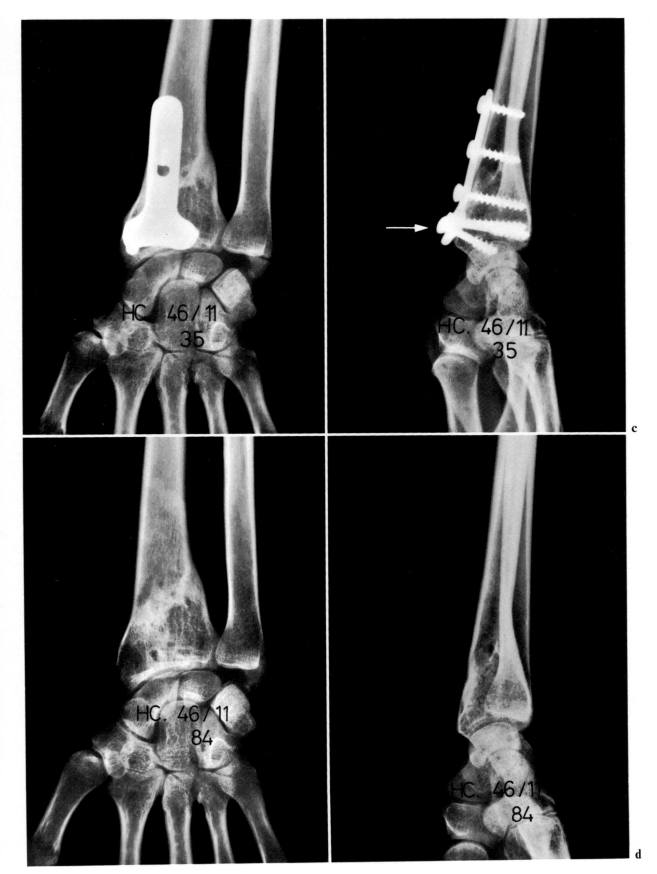

Fig. 86a–c. Clinical example: Dorsal T-plate in Colles fracture

H., R., retired school teacher aged 66 years

a Fracture of the distal metaphysis of the radius. Closed reduction and percutaneous pin fixation resulted in malalignment and shortening of the radius

b Open reduction and internal fixation with oblique T-plate after 4 days. Removable plaster splint for 2 weeks followed by functional treatment. The X-ray picture was at 15 weeks after operation. Removal of the plate after 8 months

c One year after the injury: Correct axial alignment slight shortening of the radius, no arthrosis. The patient is pain-free. Both extension and flexion are limited by 20°, whereas pronation and supination are full

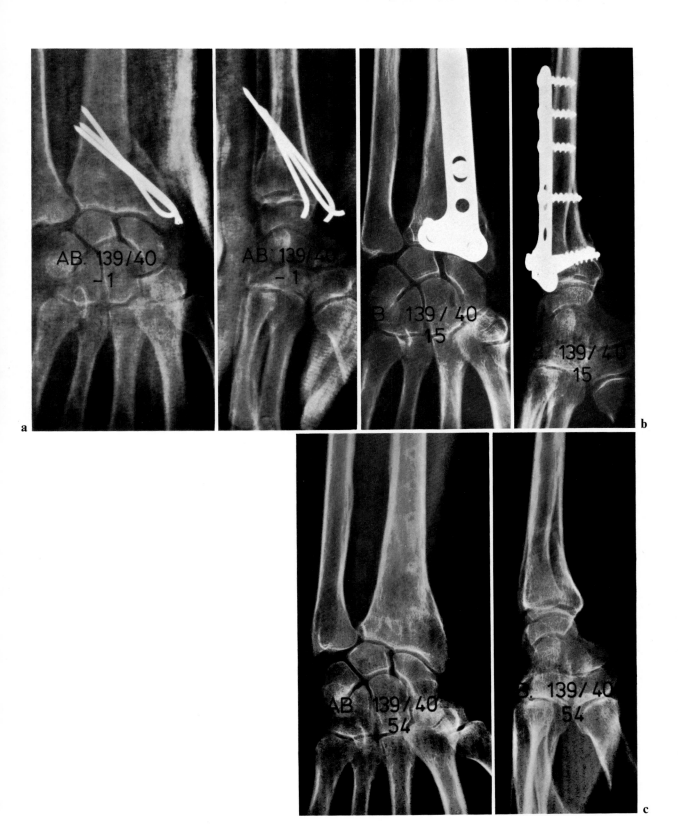

a

b

c

153

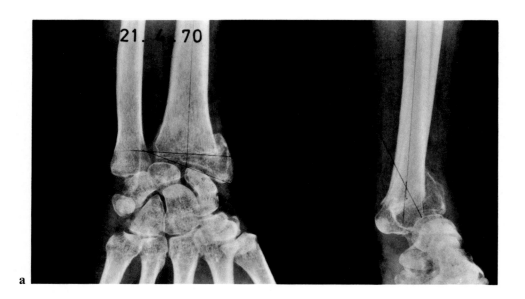

Fig. 87a–d. Clinical example: Dorsal T-plate at the radius in a case of malposition

T., Lena, 41-year-old housewife. Fracture of the distal end of the radius by a fall on the hand. Closed reduction and fixation by plaster cast. Secondary displacement of the fracture. Admission for corrective operation after 9 weeks

a Severe malposition with shortening and dorsal impaction of the radius, atrophy of the bone and trophic disorders with marked limitation of movements of the wrist and the fingers

b An osteotomy was performed with a radiodorsal approach and a corticocancellous bone graft interposed 3 months after injury. Stabilization was achieved by a dorsal buttress T-plate
No complications in the postoperative course. Functional treatment without external support. Removal of the implants after 6 months

c Review after 17 months: Slight limitation of movement of the wrist joint, the fingers being fully mobile. The trophic changes have healed, and the psychosomatic component has diminished

d 8 years after injury: Still has a slight psychological disorder. There is some swelling of the wrist joint. Palmar flexion is reduced by 25°, dorsiflexion by 10°. Pronation and supination are the same in both hands. The function of the thumb and fingers is normal. The X-ray demonstrates correct alignment and normal bone structure

154

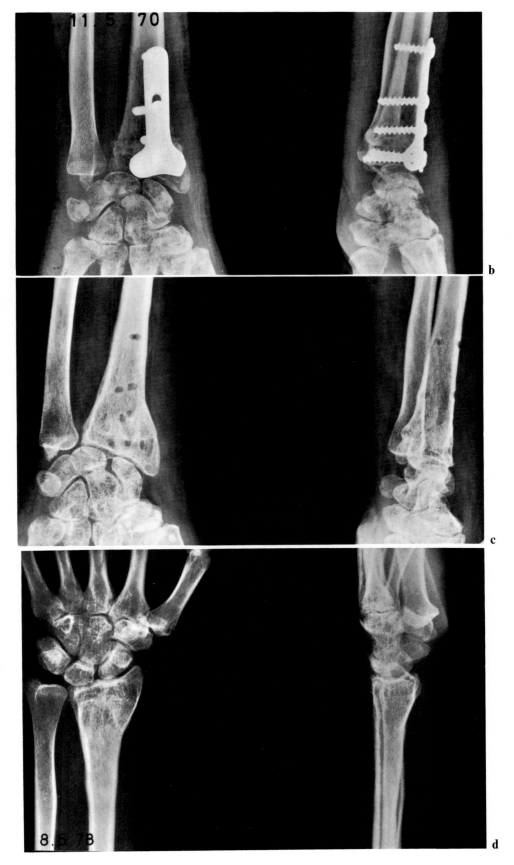

11 5 70

8.5 78

b

c

d

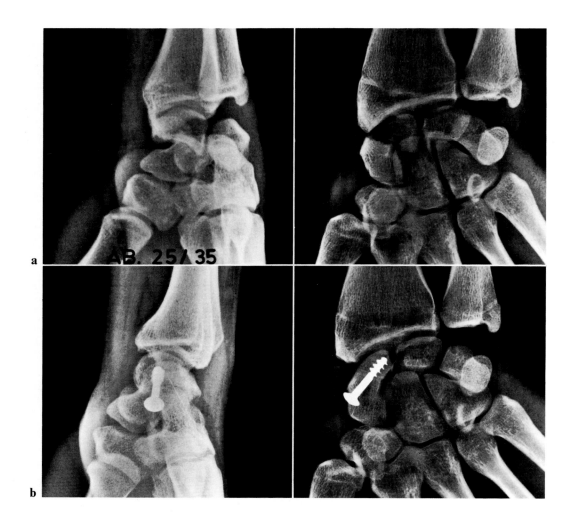

Fig. 88 a, b. Clinical example: Trans-scaphoid, peri-lunar fracture-dislocation of the scaphoid (De Quervain)

W., P., male student aged 18. Fall from small motorcycle

a De Quervain's perilunar fracture-dislocation of the scaphoid. Closed reduction of the dislocation but the scaphoid fracture remained displaced

b Screw fixation of the fracture one week after injury. Plaster cast for 4 weeks. Full weight lifting and capacity for sports after 8 weeks. Removal of the screw after 11 months.
One year after injury the patient is free of pain. There is limitation of 15° of extension, flexion, ulnar abduction and pronation of the wrist

Fig. 89 a–c. Clinical example: Fracture of trapezium

M., R., male elevator fitter aged 30. Fall from bicycle

a Vertical fracture of the trapezium

b Internal fixation after one week with 4.0-mm small cancellous screw. No external splint. Immediate functional treatment. Full working capacity after 7 weeks. X-ray was taken 40 weeks after injury

c Removal of the screw after 11 months. The patient had no complaints, full function and no arthrosis

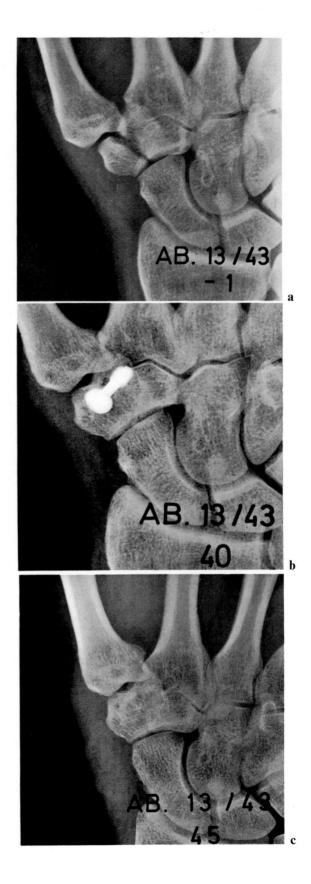

157

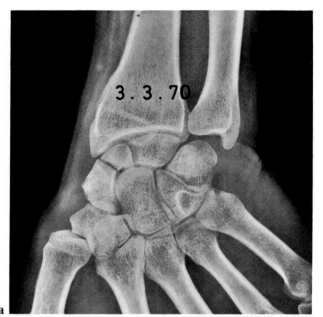

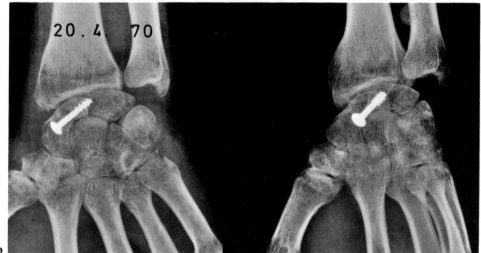

Fig. 90 a–d. Clinical example: Pseudarthrosis of scaphoid

B., Luis, merchant aged 41. Fall on his hand. Treated as a sprain

a X-ray after 10 months shows non-union of the scaphoid without displacement or cysts. The fragments are alive. Plaster cast for 3 months is unsuccessful

b 13 months after injury the pseudarthrosis is fixed with a screw and styloidectomy is done.
Uncomplicated postoperative course. Plaster cast for 4 months. Removal of the screw after 11 months

c After 2 years there were no complaints, full function and no arthrosis

d 10 years after the operation, the patient is still free of pain and has full mobility of the wrist joint. The X-ray shows regeneration of the radial styloid process and slight arthrosis

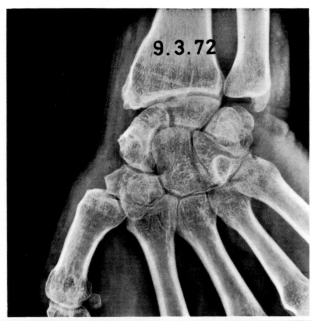

c

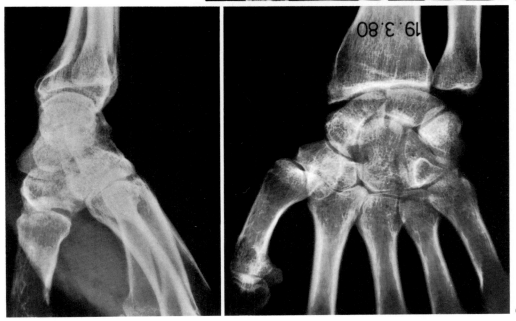

d

159

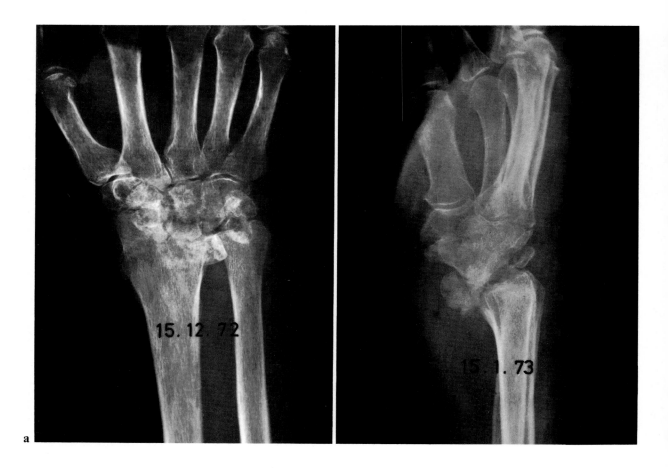

a

Fig. 91 a–c. Clinical example: Arthrodesis of the wrist joint with plate and autogenous cancellous bone graft

M., Anna, housewife aged 76. For 2 years the patient had had a painful wrist with episodes of swelling of different joints, especially the right wrist. A capsular biopsy showed chronic synovitis and *B. coli* was cultured from the synovial fluid

a The X-rays taken later showed destruction of the joint, which could not be seen before

b The carpus was then resected since it was completely destroyed and porotic. The defect of the two carpal rows was replaced by a cancellous bone graft from the iliac crest with slight shortening. Stabilization was achieved by a long one-third tubular plate (combination of one six hole plate and one eight hole plate) between the radius and the third metacarpal. The distal end of the ulna was resected.

The surprising histological diagnosis was that of tuberculosis of the bone.

Uneventful postoperative course with antituberculous treatment and protection with a removable splint. For several months the patient was treated in a sanatorium. 16 months after operation, the arthrodesis is united and the implants are removed. Infection was healed and the hand could be used reasonably

c 2 years after surgery the clinical and X-ray findings show the tuberculosis to be still healed

160

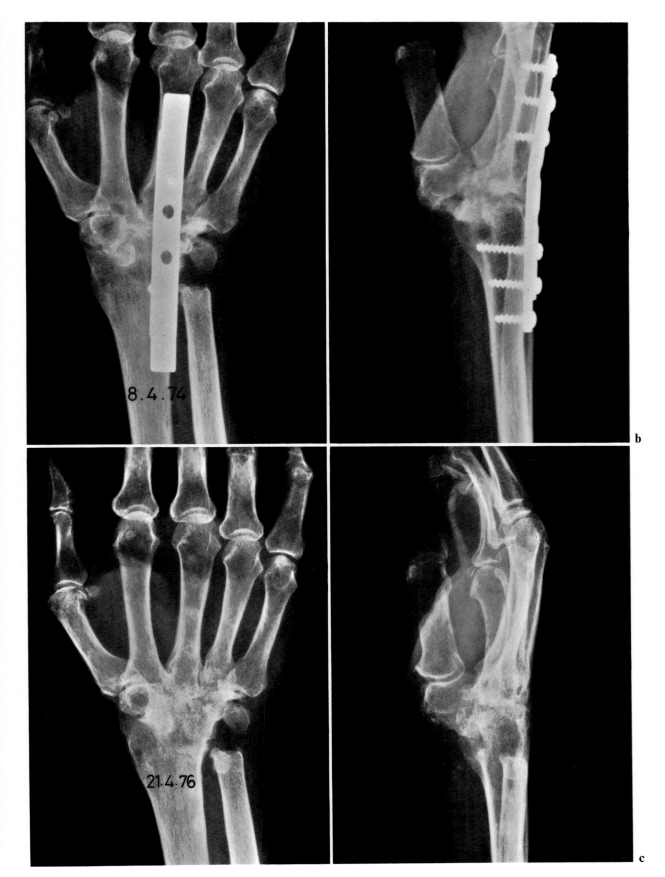

8.4.74

b

21.4.76

c

161

XIII. The Hand

A. Introduction

The technique of internal fixation of the bones in the hand is difficult, and the surgeon assumes great responsibility. A thorough knowledge of the contents of the instrument set and a good grasp of the functional anatomy of the hand are indispensable. Delicate atraumatic treatment of the soft tissues is essential to preserve full mobility. Unsuitable incisions and injury to the peritendinous layers and capsule of the joints can result in permanent stiffness. Experience has, however, shown that rigid internal fixation enables us to achieve much better results than the previously used procedures, provided that the techniques described are adhered to carefully.

This is particularly true for open fracture of the bones of the hand with injuries to the tendons, nerves or vessels. Rigid internal fixation of bony fragments aids the postoperative treatment of the soft tissues involved. Primary reconstruction of all the injured structures can thus be obtained in one step. Stabilization of the bony fragments also helps wound healing because splints and plaster casts can be dispensed with. There are, however, some limitations to the scope of comprehensive primary treatment, either because of circulatory impairment from crush injuries, especially in the finger, or because the safe tourniquet time must not be exceeded. When multiple open fractures and associated injuries of nerves, tendons, vessels or skin require time-consuming grafting procedures, the surgeon should consider whether simple Kirschner wires, inserted obliquely, axially or transversely, perhaps combined with hemicerclage wiring, should be preferred to rigid internal fixation.

Many small fragments are unsuitable for screw fixation; for these tension-band wiring can be used, either in a figure-of-eight system or by wires inserted with a pull-out method as in Bunnell's tendon sutures. Internal fixation is imperative where there are rotational deformities or articular steps which cannot be reduced.

B. Injuries and Internal Fixation of the First Ray

Special methods are needed to deal with the first or opposition ray for three reasons: (a) basal fractures of the first metacarpal and associated conditions are important; (b) fractures in the region of the metacarpo-phalangeal and interphalangeal joints of the thumb are common; (c) because the muscles and tendons are strong here, most shaft fractures are unstable so that it is difficult to employ conservative means to hold fragments firmly. Internal fixation is then often indicated and except for Bennett's fracture anatomical approaches to the thumb are relatively simple.

1. Fracture of the Base of the First Metacarpal

a) Approach to the First Carpometacarpal Joint and Operative Technique

The main problem in achieving perfect reduction and internal fixation of Bennett's fracture-dislocation is that the small proximal palmar fragment is difficult to see.

Radiopalmar Approach Described by Gedda-Moberg. This gives the best exposure and begins with a radiopalmar sickle-shaped incision at the level of the first carpometacarpal joint and extended dorsally. The tendon of abductor pollicis longus and the accompanying nerves must be carefully protected (Fig. 92). The joint is opened from the palmar surface and, if necessary, from the dorsum as well. The fracture is temporarily fixed by a fine Kirschner wire introduced from the palmar side (Fig. 94 c).

Radiodorsal Approach. A longitudinal incision is made over the radial edge of the first metacarpal bone and extended proximally to raise a Y-shaped flap on the dorsal and palmar side (Fig. 93 a). The periosteum is then incised at the radial side of the extensor pollicis brevis, preserving the insertion of abductor pollicis longus and the fine branch of the radial nerve to the back of the thumb (Fig. 93 b). The thenar muscles are elevated to expose the radiopalmar aspect of the joint, which is opened just below the abductor pollicis longus tendon. The fracture is then reduced and provisionally transfixed by a fine Kirschner wire inserted from the dorsum. Exposure of the fracture is less satisfactory using this approach but it is easier to protect the soft tissues and the capsule.

b) Bennett's Fracture-Dislocation

This is a fracture-dislocation of the first carpometacarpal joint. The shaft fragment is displaced to the dorsoradial side and is held in adduction. A small ulnopalmar fragment remains fixed to the carpus. Unless the dislocation is completely reduced, it will certainly lead to severe post-traumatic arthrosis, with pain and disability in the whole thumb. Full abduction of the thumb must be provided to allow a broad grip between the thumb and index, as emphasized by Iselin's school. Though it is uncommon, Bennett's fracture is often mentioned in the literature and many surgeons have tried to find a reliable procedure for achieving and maintaining reduction.

Our experience has convinced us that for fractures with a large proximal fragment, open reduction and rigid fixation with a screw is the best procedure, though there are some technical difficulties.

If there is a very small proximal fragment, which is unsuitable for screw fixation, we prefer closed reduction and transfixion with a fine, oblique Kirschner wire according to the technique described by Wagner.

Screw fixation is best done from the dorsal aspect whether using the palmar or radiodorsal approach (Fig. 94). A hole is drilled in the centre of the fragment with a 2-mm bit and the thread is tapped. A small cancellous screw is used in larger fragments, but in smaller ones the screw must be in proportion to the size of the fragment. A cortex screw can be used to obtain interfragmentary compression if the screw hole is drilled out to a diameter larger than the screw while the thread is tapped in the drill hole of the palmar fragment. This is difficult but important. Review of our cases has shown that post-traumatic arthrosis does not occur even if reduction is not ideal, as long as the dislocation has been corrected.

The transfixion wire is only removed after the screw has been tightened to prevent rotation of the small fragment. In some cases it may be left in place.

If for technical reasons screw fixation is not possible, because the fragment is too small or there are multiple pieces which have not been seen on X-ray, we prefer internal fixation with two or more intersecting Kirschner wires according to Moberg (Fig. 94 b–d).

c) Rolando's Fracture

This is a Y-shaped intra-articular fracture of the base of the first metacarpal and is usually comminuted. Internal fixation is technically difficult but is indicated when there is no gross displacement or instability.

Operative technique. The best exposure is provided by the Gedda-Moberg incision, which must be extended distally along the back of the first metacarpal (Fig. 92a). The extensor tendons and branches of the radial nerve must be preserved, and the joint is opened on the dorsal and radial aspect.

The dorsoradial approach may suffice in easier cases (Fig. 93). The first step is to reconstruct the articular surface. The fragments are then provisionally transfixed with fine Kirschner wires, which can be replaced in suitable cases by a transverse lag screw (Fig. 95). The articular fragment is then attached to the shaft with the neutralization plate in the form of a reversed metacarpal T-plate with 2.7-mm screws.

Comminution is common on the palmar side and defects should be filled with cancellous bone graft to accelerate consolidation. Stability is greatly helped by insertion of an interfragmentary lag screw through the plate to fix the shaft to the main basal fragment.

If absolute rigidity is not thus achieved, a plaster splint is applied with the thumb in abduction and opposition for 4–6 weeks. The distal phalanx is left free, so that active movements can be started immediately to prevent tendon adhesions.

d) Extra-Articular Fracture

This is more common than Bennett's fracture-dislocation. There is always an adduction crack in the shaft fragment which narrows the web between the thumb and the index. Maintenance of reduction by a plaster is difficult and internal fixation is often indicated. Complete rigidity is thus obtained so that early mobilization and resumption of work are possible.

Internal Fixation. We chiefly use the dorsoradial longitudinal incision (Fig. 93). It is usually unnecessary to open the carpometacarpal joint but its position is marked by a cannula introduced into the joint space. Long oblique fractures can be fixed by simple screws and in a transverse fracture a reversed T-plate with 2.7-mm screws can be used as a tension-band plate. The plate is slightly bent dorsally to allow full abduction of the thumb. The plate is first screwed to the proximal fragment; the distal fragment is reduced up against the plate with the help of bone forceps, and then

fixed to the shaft (Fig. 96). Stability can be augmented in this fracture by inserting an interfragmentary screw through the most proximal screw hole in the plate. Cancellous bone grafting is recommended as a primary measure for defects on the palmar surface. Consolidation usually allows safe load bearing after 6 weeks.

e) Removal of the Implants

The original wounds are incised to remove the implants but on the dorsum of the thumb the fine branch of the radial nerve must be protected, though it may be hard to identify in the subcutaneous scar tissue. As prolonged disability may result from its division, removal of implants is not an operation for inexperienced surgeons.

2. Distal Fractures

a) Articular Fractures

Fractures of the metacarpophalangeal and interphalangeal joints of the thumb are quite common, and may be open and combined with injuries to tendons, nerves and vessels. There are usually small fragments which can be fixed by an appropriately sized screw (Fig. 97c).

b) Fractures of the Shaft of the First Metacarpal and the Proximal Phalanx

Internal fixation has become an approved method here, especially with associated soft tissue injuries. It facilitates early mobilization, which is very important in the first ray and makes external support unnecessary. A plate provides better rigidity (Fig. 97b).

Approach: A dorsolateral incision is made to expose the fracture, taking care to protect the extensor tendon and its paratenon (Fig. 97a). The plate is applied in the normal way.

3. Secondary Operations on the First Ray

a) Carpometacarpal Joint

The main indication for secondary operations is arthrosis, be it subsequent to an inadequately reduced Bennett's fracture or to instability after a ligament injury or rheumatoid disease. The condition is painful and almost completely incapacitate the thumb. Different approaches to treatment are available:

Excision of the trapezium is often undertaken for rheumatoid arthritis in the female hand. The resulting defect may be filled in by rolling up part of the longitudinally split tendon of flexor carpi radialis. This acts as a space filler but some strength of the thumb is usually lost.

Replacement of the trapezium with a prosthesis: Swanson's silastic prosthesis, which has a stem in the shaft of the first metacarpal, is used for this purpose. It must be protected from dislocation by means of tendon transfers. Another method is to hold the joint apart with crossed Kirschner wires and to insert a liquid silastic mass as described by Wilhelm. In addition a total joint replacement on the lines of the hip prosthesis has been described, in which a metallic head is cemented to the first metacarpal and a socket of synthetic material joined to the remains of the trapezium.

Arthrodesis is preferred in young patients, where strength of grip is the chief requirement. It only relieves pain, however, in the absence of arthrosis in the trapezioscaphoid joint, which must be checked on X-ray. In our experience functional limitation is often over-estimated; postoperative treatment without external fixation allows exercises of the neighbouring joints because of the high degree of stability. The most important thing for the patient is the loss of pain, especially in a manual worker.

Operative Technique. The approach is similar to that for Rolando's fracture and involves an accurate exposure of the carpometacarpal joint and the trapezium. The joint must be excised with an osteotome and the defect filled with cancellous bone graft. Special attention must be paid to placing the thumb in a proper degree of opposition. A compressed bridging graft of corticocancellous bone is used, bedded in the trapezium and the base of the first metacarpal. Rigid fixation is achieved by using a reversed small T-plate. The proximal two screws, of the 3.5 mm size, must be placed precisely in the centre of the trapezium (Fig. 98).

Alternatively, a figure-of-eight tension-band wire may be used with two parallel Kirschner wires. Either techniques gives excellent stability, but consolidation may take many months and the implants should not be removed too soon.

b) Metacarpophalangeal Joint

This joint of rather simple structure has the least physiological range of movement of the joints in the hand but individual differences are frequent. Arthrodesis in a position of less than 10° of flexion results in very little functional disturbance. The following operation works well: The joint is excised and a tension-band plate applied alone or together with a compressed bridging graft (Figs. 35, 36).

c) Interphalangeal Joint

Comminuted fractures of this joint may require either primary or secondary arthrodesis, and retrograde screw fixation has proved best for this purpose (Fig. 38). The appropriate position of the joint is extension to neutral position or very slight flexion. In patients whose occupation requires a tip-to-tip pinch, flexion may be as much as 15°. When the metacarpophalangeal and carpometacarpal joints are uninjured, functional limitations are insignificant.

d) Malposition of the First Ray

A major adduction malposition may require osteotomy of the first metacarpal, but this is seldom indicated for the proximal phalanx. Osteotomy is carried out using a compressed bridging graft fixed with a tension-band plate (Fig. 35). The resulting stability is enough to allow early mobilization.

e) Pollicization

In transposing a finger ray to the remainder of the thumb, the use of a small plate for fixation has become accepted. Postoperative treatment can then be concentrated on the soft tissues.

4. Clinical X-ray Examples
(Figs. 99–108)

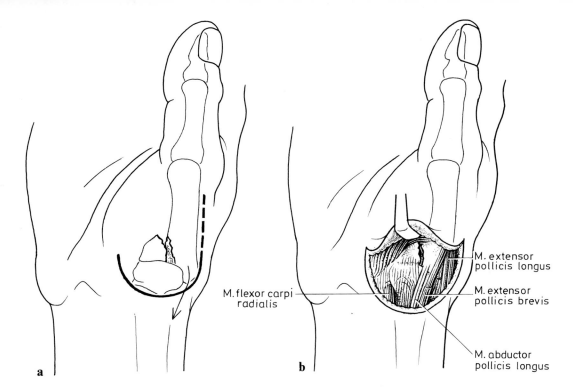

Fig. 92 a, b. Gedda-Moberg's approach to the base of the first metacarpal bone

a Bennett's fracture: Incision and its possible extension

b Topography: Aspect of the articular fragment from palmar side with the tendons

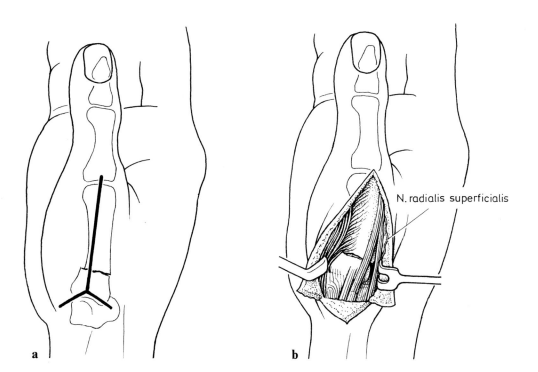

Fig. 93 a, b. The radiodorsal approach to the base of the first metacarpal bone

a Longitudinal incision at the dorsoradial border of the first metacarpal with Y-shaped proximal extension

b Topography of an extra-articular transverse fracture. The branch of the radial nerve to the thumb is retracted to the dorsal side

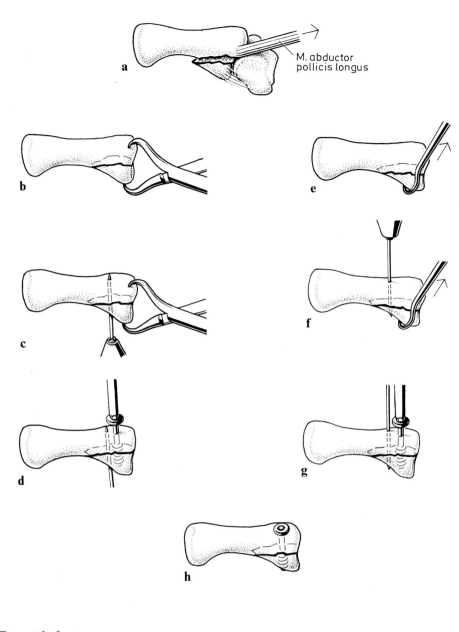

M. abductor
pollicis longus

a

b

e

c

f

d

g

h

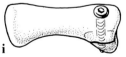

i

Fig. 94a–i. Screw fixation of Bennett's fracture

a Initial situation

b–d Internal fixation using Gedda-Moberg's approach: Reduction with forceps, temporary fixation with a Kirschner wire from the palmar aspect, screw fixation from the back

e–g Internal fixation using the dorsoradial approach: Reduction with a small hook, temporary fixation with Kirschner wire from the dorsal surface and screw fixation also from this aspect

h, i Completed internal fixation: Large fragments require small cancellous screws, small fragments small cortex screws, but in this case a gliding hole must be made in the shaft fragment

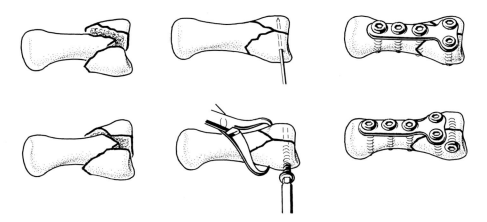

Fig. 95. Internal fixation of Rolando's fracture

Depending on the type of fracture, either using a T-plate alone or combined with preliminary lag screw fixation of the joint fragments

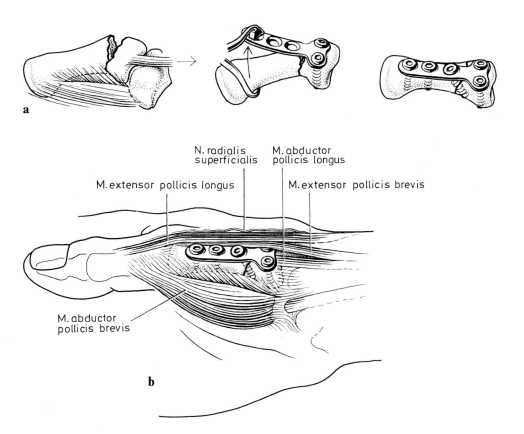

Fig. 96a, b. Extra-articular fracture of the base of the thumb metacarpal: internal fixation

a The T-plate is first fixed to the proximal fragment and then used as a lever to achieve reduction

b Topography of the internal fixation using a plate on the base of the first metacarpal. The branch of the radial nerve to the thumb must be preserved by any means

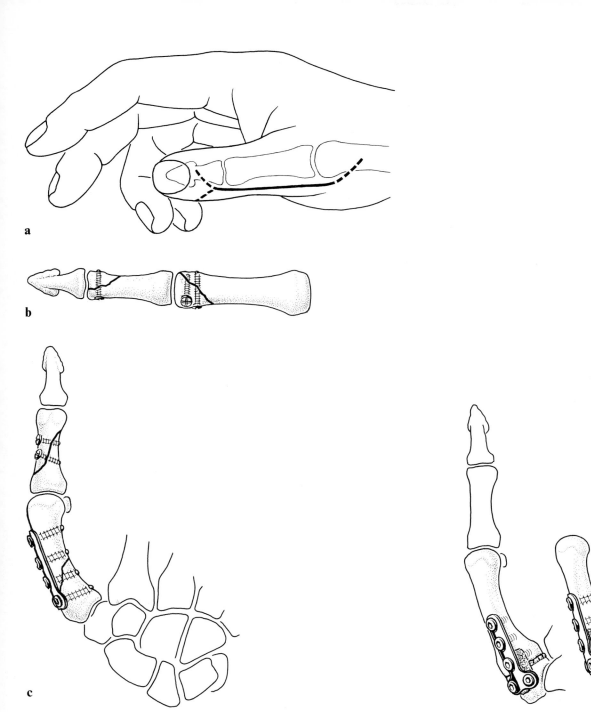

Fig. 97 a–c. Peripheral internal fixations of the thumb

a Longitudinal, dorsoradial incision. The extension at the proximal end is curved, at the distal end V-shaped

b Internal fixation of articular fractures

c Internal fixation of the shaft. For better stability, plate fixation is usually preferred at the proximal phalanx of the thumb to simple screw fixation

Fig. 98. Arthrodesis of the first carpometacarpal joint

Excision of the joint, compressed bridging graft and fixation with tension-band plate

171

Fig. 99 a–c. Clinical example: Screw fixation of Bennett's fracture

W., B., car mechanic, aged 20

a Bennett's fracture-dislocation caused by handball injury

b Internal fixation after 4 days with 4.0-mm small cancellous screw.
Immediate mobilization without weight lifting. 50% working capacity after 7 weeks, 100% after 9 weeks. X-ray taken after 1 year

c Radiological aspect after removal of the screw. Strength and range of motion was the same in both hands. He continued to play handball competitively after 3 months

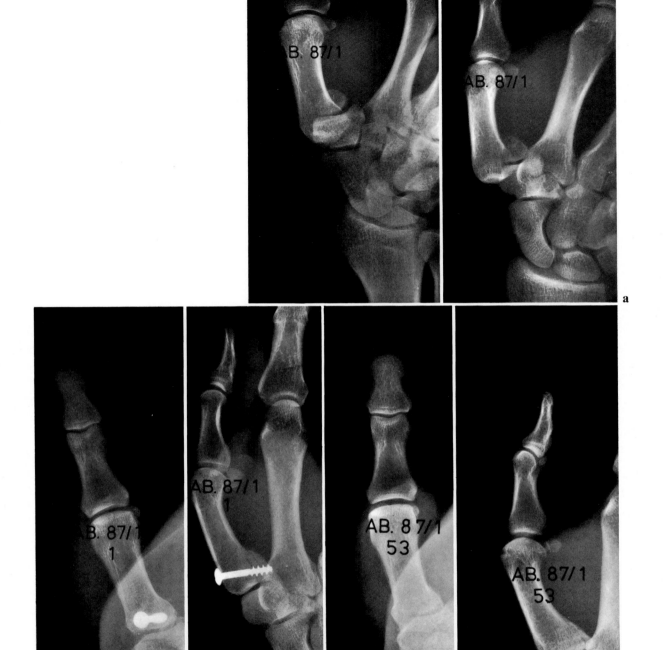

Fig. 100 a–d. Clinical example: Rolando's fracture

V., K., male motor mechanic, aged 46

a Intra-articular fracture of the base of the first metacarpal due to impaction of the thumb at work

b Internal fixation the same day with 2.7-mm interfragmentary lag screw and neutralization T-plate. A second interfragmentary 2.7-mm screw is placed through the plate in the medial basal fragment. Reduction of the palmar comminuted zone is insufficient. Nevertheless an external splint was not applied and functional treatment started instantly without weight lifting. The working capacity was 50% at 8 weeks and 100% at 12 weeks

c 17 weeks after injury a stable fixation callus is seen at the comminuted area of the palmar cortex

d The implants have been removed after 23 weeks, the patient being pain-free, with equal function of both hands. No arthrosis can be seen

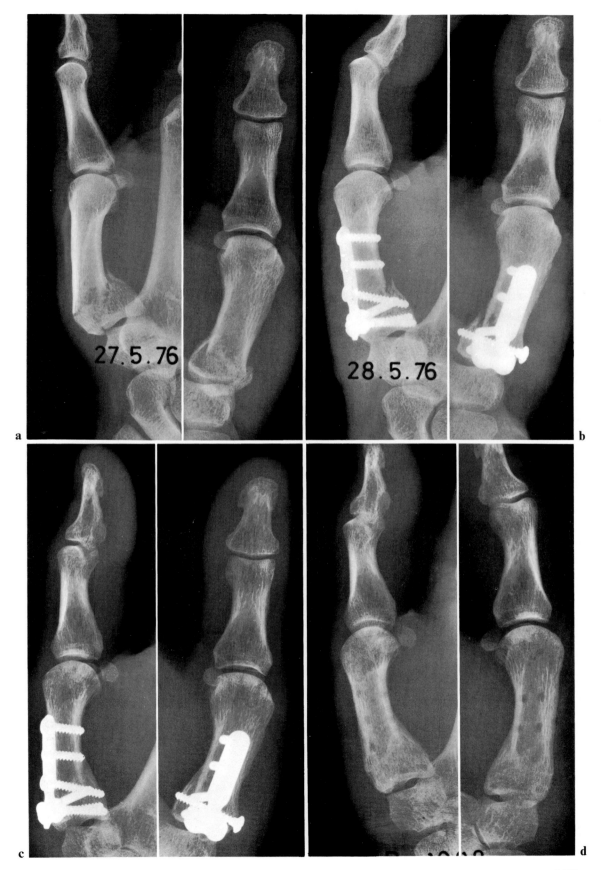

a

b

c

d

Fig. 101a–d. Clinical example: Comminuted fracture of the base of the first metacarpal with defect

R., Matteo, bricklayer aged 46. Accident at work: in an explosion his hand was hit by a piece of metal

a Comminuted fracture of the joint surface of the first metacarpal of the left hand (atypical Rolando's fracture). Marked swelling of the hand and scratches on the skin. The hand was immobilized and elevated

b Internal fixation after 3 weeks with a T-plate and cancellous bone graft from the iliac crest. Primary wound healing. Dorsal plaster splint for 4 weeks

c After 6 weeks the bone graft is healed. Thus mobilization was started and the patient was able to work partially. The implants were removed after $3^1/_2$ months

d Final check 5 months after injury. The patient has no complaints, the scar is linear, extension is complete, flexion of the MP joint is slightly reduced

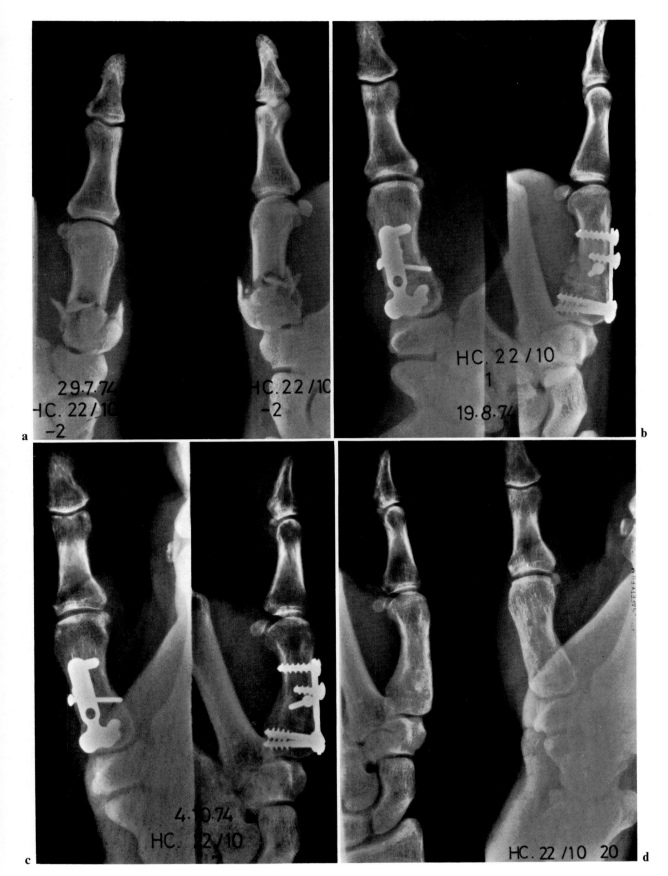

29.7.74
HC. 22/10
-2

a

HC. 22/10
-2

HC. 22/10
1
19.8.74

b

4.10.74
HC. 22/10

c

HC. 22/10   20

d

177

Fig. 102 a–c. Clinical example: extra-articular fracture of the base of the first metacarpal

K., M., post office employee aged 56

a Transverse fracture of the base of the first metacarpal due to a fall from a motorcycle

b Primary internal fixation with a 2.7-mm tension-band T-plate. An oblique interfragmentary lag screw was introduced through the plate. Functional postoperative treatment without weight lifting was started at once. In spite of this, dystrophy occurred on the base of a pre-existing, marked carpal tunnel syndrome

c At 20 weeks the implants were removed and at the same time the median nerve decompressed with endo-neurolysis.
5 months after injury the patient has full working capacity, he is pain-free and the function of both hands is the same

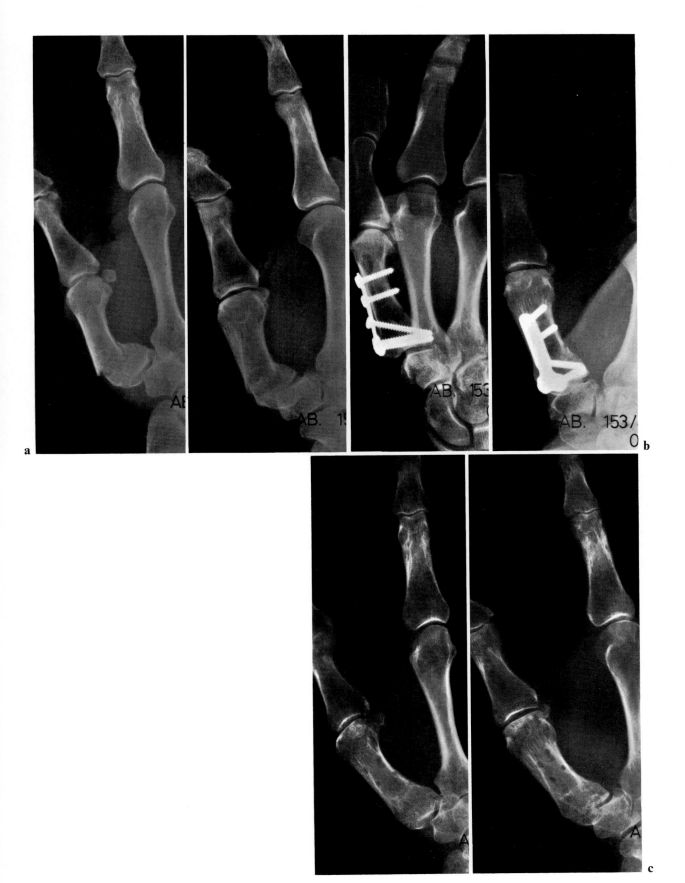

a

b

c

179

Fig. 103 a–d. Clinical example: Multiple fractures of metacarpals

C., A., building worker aged 29. His hand was caught in the gears of a crane

a Open fractures of all metacarpals together with lacerations of the first web space, avulsion of adductor pollicis and of dorsal interosseous muscle from their origin

b Primary internal fixation: 2.7-mm T-plate applied to the thumb metacarpal and fixation of all the other metacarpals by double Kirschner wires following the "Eiffel Tower" method. Functional treatment started the first postoperative day. In spite of this measure marked dystrophy occurred, which is shown by the spotted osteoporosis

c Removal of the Kirschner wires after 2 months. 50% working capacity was obtained after 5 months and 75% after 7 months

d After 1 year the plate was removed and a Z-plasty for the first web space undertaken.
End of treatment after 14 months. The patient was pain-free but he had loss of strength of his hand and loss of extension of the PIP joint of the little finger of 40° and some contracture of the first web space remained

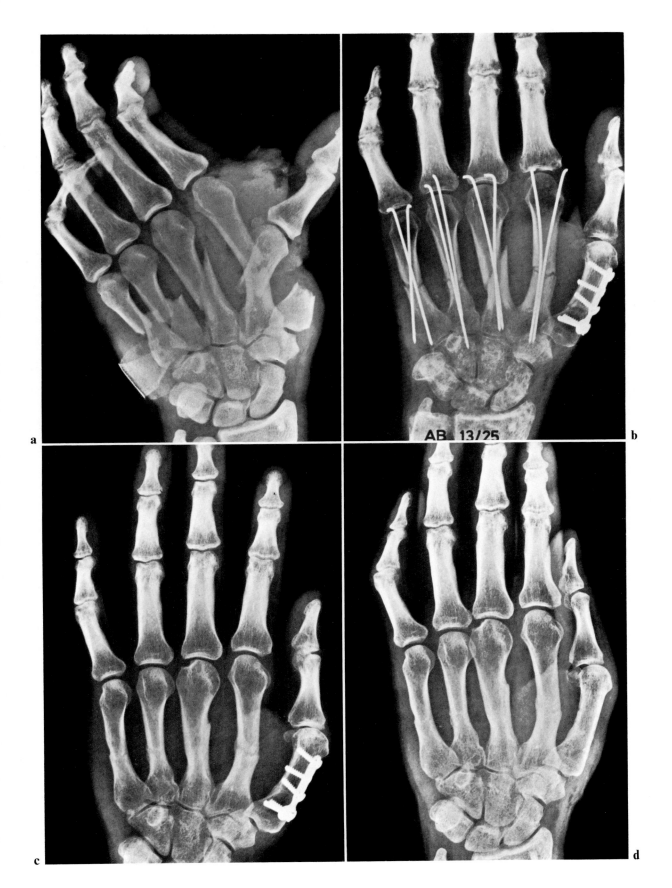

a

b

AB 13/25

c

d

181

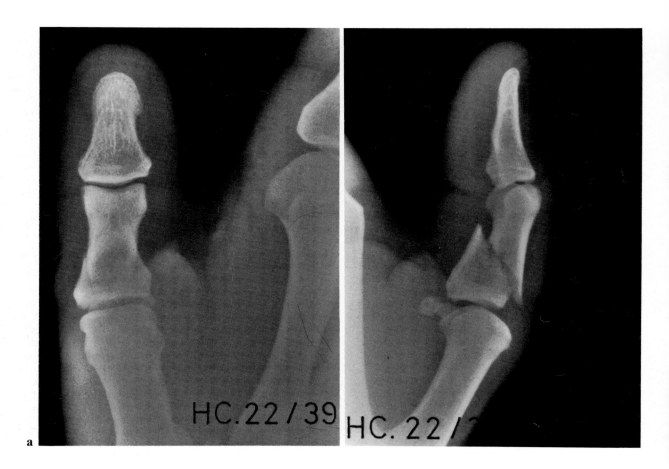

a

HC.22/39

HC.22/

Fig. 104 a–c. Clinical example: Open fracture of the proximal phalanx of the thumb

A., Caspar, 27-year-old factory labourer. Squeezed his left thumb between a fork lift and a truck

a 2nd degree open oblique fracture of the proximal phalanx of left thumb

b Immediate internal fixation by mini T-plate applied to the dorsolateral aspect.
Primary wound healing and uneventful course. Postoperative treatment without external support. Active exercises and weight lifting were started the second week. After 7 weeks, full work in the factory. Removal of the implants after 4 months

c At review after $4^{1}/_{2}$ months the patient was pain-free and had full function of his thumb

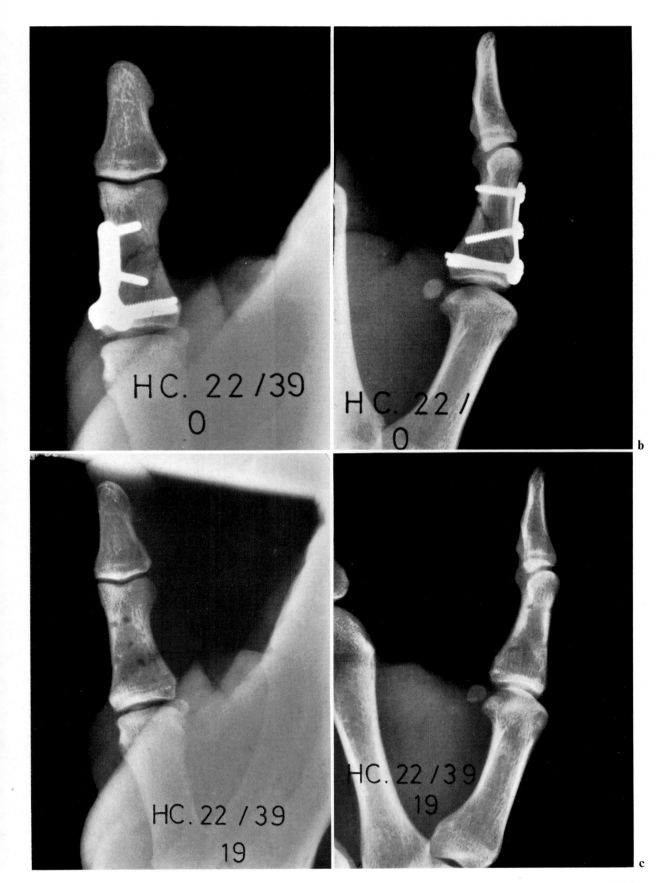

HC. 22 /39
0

HC. 22 /
0

b

HC. 22 /39
19

HC. 22 /39
19

c

183

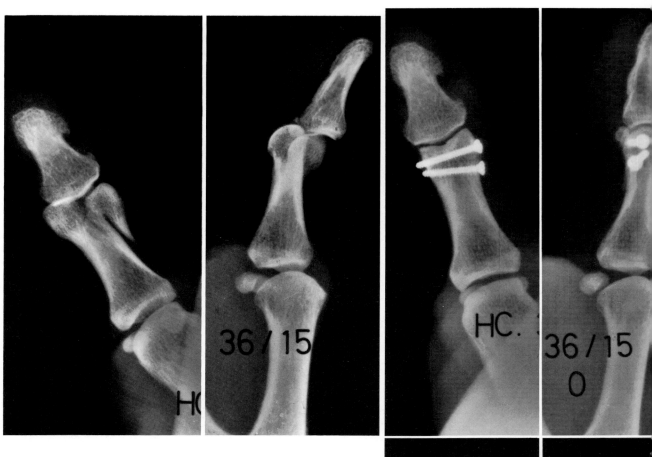

a, b

Fig. 105a–c. Clinical example: Monocondylar fracture of the proximal phalanx of the thumb

H., Margrit, housewife aged 50. Fall while skiing

a Monocondylar fracture of the proximal phalanx of the thumb with much displacement and an articular step

b Internal fixation with two 1.5-mm lag screws the same day.
Uneventful course. Discharge with a protective splint

c Review at $2^{1}/_{2}$ years: Recently the patient had some pain at the fracture level, where a small protrusion could be seen. The X-ray showed loosening of one screw which was responsible for the symptoms. Limitation of flexion 20° and extension 10°, compared to the healthy thumb. The patient now agreed to removal of the screws, which was done 2 weeks later

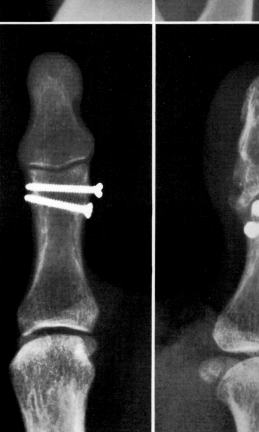

c

184

Fig. 106a–c. Clinical example: Arthrodesis of the first carpometacarpal joint

A., Elisabeth, 39-year old laundry worker. Fell on her hand sustaining a Bennett's fracture. Conservative treatment with plaster cast

a 1$^1/_2$ years later she was referred to us because of painful pseudarthrosis

b Arthrodesis in the carpometacarpal joint using joint resection and compressed bridging graft, as well as a T-plate. Uneventful course. No external fixation. Bony union and full working capacity after 3 months

c Removal of metal and final check after 8 months. Minimal discomfort. Rigid arthrodesis; unlimited function of the peripheral joints

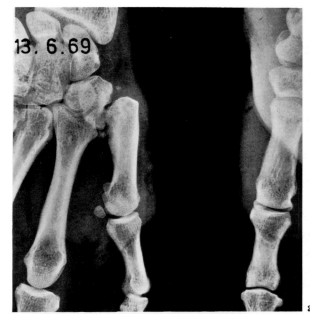

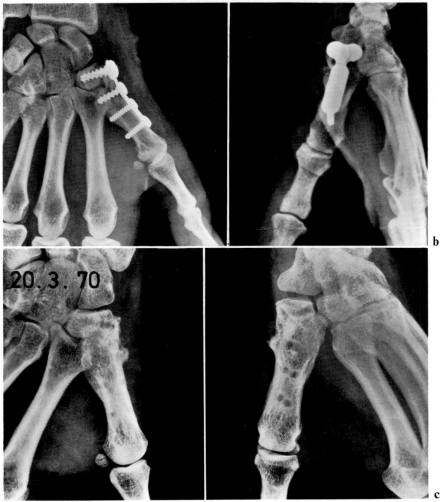

Fig. 107a, b. Clinical example: Arthrodesis of the first MP joint with a plate

K., M., female warehouse worker aged 47. Painful arthrosis of the MP joint of the thumb after dislocation of the joint some years before

a Arthrodesis by joint excision and a 2.7-mm tension-band plate. Dorsal plaster splint for 4 weeks. Full working capacity after 2 months

b Removal of the plate after 13 months. At the end of treatment after 14 months the patient was free of pain. She had 20° limitation of flexion of the interphalangeal (IP) joint

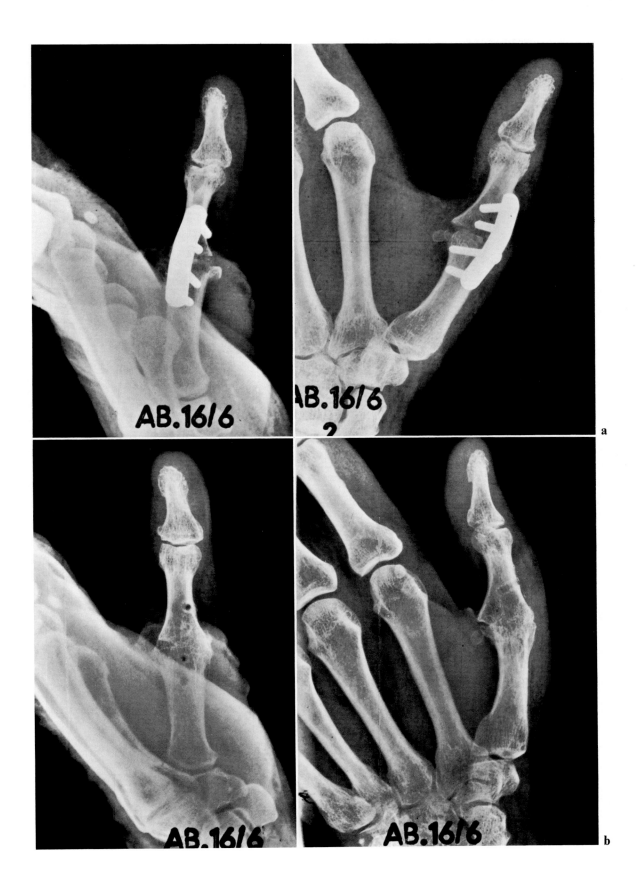

187

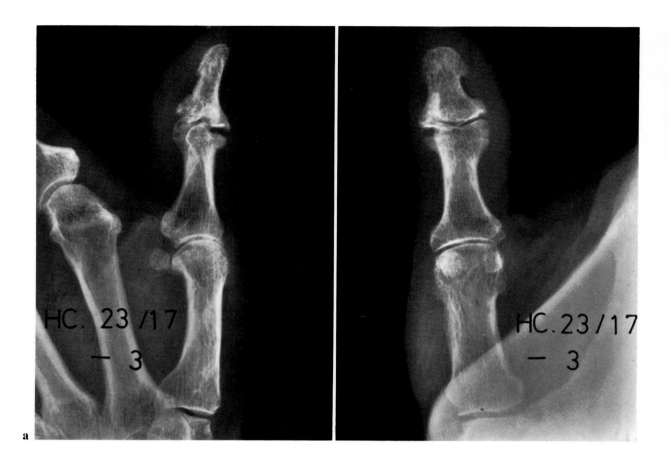

a

Fig. 108 a–c. Clinical example: Screw arthrodesis of the IP joint of the thumb

M., Klara, housewife aged 67

a One year after articular fracture, the patient had a painful arthrosis of the IP joint

b Classic retrograde arthrodesis with a screw of extra length. Primary wound healing. Immediate mobilization

c Review and removal of the screw after 7 months: Bony healing of the arthrodesis. The thumb is used without pain

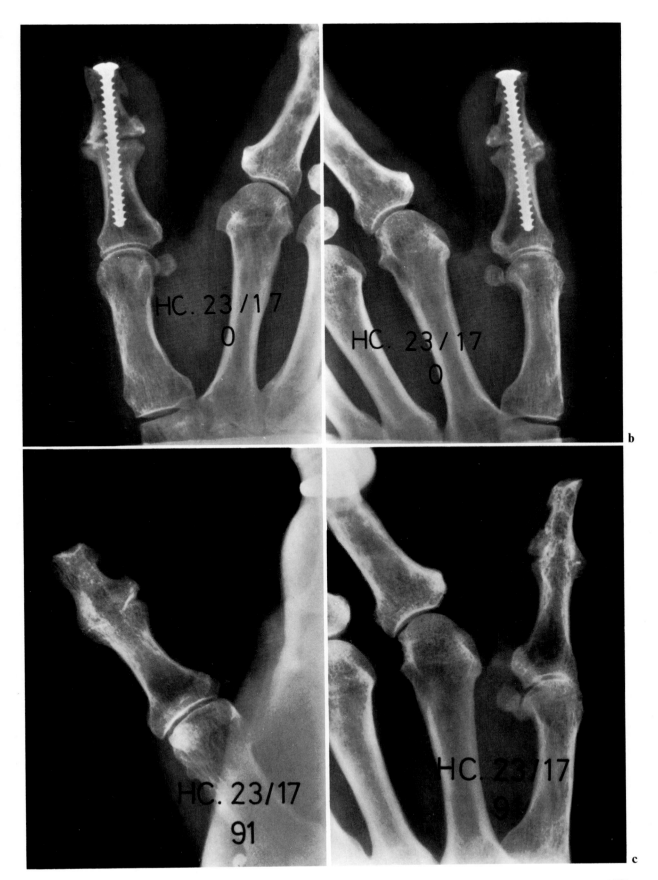

HC. 23 / 17
0

HC. 23 / 17
0

b

HC. 23/17
91

HC. 23/17
91

c

189

C. Injuries and Internal Fixation of the Second to Fifth Rays

These rays are also called the palmar rays as they form the palm proximally and emerge from it distally. They form a distinct functional unit, and this chapter therefore deals with them collectively. Greater detail is provided for the second and fifth rays, as they are more exposed to injury than the others.

The SFS has acquired an important place in the management of metacarpal fractures as they are easy to reach and not very difficult to treat. Good final results can be obtained by functional treatment after operation.

The indications for internal fixation of fractures of the phalanges, however, are more debatable. In most cases the approach inflicts additional trauma to tendons, and the extensor tendons in particular tend to adhere to underlying bone. For these reasons, the functional postoperative treatment cannot guarantee a perfect result in every case, and the operation itself can be very difficult. Careful assessment, both of the indications and of one's own surgical skill, is therefore the chief requirement.

1. Approaches

As the approaches are little known, they are described here in detail.

a) The Second and Fifth Metacarpals

A posterolateral longitudinal incision is made with a curve at the distal or proximal end. Fine nerve fibres, especially over the fifth metacarpal, are carefully retracted and the extensor tendons must be elevated, preserving their paratenon. The periosteum is incised and the bones easily exposed (Fig. 109). The plates are usually placed on the dorsal aspect of the metacarpals. Because of the convergence of the tendons there are no difficulties with the extensors.

b) The Third and Fourth Metacarpals

We now prefer longitudinal incisions for operations on these two bones, and for internal fixation of combinations of metacarpals when several are involved. They are usually placed between the metacarpal rays and may be extended distally or proximally by Y-shaped prolongations. Extending the approach onto a finger is then possible without crossing the web space. A good approach to two or even three metacarpal bones is provided by this procedure (Fig. 109). We have abandoned transverse incisions on the dorsum of the hand.

It is important to preserve the small nerves and especially the veins, since the latter transmit most of the blood from the hand. To protect the paratenon, exposed tendons must be drawn back with small Hohmann retractors (Fig. 110). In rare cases, the peripheral intertendinous connection has to be divided, but it should then be sutured at the end of the operation.

c) The Metacarpal Heads

Fractures into the joint and fractures of the neck of the metacarpals need special approaches (Fig. 109):
- For the heads of the second and fifth metacarpals the incision must be extended in a curve beyond the joint.
- An interdigital Y-shaped extension of the incisions gives good exposure to two neighbouring metacarpal heads and does not violate the web space.
- If necessary the extensor hood may be incised at its proximal edge but it should be reconstructed with fine sutures at the end of the operation.

d) The Metacarpophalangeal Joint

A slightly curved, longitudinal, paramedian incision is made over the joint (Fig. 112a). The extensor tendon is then split longitudinally for an adequate distance and the joint capsule incised separately. If possible the capsule is sewn back separately at the end of the operation. The extensor tendon is repaired by a running suture or by interrupted sutures of atraumatic, absorbable material (Fig. 112 b). This allows immediate functional exercises.

e) The Proximal and Middle Phalanges

In most operations on the fingers, we use long, dorsolateral incisions with curved ends (Fig. 113). It is important that the incisions extend well beyond the neighbouring joints to prevent damage to the skin blood supply. The dorsal venous network has to be preserved whenever possible. The palmar neurovascular bundle is preserved by keeping it continuously connected to the skin flap. This standard incision provides different approaches to the bone, the choice of which is dependent on the type and site of the fracture.

– A dorsal longitudinal incision through the extensor tendon exposes the proximal part of the proximal phalanx (Fig. 114 a).
– The lateral approach with careful elevation of the interosseous tendon exposes the distal part of the proximal phalanx (Fig. 114 b). The paratenon and periosteum must be carefully preserved to prevent adhesions developing between the tendon and the bone.
– A palmar approach through the dorsolateral incision with the finger in flexion, exposing and incising the flexor tendon sheath. The flexor tendons are then retracted with a blunt hook and this exposes the lateral and palmar aspect of the phalanges. The tendon sheath must not be sutured and early movement will prevent tendon adhesions.

f) The Proximal Interphalangeal Joint

This can be exposed by either of two approaches:
– Between the insertion of the extensor communis tendon and the interosseus tendon.
– Between the interosseus tendon and the collateral ligament of the joint.
In certain circumstances the collateral ligament must be divided to complete the expo-

sure of the proximal interphalangeal (PIP) joint. It is divided at its proximal insertion, which must be reattached at the end of the procedure using a transosseous wire suture (Fig. 114 d, e) which is fixed on the opposite side of the finger under tension over a rubber plate.

g) The Distal Interphalangeal Joint

A dorsal approach through a Z or H-shaped incision has proved adequate (Fig. 113 b). The incision may be extended if necessary because of the good blood supply of the skin. It provides a good exposure of the extensor aponeurosis and the distal part of the middle phalanx. In some cases the extensor aponeurosis must be divided in a Z-shaped manner, and it can be sewn back at the end of the operation. In most cases it is unnecessary to divide the collateral ligament.

The approach to the interphalangeal joint of the thumb is the same.

2. Fractures of the Second to Fifth Metacarpals

a) Basal Fractures

Today these fractures are more often seen as a result of road accidents; they are sometimes multiple or combined with dislocation. Transverse or oblique fractures of the base of the fifth metacarpal are common and because the fifth ray is so mobile, they pose special problems. Internal fixation has proved to be successful with the reversed small T-plate (Fig. 111 b). The rare avulsion fracture of the insertion of the extensor carpi radialis longus, at the base of the second metacarpal, is best fixed with a screw or a tension-band wire loop.

b) Shaft Fractures

Spiral fractures of the central metacarpals may lead to rotation deformity and are best treated by internal fixation. If there is a long fracture line this can be done by screws alone, but reinforcement with a neutralization plate is sometimes necessary. In the second and fifth metacarpals, which are more exposed to mechanical stress, a plate is the best form of internal fixation. Depending on the type of fracture, a tension-band or neutralization plate is combined with lag screw fixation (Figs. 111, 115).

c) Fractures of the Metacarpal Neck

A palmar angulation of the neck of the fifth metacarpal with impaction is common. It is usually a stable fracture and is best treated conservatively if there is not too much angulation. An oblique X-ray may not show the whole extent of the angulation and if there is much axial deviation we advocate closed reduction with fixation using an axial Kirschner wire, or open reduction followed by fixation with a tension-band wire loop (Fig. 116). The percutaneous Kirschner wire is removed after three weeks and exercises begun immediately afterwards.

The same treatment is recommended in fractures of the necks of the other metacarpals. These should always be reduced since the heads protrude into the palm and cause pain when the fist is clenched because of the restricted mobility of the carpometacarpal joints, which makes it impossible to compensate the malposition.

Internal fixation with plates has been abandoned.

3. Articular Fractures

a) The Metacarpophalangeal (MP) Joints

Fractures of the metacarpal heads are often open fractures combined with tendon injuries and require internal fixation, which is usually carried out with screws. Postoperative treatment depends on the injury to the soft tissues (Fig. 115).

Displaced fractures of the base of the proximal phalanx are indications for open reduc-

tion and internal fixation. Impaction of the joint surface is frequent and the resulting bony defects must be filled in with cancellous bone. Screws alone may not be enough to get a good fixation and additional Kirschner wires may be necessary. Mobilization must sometimes be postponed if stability is uncertain.

b) The Proximal Interphalangeal Joint

Typical fractures of the PIP joint are:
– A fracture dislocation with avulsion of a palmar fragment at the base of the middle phalanx. Open reduction is recommended here. The volar lip fragment is exposed and fixed with a small screw applied directly or – if it is large enough – indirectly, i.e. from the dorsum (Fig. 117).
– Displaced fractures with impaction and axial malposition may require open reduction and screw fixation.
– Condylar fractures of the proximal phalanx are classic indications for internal fixation. In bicondylar fractures, the two articular fragments are first screwed together and then the joint complex is connected to the shaft either with a screw or a Kirschner wire (Fig. 118).

c) The Distal Interphalangeal Joint and Interpahalangeal Joint of the Thumb

Fractures of the condyles of the middle phalanx may occur, and at the distal phalanx avulsion of the insertion of the extensor tendon or occasionally impaction of the joint surface may be seen. The presence of a large fragment or dislocation of the joint may provide indications for operation. The methods include transosseous pull-out wire fixation, fixation with a small Kirschner wire, a small tension-band wire loop, or a fine screw. None of these procedures give good stability, so that it is wise to add a temporary arthrodesis with a fine Kirschner wire which is drilled through the joint in an oblique direction (Fig. 118).

d) Comminuted Articular Fractures

For these fractures of the PIP or distal inter-phalangeal (DIP) joints, primary arthrodesis is the best method. This can be performed either with a screw or by tension-band wiring combined with parallel Kirschner wires (Figs. 36–38). In cases with large bony defects, the combination of screw fixation, tension-band wiring and a corticocancellous graft may be considered.

In the rare cases when reconstruction of the extensor apparatus seems possible, a silastic prosthesis of the Swanson type may be implanted at the PIP joint. A later arthrodesis may be needed if this fails.

4. Fractures of the Shafts of the Phalanges

There is a danger of axial and rotational deformity in such fractures, and internal fixation is indicated if reduction is not possible or cannot be held in a splint. Screw fixation is best in the proximal phalanx because internal fixation with a plate sometimes gives an unsatisfactory functional result.

Transverse fractures of the base of the proximal phalanx are often displaced and the treatment of choice is closed reduction followed by transarticular medullary Kirschner wire fixation (Fig. 116c). This method may also be used in some spiral fractures of the proximal phalanx. The flexed proximal fragment is pierced by the pin and then reduced, after which the distal fragment can be threaded on the pin.

Displaced fractures of the middle phalanx may pose considerable technical difficulties. Retention of the fractures with splints can be impossible, since the pull of the tendons can angulate the fracture. Transverse fractures are still best fixed by oblique or crossed Kirschner wires, which may be combined with a wire suture for compression. Transfixion of the neighbouring joints must be avoided if possible.

In contrast to fractures in the tuft of the distal phalanx, which can be reduced and fixed with the help of the finger nail, transverse fractures of the proximal shaft of the distal phalanx may be distracted and resist closed manual reduction. Stability can then be achieved with an axial Kirschner wire inserted from the finger tip and passed through the DIP joint into the middle phalanx (Fig. 118f).

5. Secondary Operations on the Second to Fifth Rays

a) Pseudarthrosis

Pseudarthroses of the second and fifth metacarpals are commoner than those of the third and fourth. There is always a palmar crack in the distal fragment which can be felt within the palm, and the grip becomes painful. Rotational deformity is not uncommon. After correcting the malalignment, stabilization can be obtained by a bone peg together with a tension-band plate, or with a compressed bridging graft (Figs. 33, 35). Early movement guarantees a rapid return to full function.

The same treatment can be used for pseudarthrosis of the phalanx, though smaller implants should be used. Plates are placed laterally to avoid disturbance of the extensor aponeurosis.

b) Osteotomy

When conservative treatment has resulted in a rotational deformity, or where there is a palmar crack and relative shortening, osteotomy of metacarpals or phalanges is indicated. The technique is similar to that for a pseudarthrosis. In the case of metacarpals, functional results can be excellent but in phalanges they are often disappointing.

c) Arthrodesis

Arthrodesis of a metacarpophalangeal joint should be avoided if possible as it leads to severe disturbance of the finger function. Arthroplasty may be an alternative, though the whole-joint prostheses which have been useful in rheumatic disease surgery are not so successful in traumatic cases, since there are often additional scarring lesions of tendons and ligaments. Nevertheless they provide a pain-free and stable, though limited, function which may be useful.

Arthrodesis of the PIP and DIP joints is performed more frequently. In the proximal joints stabilization is achieved by screw fixation or a tension-band wire combined with parallel Kirschner wires. The angle of flexion must be chosen according to the occupational requirements of the patient and varies from 20° in the index to 50° in the little finger. Arthrodesis of the DIP joint is usually achieved by a retrograde screw (Fig. 38). A neutral position or slight flexion is usually best.

6. Clinical X-ray Examples
(Figs. 119–133)

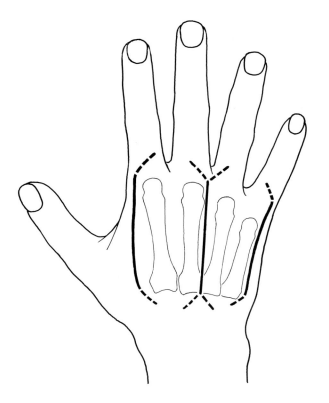

Fig. 109. Exposure of the metacarpals: Incisions

Two metacarpal bones may be exposed by interosseous longitudinal incisions which are provided with V-shaped or "leaf of a door" expansions at the proximal and the distal end

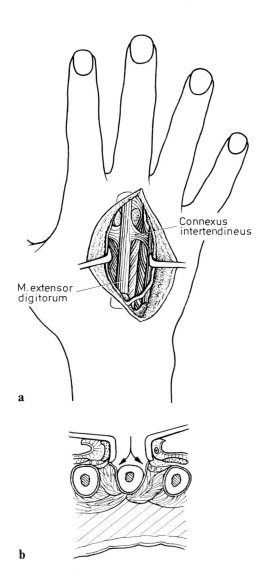

a

b

Fig. 110 a, b. Exposure of the metacarpals: deep layer

a Careful retraction of the extensor tendons with the paratenon, and of the nerves and veins. The periosteum is incised over the fracture in the longitudinal direction

b Cross-section: The periosteum is carefully reflected preserving the insertions of the muscles. After internal fixation the periosteum can usually be sutured over the implants

195

Fig. 111 a–c. Functional effects of displaced meta-carpal fractures and biomechanically correct stabilization with different plates

a Metacarpal shaft fracture with palmar crack of the distal fragment. Shortening by the pull of the flexor tendons and the intrinsic muscles. The extensor tendons are in danger of being speared by the tips of fragments.

Correct internal fixation: in the distal area with 2.7-mm tension-band plate, in an oblique fracture of the shaft with a 2.7-mm neutralization plate and an interfragmentary lag screw. In a very heavy skeleton internal fixation can be done with a one-third tubular plate with four holes

b A fracture-dislocation of the metacarpal base may be disguised by much swelling of the soft parts. The extensor tendons which are bunched at this level are picked up more frequently. In large fragments internal fixation is achieved by a T-plate placed extra-articularly. In a fracture-dislocation with a small palmar fragment, the use of a straight plate may be necessary with temporary immobilization of the carpometacarpal joint

c The typical displacement of a fracture of the base of the fifth metacarpal with axial malalignment and internal rotation. Fixation with a T-plate applied dorsally

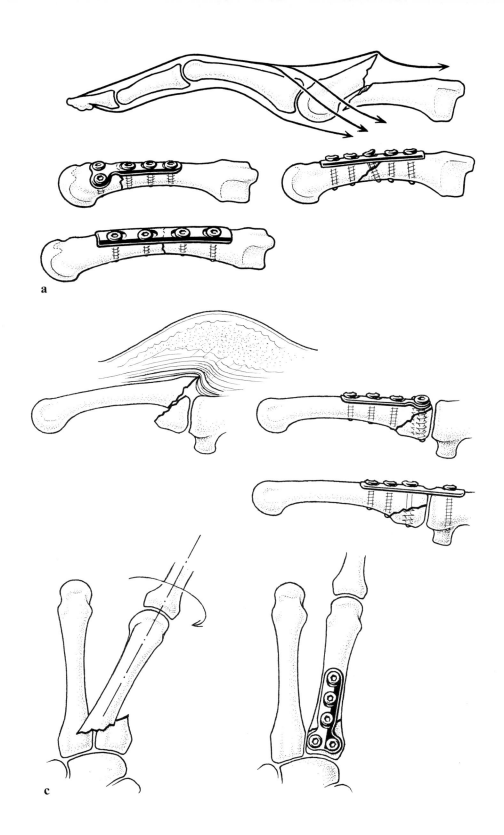

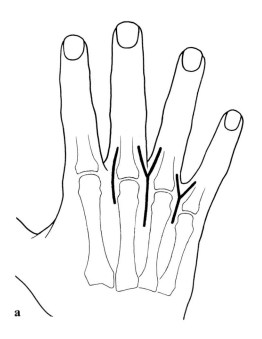

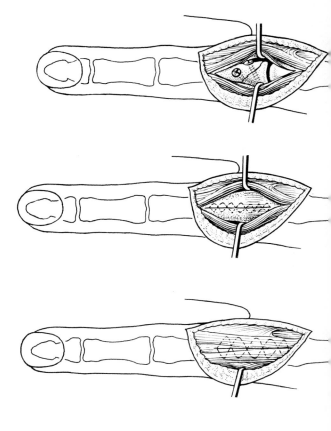

Fig. 112 a–c. The exposure of the MP joints

a The skin incisions: Curved, dorsolateral incision for exposure of one joint, longitudinal intermetacarpal incision with V-shaped expansion at the distal end for exposure of two neighbouring joints

b Deep layer: Longitudinal incision and retraction of the extensor aponeurosis. The longitudinal division of the joint capsule provides a good exposure of the joint. At the end of the operation both layers are closed with fine, atraumatic, running sutures

c Cross-section: skin incision, extensor aponeurosis, joint-capsule

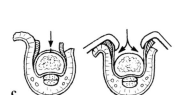

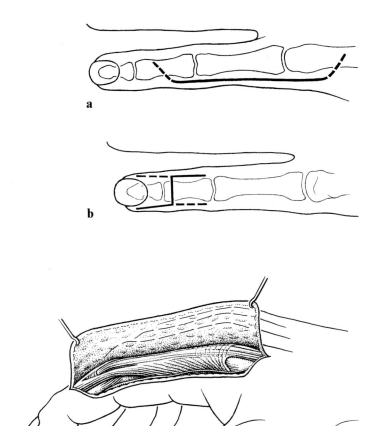

Fig. 113a–c. Exposure of the phalanges, superficial layer

a Dorsolateral incision for exposure of the proximal phalanx and the PIP joint

b Z-shaped incision transformed to an H-incision for exposure of the DIP joint

c Simplified topography of the extensor apparatus

199

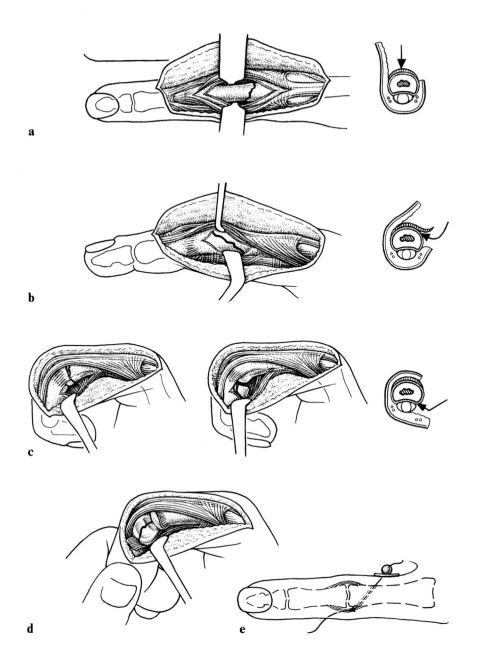

Fig. 114a–e. Exposure of the phalanges, deep layer

a Longitudinal incision of the extensor tendon, which is an extension of the approach to the MP joint

b Retraction of the interosseous aponeurosis for exposure of the shaft of the proximal phalanx

c Approach to the PIP joint and the middle phalanx in flexion

d Wide exposure of the base of the middle phalanx by division of the collateral ligament and incision of the palmar plate

e Reconstruction of the collateral ligament at the end of the procedure by transosseous pull-out wire suture

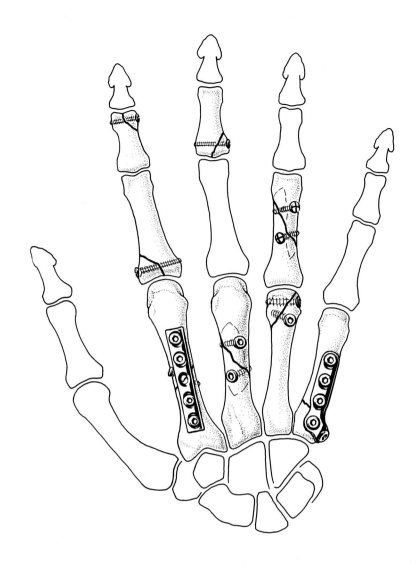

Fig. 115. Typical internal fixations in metacarpals and phalanges

Fractures of the second and fifth metacarpals are fixed by 2.7-mm screws and tension-band plates. Spiral fractures of the third and fourth metacarpals can be stabilized by lag screw fixation alone.
Internal fixation of different phalangeal fractures by 1.5- and 2.0-mm lag screws

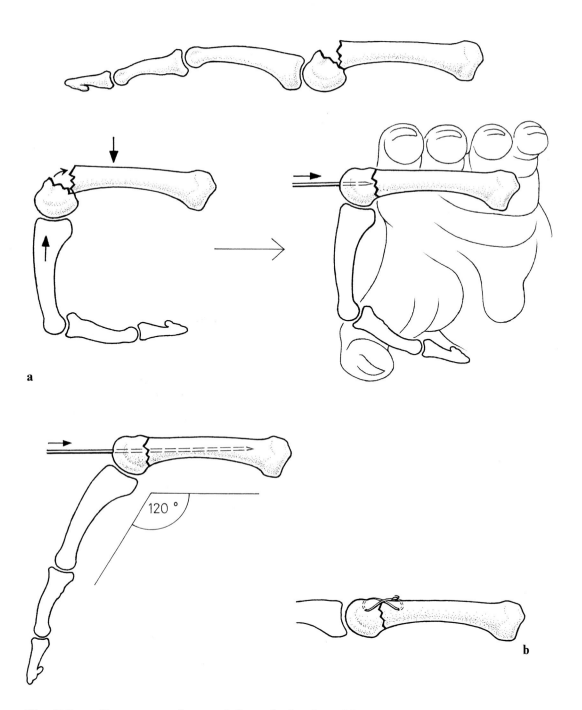

Fig. 116a–c. Percutaneous intramedullary pin fixation of fractures near the MP joint

a Fracture of the metacarpal neck: Reduction of the metacarpal head by compression of the metacarpus and the flexed PIP joint. Insertion of a Kirschner wire in the medullary cavity with the small chuck (Fig. 10, No. 34)

b Alternative procedure: Figure-of-eight tension-band wire on the dorsal aspect

c Percutaneous pin fixation of a fracture of the base of the proximal phalanx with a dorsal crack:

Insertion of an axial Kirschner wire with the help of the small air drill through the metacarpal head into the proximal fragment. The joint must be flexed to 80°. Reduction is achieved by flexion of the finger until the pin can be advanced to the distal fragment. A well-padded dorsal splint is applied, which fixes a neighbouring finger as well to prevent rotational deformity

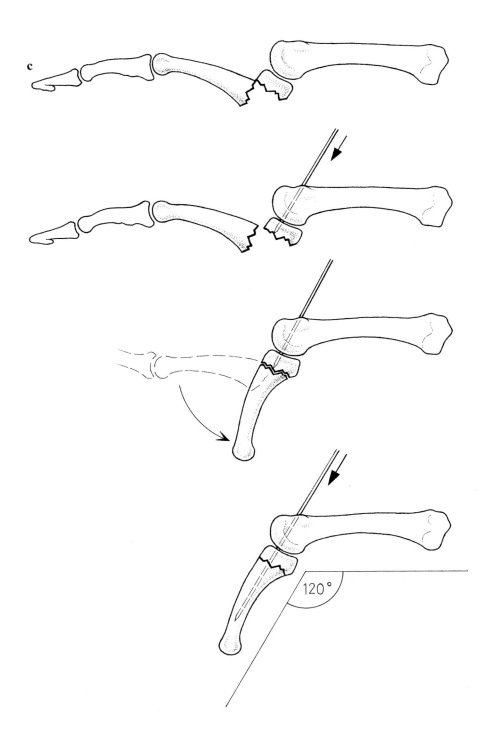

c

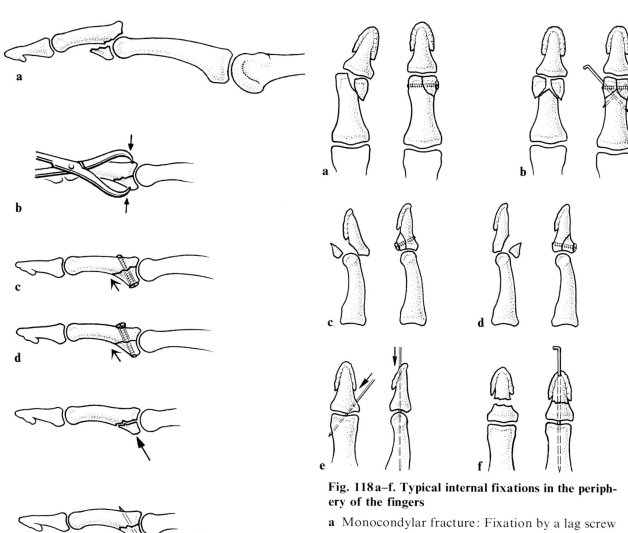

Fig. 117a–e. Internal fixation of the fracture-dislocation of the base of the middle phalanx

a Typical fracture with dorsal dislocation of the distal fragment

b Temporary fixation and compression of the fracture with a forceps

c Direct screw fixation from the palmar aspect

d A larger fragment may be fixed by a lag screw from the dorsal aspect

e Small fragments may be fixed with a Kirschner wire from the palmar side

Fig. 118a–f. Typical internal fixations in the periphery of the fingers

a Monocondylar fracture: Fixation by a lag screw

b Bicondylar fracture: Screw fixation of the condyles and connection with the shaft by fine Kirschner wires. The wire next to the screw head is buried; since the bone is exposed, the second wire is inserted percutaneously and can be removed early

c Avulsion fracture of the insertion of the flexor profundus tendon from the distal phalanx: fixation by a lag screw

d Screw fixation of a large avulsion fragment of the insertion of the extensor aponeurosis

e Additional temporary arthrodesis of the DIP joint is frequently necessary in these internal fixations. The fine Kirschner wire may be inserted in the long axis of the phalanx but the oblique insertion is preferred

f Displaced fracture of the distal phalanx at the level of the nail matrix: Reduction and stabilization by an axial Kirschner wire also acting as a temporary arthrodesis of the DIP joint

204

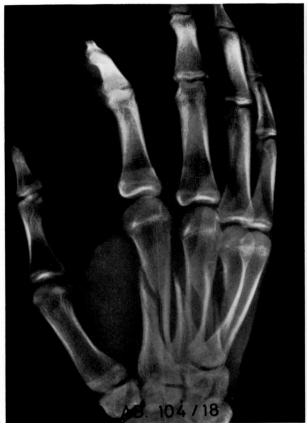

a

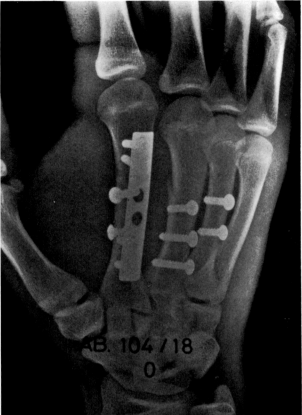

b

Fig. 119 a–c. Clinical example: Multiple metacarpal fractures

N.P., apprentice gardener, aged 17

a Multiple fractures of the metacarpals of the right hand in a fall while playing football. The second metacarpal shows a spiral fracture with a butterfly fragment; the third and fourth have pure torsion fractures

b Primary internal fixation:
Second metacarpal: Stabilization of the butterfly fragment with two 2.7-mm lag screws and for neutralization a one-fourth tubular plate with six holes is applied and fixed with four screws.
Third and fourth metacarpals: Internal fixation with 2.7-mm lag screws alone.
Because of the difficulties of exposure of the palmar aspect of the metacarpals without excessive stripping of the periosteum and the muscle insertions, reduction of the third metacarpal is not perfect in the distal palmar cortex.
Immediate functional treatment without external support. After 8 weeks working capacity is full. Removal of the implants after $5^{1}/_{2}$ months

c Review after 44 weeks: The patient is pain-free and has a full range of movement of the fingers and equal strength of both hands

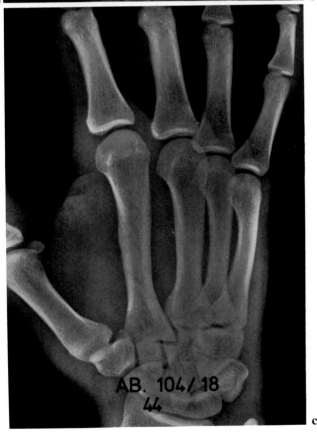

c

Fig. 120 a–c. Clinical example: Oblique fracture of the metacarpal neck

J.W., labourer at a chemical factory, aged 36. He had his hand crushed in a conveyor belt

a Open fracture of the second metacarpal, an additional fracture of the proximal phalanx of the thumb, and injury to the extensor tendon of the middle finger

b Primary internal fixation of the second metacarpal with a 2.7-mm T-plate. Plaster cast for 4 weeks. As a complication, trophic disorders occurred. After 4 months working capacity was partial and was restored 100% after only 7 months

c Removal of the plate after 6 months. After 7 months the patient was pain-free but there was a reduction of flexion at the index and middle finger with a distance of 3 cm between finger and palm and some loss of strength

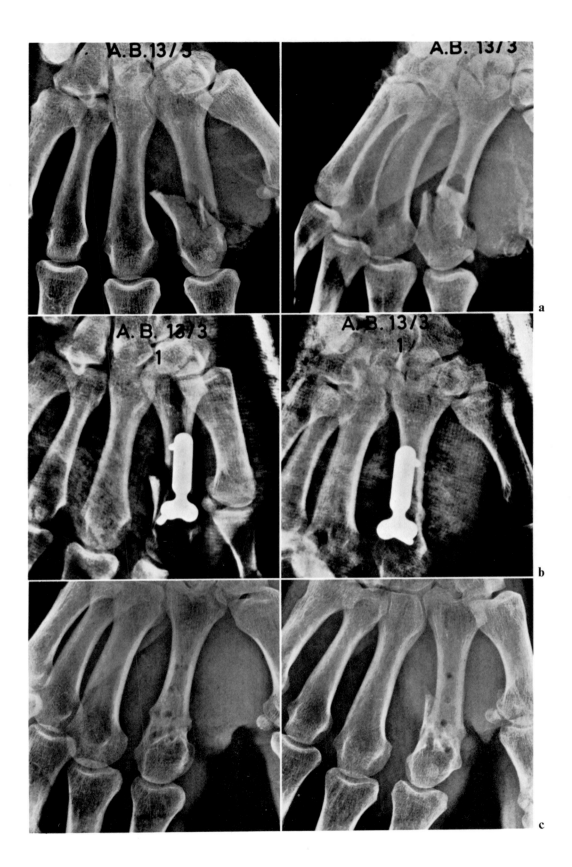

207

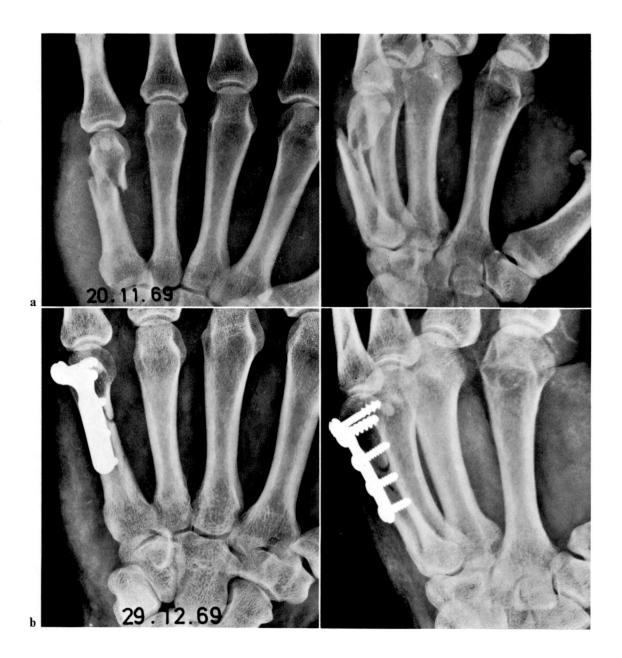

Fig. 121 a–d. Clinical example: Open fracture of the distal shaft of the fifth metacarpal

Sch., Ernst, mechanic, aged 39. His hand had been crushed in a roller

a Open fracture of the fifth metacarpal with skin loss

b Internal fixation with L-plate after 4 days. Skin loss was treated by a thick split-thickness skin

graft. Postoperative course without complications. Functional treatment from the beginning

c Check and removal of the metal after 7 months. No complaints and full function

d After 11 years the scar is quite invisible. The fracture line is just visible on the X-ray

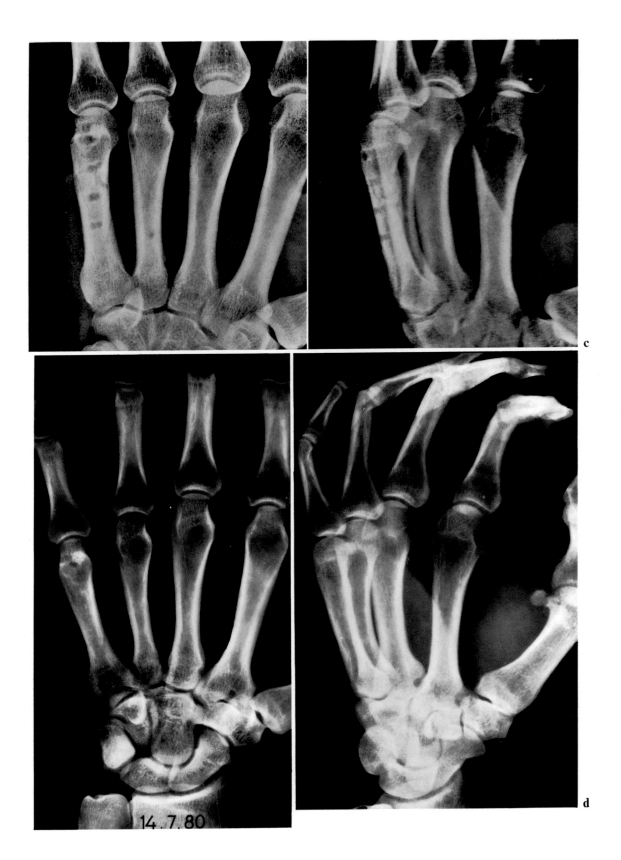

c

d

14.7.80

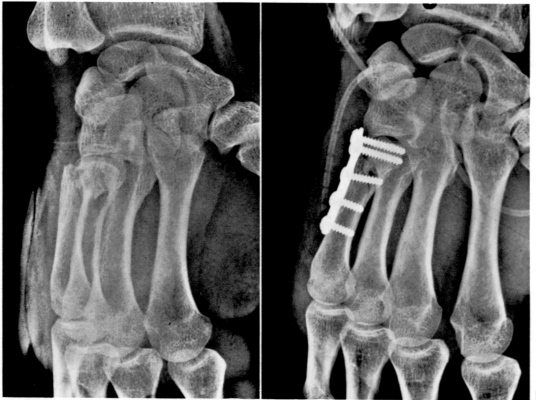

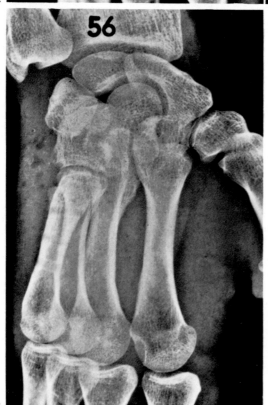

Fig. 122a–c. Clinical example: Fracture of the base of the fifth metacarpal

V., Ramon, 36-year-old labourer. He had fallen on his hand

a Extra-articular oblique fracture of the base of the fifth metacarpal with shortening

b Primary osteosynthesis with L-plate. Uneventful course. Full working capacity after 40 days

c Removal of metal and final check after 13 months. The patient was pain-free, had a full range of motion, and had equal power in both hands

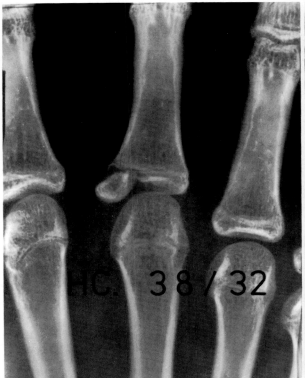

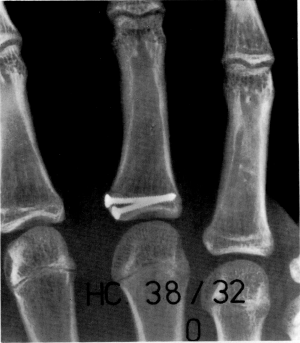

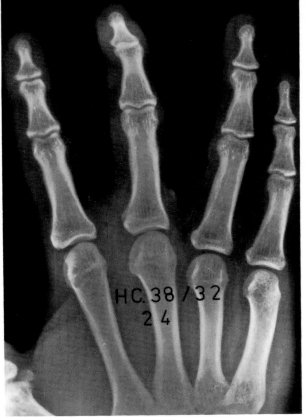

Fig. 123a–c. Clinical example: Avulsion fracture of the base of the proximal phalanx

B., Dominik, apprentice aged 16. Fall from a motorcycle on the right hand

a Avulsion at the base of the proximal phalanx on the radial side, the epiphysis still being open

b Internal fixation with two 1.5-mm screws on the day after injury

c Removal of the screws after 5 months. The fracture is united, the patient is pain-free and has a full range of motion

211

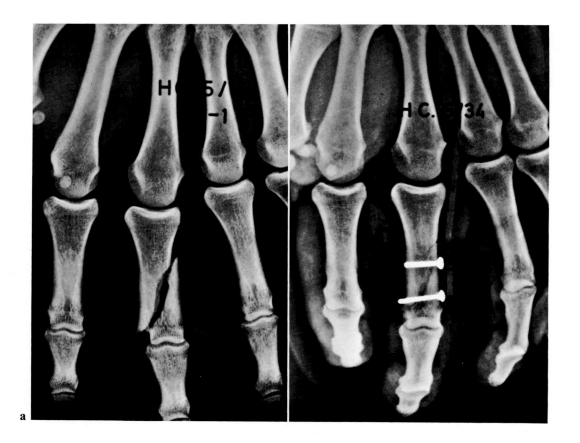

a

Fig. 124a–d. Clinical example: Screw fixation of a spiral fracture of the proximal phalanx

G., Christian, postman aged 31. Fall into a crevasse

a Spiral fracture of the proximal phalanx of the middle finger with rotational deformity. Closed treatment failed

b Internal fixation with two 2.0-mm lag screws after 1 week.
Uneventful course. Functional treatment. Removal of the screws after 5 months

c Check after 5 months: Linear scar, flexion is slightly reduced, the fracture is healed. A small cyst in the cortex at the distal screw proves necrosis of the tip of the fragment

d After 9 years the patient has no complaints and a full range of movements. The cyst is still visible on the X-ray

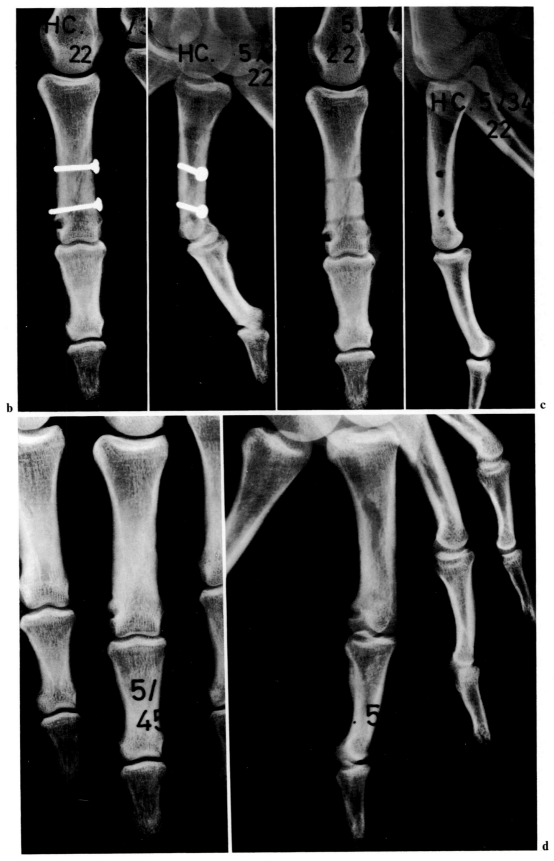

b

c

d

213

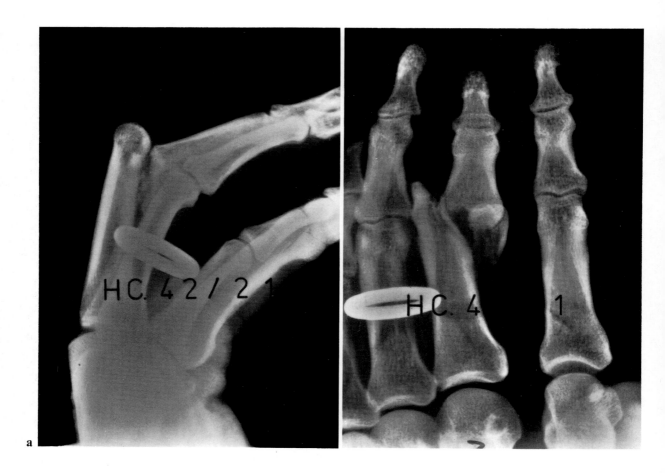

a

Fig. 125a–c. Clinical example: Open articular fracture of the proximal phalanx

L., Bartholomäus, a civil servant aged 51. Suffered a blow from a hatchet when chopping wood

a Incomplete amputation of the left middle finger with articular fracture of the proximal phalanx and division of the extensor tendon

b Primary internal fixation with two screws, suture of the extensor tendon, temporary arthrodesis of the PIP and DIP joints with fine Kirschner wires. Uncomplicated wound healing. The Kirschner wires have been removed after 3 weeks. The fracture has healed but the extensor apparatus is defective

c The fracture is united. The screws are removed after $3^1/_2$ months. At the end of treatment at 4 months there remains a loss of extension of the PIP of 50°, the flexion being 90°. The patient is back at work and he is not disturbed by the loss of extension

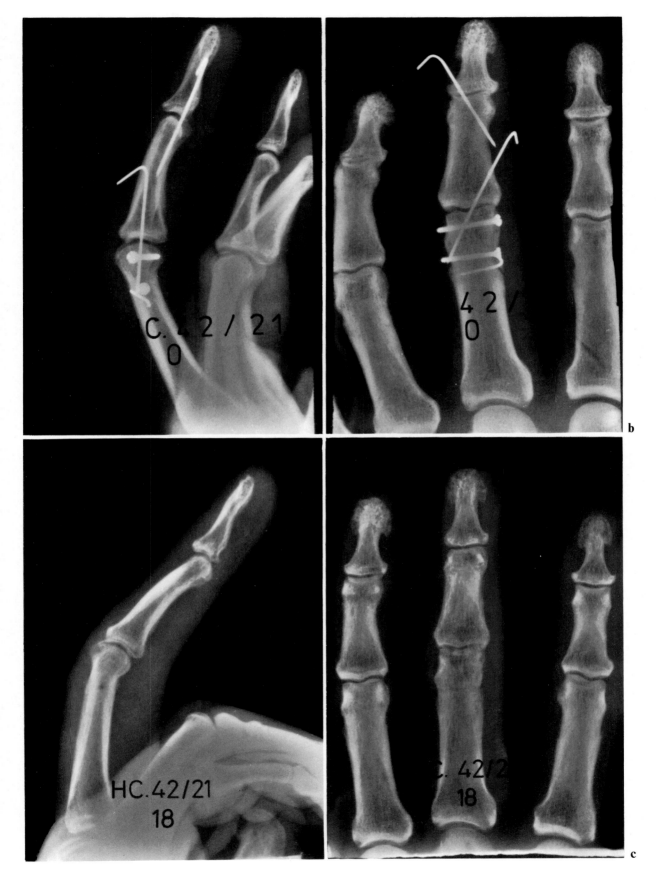

C. 42 / 21
0

4 2 /
0

b

HC.42/21
18

C. 42/2
18

c

215

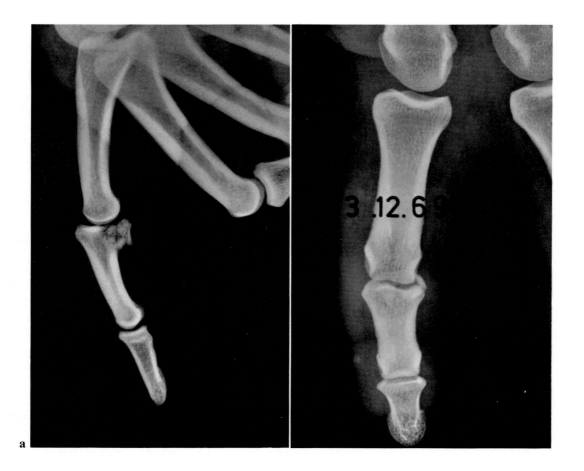

a

Fig. 126a–d. Clinical example: Fracture-dislocation of the base of the middle phalanx

M., Peter, farmer aged 32. He had a blow from a motor crank on his index finger

a Comminuted articular fracture of the base of the middle phalanx of the index finger, with partial dorsal dislocation. Ulnar deviation of the finger. No improvement was obtained with closed treatment in plaster

b Secondary internal fixation at 2 weeks: By a palmar approach, the comminuted area was compressed with a screw and a washer.
No complications postoperatively. Practically full weight bearing after healing of the wound. Removal of the metal after 4 months

c Review after 12 months: full working capacity as a farmer, he has minimal disturbances and mild arthrosis. Dislocation of the joint is reduced and axial malalignment is improved

d After $10^1/_2$ years the patient works without pain as a farmer. Ulnar deviation has not changed. Active flexion of the joint is 80°. The arthrosis is no worse

216

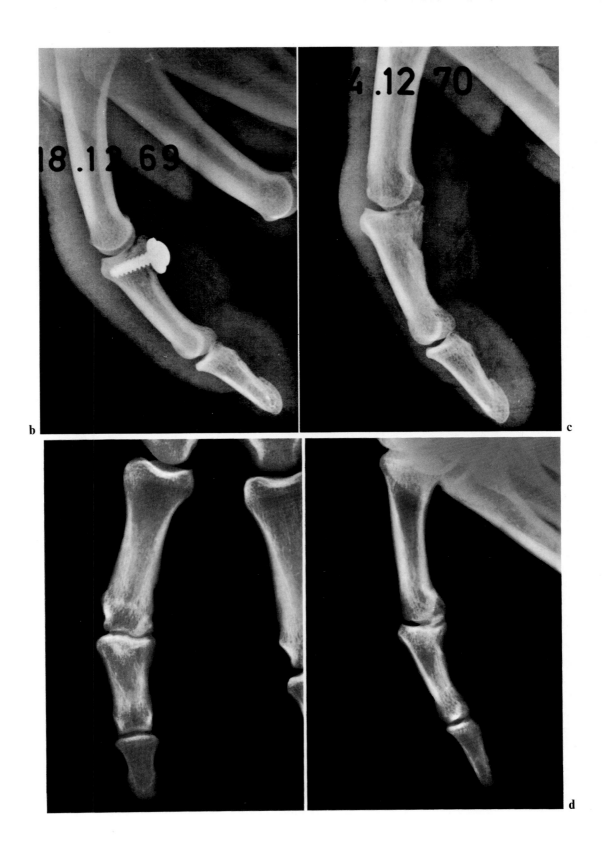

b

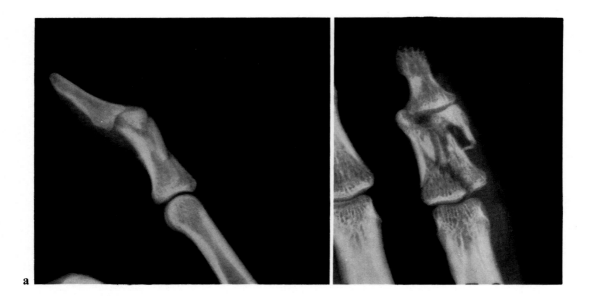

a

Fig. 127 a–c. Clinical example: Open, comminuted, biarticular fracture of the middle phalanx

I., Giovanni, a mechanic aged 30. He sustained a crushed right index finger in a machine

a Third degree open, comminuted fracture of the middle phalanx of the index finger with involvement of the PIP and DIP joints and laceration of the extensor aponeurosis. Additional open fracture of the distal phalanx of the ring finger

b Emergency operation: Internal fixation of the fragments with six 1.5-mm mini screws, partial suture of the extensor aponeurosis, open treatment of the wound.
Immobilization with a splint, healing of the wound by second intention without complications. Active mobilization was started at 6 weeks and the patient was back at work after 7 weeks. The screws were removed at 3 months

c After 8 months the scar is somewhat hypertrophic. Flexion of the DIP joint is reduced, but the function of the PIP joint is normal. The patient has no complaints

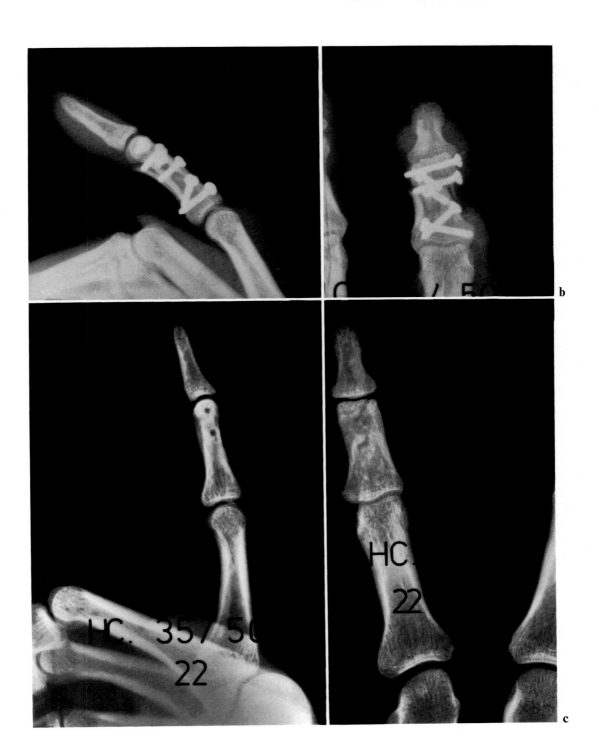

b

HC. 35/56
22

HC.
22

c

219

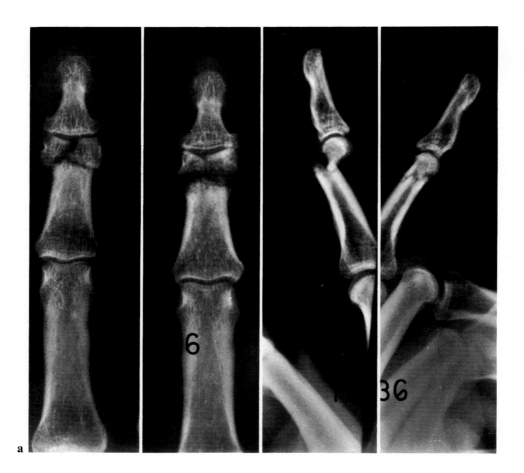

Fig. 128 a–c. Clinical example: Bicondylar fracture of the middle phalanx

Sch., Anton, 57-year-old bricklayer. His left hand was crushed between two cement tubes. He was admitted the next day

a Bicondylar displaced Y-shaped fracture of the middle phalanx of the middle and ring finger of the left hand. Operation was postponed because of contusion of the skin

b Internal fixation after 4 days: combination of screw fixation of the condyles with Kirschner wire pinning. One wire was introduced through the incision and buried. The other one was introduced percutaneously. In the middle finger the extensor aponeurosis was divided for better exposure. Im-

mobilization with a splint. Wound healing was uncomplicated. After 5 weeks the percutaneous Kirschner wire and the tendon wire were removed and active exercises started. After 3 months the remaining metal was removed. After 6 months the patient was back at work

c Review after 6 years: There is a slight flexion deformity of the DIP joints and some axial malalignment to the ulnar side of the ring finger. Flexion is reduced in both DIP joints. There is a good strength of the fist in spite of moderate symptoms. The X-ray shows arthrosis of the middle finger

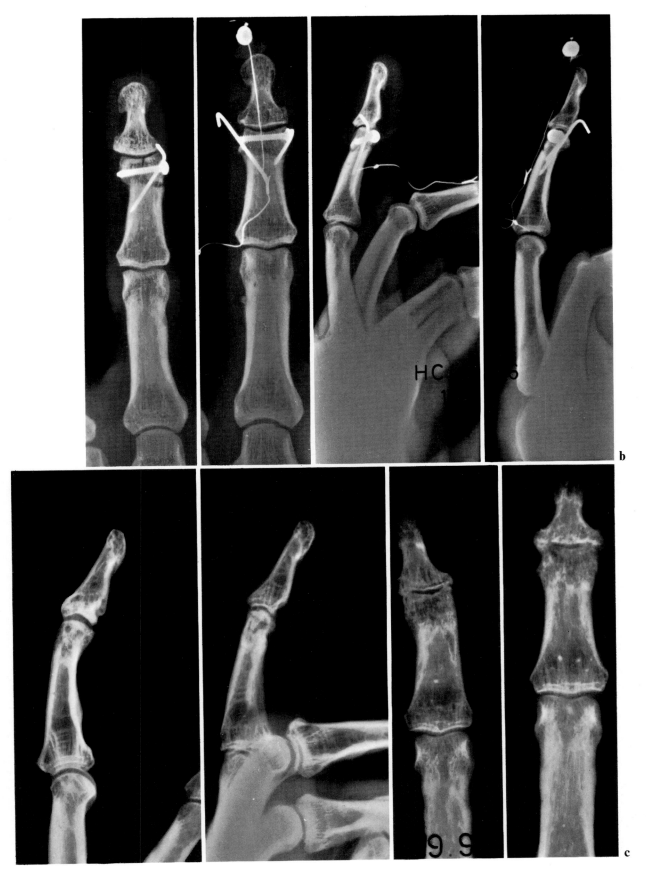

b

c

221

Fig. 129 a–c. Clinical example: Avulsion fracture of the base of the distal phalanx

Sch., Heinz, engineer aged 44. Ring injury of the right ring finger by a sudden pull of a dog on its lead

a Grossly displaced avulsion fracture of the base of the distal phalanx

b Primary internal fixation: Reinsertion of the flexor tendon by reduction of the avulsed fragment and fixation with a 1.5-mm screw. Reconstruction was achieved through a radiopalmar approach.
No complications. The DIP joint was immobilized by a plastic splint for 4 weeks, followed by active mobilization. Removal of the screw after 5 months

c After 3 years, no complaints, full range of motion, no arthrosis

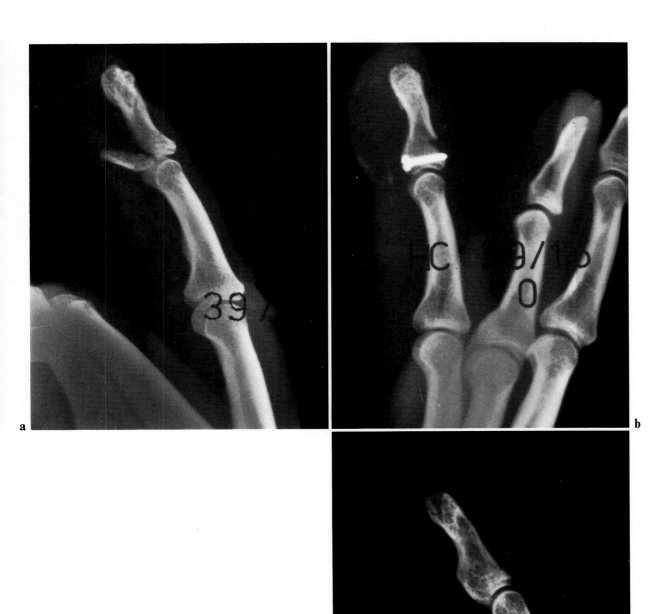

223

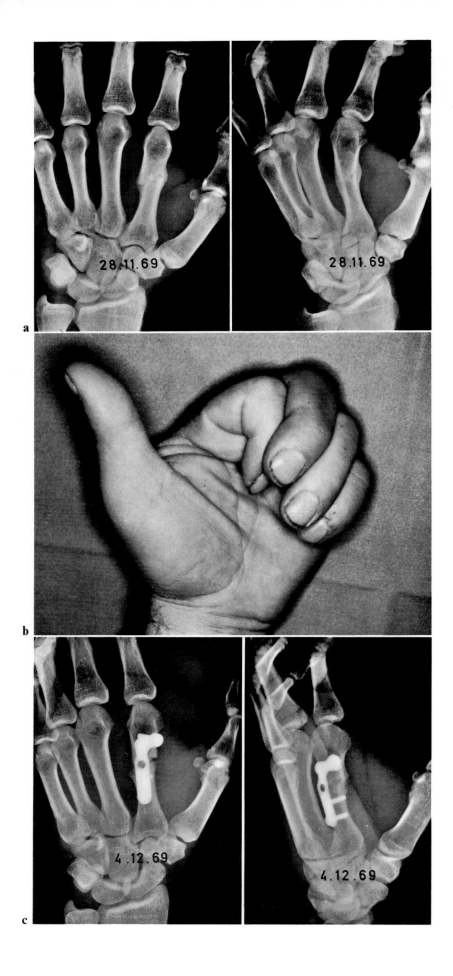

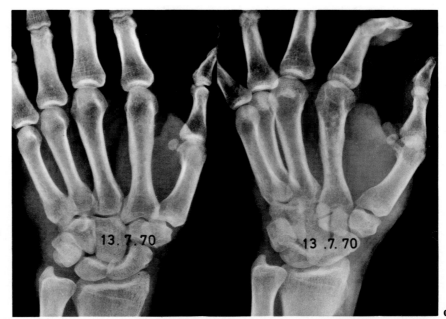

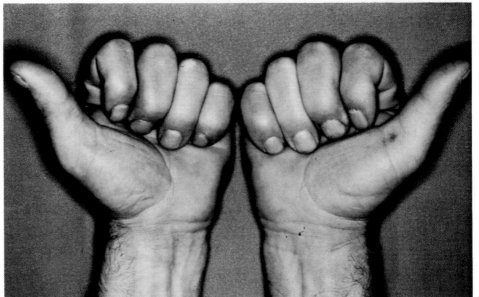

Fig. 130a–e. Clinical example: Osteotomy of the second metacarpal

C., Antonio, iron bender ages 29. Crush injury of the hand. Open fracture of the shaft of the second metacarpal

a Non-union resulted from closed treatment in plaster

b Rotational deformity of the index finger

c Rotation osteotomy with bone peg and tension-band plate applied 4 months after the accident.

No complications. Functional postoperative treatment without external support. Full working capacity after 3 months

d Removal of the implants after 8 months

e Final review after 10 months: Symptom-free, full function, flexion identical in both hands

225

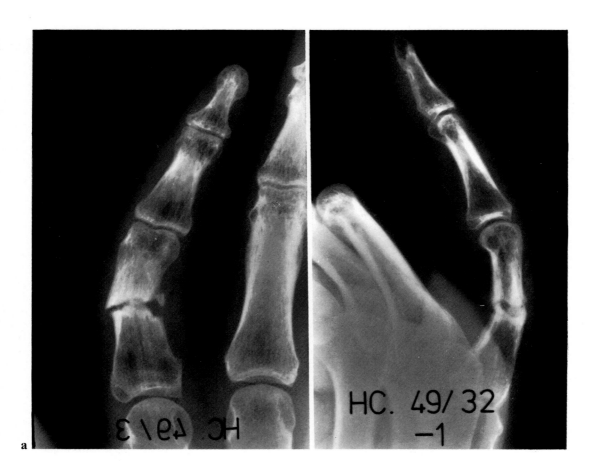

a

HC. 49/32
—1

Fig. 131 a–c. Clinical example: Pseudarthrosis of the proximal phalanx

H., Hugo, labourer aged 20. He had an accident in the construction of a cable railway. Open fracture of the proximal phalanx of index finger. Primary treatment with crossed Kirschner wires without consolidation of the fracture

a Painful pseudarthrosis after 4 months. Axial malalignment of the fracture to the ulnar side. Partial stiffness of all the finger joints and trophic disorders

b Internal fixation at 4 months. An autogenous cancellous bone graft and a six-hole plate have been applied laterally (the plate being a special construction for the use of mini screws according to the DCP principle). The scar was corrected as well.

Uneventful course. In spite of intensive exercises the mobility of the PIP joint remained reduced. The pseudarthrosis healed within 4 months

c After 8 months removal of the plate and tenolysis. Review after 11 months: Full working capacity and no complaints. The MP joint is freely mobile. Active motion of the PIP and DIP joints is 35° with some lack of extension

226

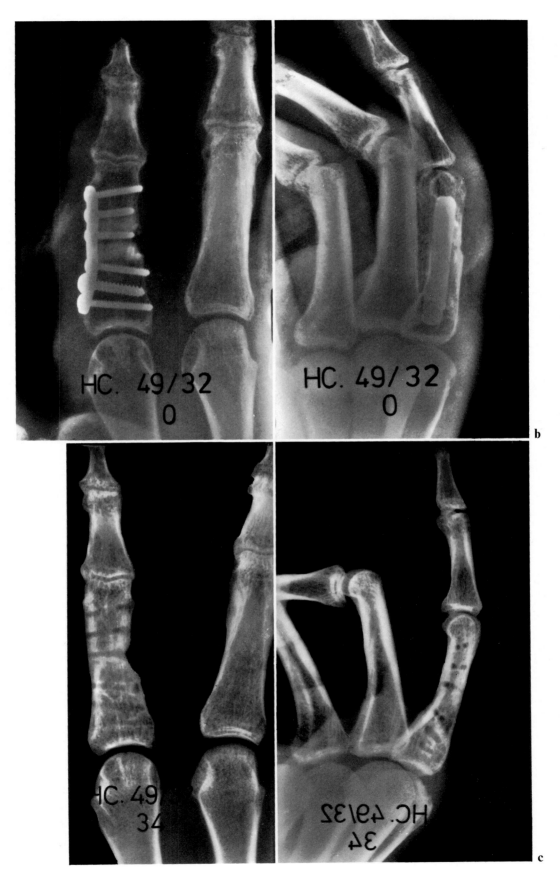

HC. 49/32
0

HC. 49/32
0

b

HC. 49
34

HC. 49/32
34

c

227

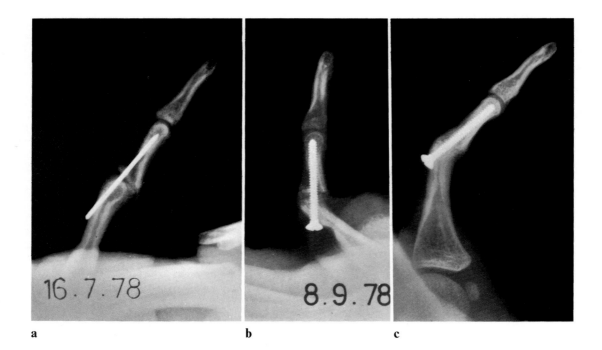

a   b   c

Fig. 132a–c. Clinical example: Arthrodesis of the PIP joint with a screw

Z.U., a 20-year-old painter had a crash with a car while on his motorcycle

a Open fracture dislocation of the base of the middle phalanx of his left little finger with a bone defect and disruption and defect of the extensor tendon. Provisional fixation with a Kirschner wire, debridement and suture of the tendon and the wound

b Definitive arthrodesis of the PIP joint after 6 weeks. Because of the very narrow medullary canal of the middle phalanx, fixation was achieved with a 2.0-mm screw at this level. The defect was filled in with a cancellous bone graft. Immobilization with a metal splint for 2 weeks. Partial working capacity at 3 weeks, full capacity at 4 weeks

c Fifteen months after the arthrodesis: The screw head was slightly painful on the back of the finger and was removed later. No other complaints; closure of the fist unlimited, mobility of the DIP joint slightly reduced

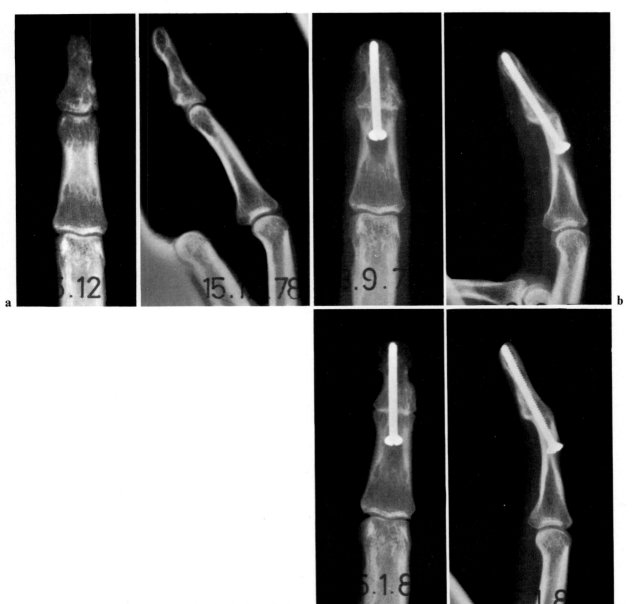

Fig. 133a–c. Clinical example: Arthrodesis of the DIP joint with screw from the proximal end

K.R., a female secretary, aged 36

a Painful arthrosis of the DIP joint of the right ring finger after two operations elsewhere for a mucoid cyst

b Arthrodesis by excision of the joint and fixation with a 2.0-mm lag screw. Functional postoperative treatment. The patient was back at work after 4 weeks

c The X-ray after 16 weeks shows bony healing. Since the patient was somewhat disturbed by the screw head, the screw was removed after 20 weeks. Thereafter the patient was pain-free and had full mobility of the proximal joints

XIV. The Knee Joint

Major fractures of the complicated knee joint involving the femoral condyles and the tibial plateau are fixed with the larger implants of the standard set. Use of the SFS is limited to small fractures, components of major fractures and avulsions of the ligaments. Since knee injuries have increased considerably in recent years it is sensible to consider these lesions in a separate chapter.

1. Patella

The transverse fracture of the patella is treated by the standard double tension-band wire loop (*Manual of Internal Fixation,* 2nd edn. 1979, p. 252). In recent years there has been greater use of the wire loop with Kirschner wires, as it has been observed that necrosis caused by the pull of the wire loop can result in shortening of the patellar ligament or a high-riding patella. Indications for the use of the SFS are limited to longitudinal fractures and to reconstruction of the lower pole of the patella.

a) Longitudinal Fracture

This type of fracture, which is not uncommon, can be difficult to see on the standard X-ray film and is often only detectable in an axial X-ray. Fixation with two transverse small cancellous screws can be used as a primary or secondary procedure. The screws get an excellent grip in the strong cancellous bone and provide perfect interfragmentary compression. To fix small fragments, washers should be used with the screws to prevent any additional fissure formation (Fig. 134a).

b) Comminuted Fractures with a Longitudinal Component

Longitudinal fissure lines are frequently seen in fragmented fractures of the patella. These fissures should be compressed by screws before the tension-band wire is applied and tightened (Fig. 134b).

c) Fractures of the Lower Pole

Avulsions and fractures of the lower pole of the patella are most often seen after road accidents. They correspond to a rupture of the patellar ligament and may be transverse or comminuted in shape. A large proximal fragment without injury to the femoropatellar cartilage is a contra-indication to partial patellectomy. The distal fragment can be brought into a broad contact with the main fragment with the help of screws but the fixation is not strong enough to resist the pull of the quadriceps. Small fragments must sometimes be removed from the fracture area (Fig. 134).

d) Systems to Resist the Effects of Muscle Pull

In such a case additional strength must be given to the patellar ligament by using a figure-of-eight tension-band wire loop. This is anchored in the tibial tuberosity and there are different methods of fixation.
- Wire may be passed around the proximal pole of the patella through the quadriceps tendon as in the usual tension-band wiring of a fractured patella.

- A drill hole may be made in the proximal pole of the patella through which the wire can pass.
- The wire can be passed through a drilled hole in the tibial tuberosity and crossed over in front of the tuberosity. A loop of wire should be made on one side which can be twisted up to provide equal tension to the opposite side, where the wire ends are twisted together.
- The wire may be passed round a screw placed transversely in the tibial tuberosity (Fig. 134e). A malleolar screw is suitable.

The choice of procedure can be made according to the anatomical situation, which can vary from case to case. Care must be taken to avoid pressure necrosis of skin or patellar tendon by the wire loop or screw heads crossing the wire in front of the ligament. Position of implants, length of the wire loop, and tension of the wire must be checked with the knee flexed before the wire is tightened and twisted.

2. Tibia

a) Avulsion Fractures of the Tibial Spines

Avulsion fracture of the intercondylar eminence corresponds functionally to rupture of the tibial insertion of the anterior cruciate ligament. This used to be seen especially in juveniles but now it may also occur in winter sports accidents. The avulsion is usually isolated but may be a component of a complex ligamentous injury. The fragment must be reimplanted and fixed accurately to its bed in order to obtain rapid revascularization. The extent of the injury is often underestimated as it is not easily seen in X-ray films. The indications for operation are rupture of the periosteum and pronounced displacement (Fig. 135).

The approach is by a classic parapatellar medial incision. The medial aspect of the upper end of the tibia along the edge of the pes anserinus is exposed. The avulsed frag-

ment is reduced with a hook and held with reduction forceps. Stable screw fixation is usually possible with the help of a pointed drill guide, and two 3.5- or 4.5-mm cancellous screws are used. The direction of the screws should be the same as that of the cruciate ligament and they may protrude for a few millimetres in the substance of the ligament. As they lie in the intercondylar fossa they do not interfere with movement. After operation a plaster cast must be used. On occasions a small cancellous screw may be inserted from the upper end into the eminence if there are very large fragments. It does not lie in the direction of the curciate ligament but it may improve interfragmentary compression (Fig. 135).

b) Avulsion Fracture of the Tibial Tuberosity

This rare injury is usually treated with a tension-band wire loop but alternatively a well contoured one-third tubular plate may be used to compress the fracture area and act as a tension band (Fig. 136b).

3. Repair of Ligaments

To reinsert an avulsed collateral ligament of the knee, a screw and spiked washer can be used instead of transosseous sutures (Fig. 136a). The spiked polyacetal resin washers incorporating a metallic ring, which may be fixed with 4.0- and 3.5-mm screws, have proved excellent for this purpose. Smaller sizes have recently been made available to be fixed with a 2.7-mm cortex screw.

Screws must be inserted with the ligament under tension and must be placed in the point of ligament insertion, which is easily seen on the naked bone where the fibres converge to one point. If the screws are inserted into the free part of the ligament, this will produce adhesions within the gliding surfaces and interfere with joint movement.

4. Avulsion Fractures of the Head of the Fibula

This injury produces the same functional disorder as rupture of the lateral, collateral ligament (Fig. 136a). The strong biceps tendon is inserted here and anatomical reconstruction and fixation is therefore important for function. Stability may be achieved by parallel Kirschner wires and a tension-band wire loop or by screw fixation. The lateral popliteal nerve is nearby and must be identified for security. As a rule additional ruptures of the joint capsule of the knee and other ligamentous injuries are associated with this lesion. Tears of these soft tissues should be sutured at the same time.

5. Shearing of Osteocartilaginous Fragments

In recent years this type of injury has frequently been reported. The fragments usually come from the femoral condyle, and occasionally from the back of the patella, and may remain as loose bodies in the joint, kept alive in the synovial fluid. If large enough these fragments can be reimplanted and fixed with small screws, the heads of which must be countersunk so that they are flush with the surface of the cartilage. The screws can be removed after 5–6 months.

6. Secondary and Orthopaedic Operations

a) Non-Union of the Patella

Real non-union of the patella is rare but when it occurs it can be treated with cancellous bone graft and screw fixation. More common is the separation of one fragment of a bipartite patella. Here also, screw fixation and a cancellous bone graft may be indicated.

b) Osteochondritis Dissecans

Smillie has advocated the refixation of large detached fragments. The appropriate treatment depends on the state of the disease when the diagnosis is made. If the separate fragment is still lying in its bed it can be fixed by a screw, which holds it in place and compresses it so that it becomes consolidated into the main bone (Fig. 137a). A slight unevenness of the surface is not of importance but the screw head should be countersunk more than is usually necessary, to stop any damage to the opposite articular cartilage. Monthly X-rays should be taken to monitor the bone healing. Weight bearing should be postponed for several months and the screws can be removed after the first year.

When a dissected fragment is entirely loose the same procedure may be appropriate; the loose body is replaced in its bed and fixed with a screw. In some cases the bed has been altered by degenerative change and filled with connective tissue so that the fragment will not fit snugly. In such a case the bed must be scraped clean and filled in with cancellous bone before replacing the fragment, which then projects slightly above the joint level. Screw fixation and postoperative treatment are then the same as described above (Fig. 137b).

If there is a major defect of the cartilage and if the fragment is necrotic, a combined graft of cartilage and bone must be considered. The graft is raised from the dorsal side of the femoral condyle which does not take much weight.

It may be difficult to find the heads of the screws when embarking on their removal, as they may become covered by newly formed cartilage.

c) Osteotomy of the Tibial Tuberosity

Osteotomy of the tibial tuberosity (Fig. 138) to move it downwards and medially has gained in popularity. It is indicated in arthrosis of the femoropatellar joint or in severe chondromalacia of the patella in adults. Only occasionally is it correct to move the tuberosity distally in a case of patella alta. A cortico-cancellous bone graft must then be placed under the osteotomized tuberosity to move it forward.

To osteotomize the tuberosity it is chiselled proximally and on both sides. The distal cortex is then weakened by drilling several holes without destroying the continuity of the soft tissue. The cortex is broken with a hammer-blow, leaving the strong fibres which connect the patellar ligament to the periosteum in continuity. The tuberosity can now be displaced 1–1.5 cm medially. If the corticocancellous bone graft is now placed deep to the tuberosity in this position, the tuberosity is displaced medially and forwards without interrupting the periosteum and tendon fibres. A Kirschner wire provides provisional fixation and when it is certain that the right position has been obtained, fixation can be achieved with a tension-band plate. A well-bent one-third tubular plate with four holes is adequate and compresses the tuberosity and the underlying bone graft firmly to the tibia, opposing the traction force of the patellar ligament. The plate must be placed in the line of the patellar ligament. After contouring, it is placed with its proximal hole over the Kirschner wire and first fixed with screws through the distal holes. The Kirschner wire is removed and replaced with a 5-cm long small cancellous screw. The tap is not used as it would tear off the fibres of the patellar tendon.

In most cases stability is good enough to allow active movement as soon as the inflammatory reaction of the wound has settled. The implants may be removed after 4–5 months.

7. Clinical X-ray Examples
(Figs. 139–144)

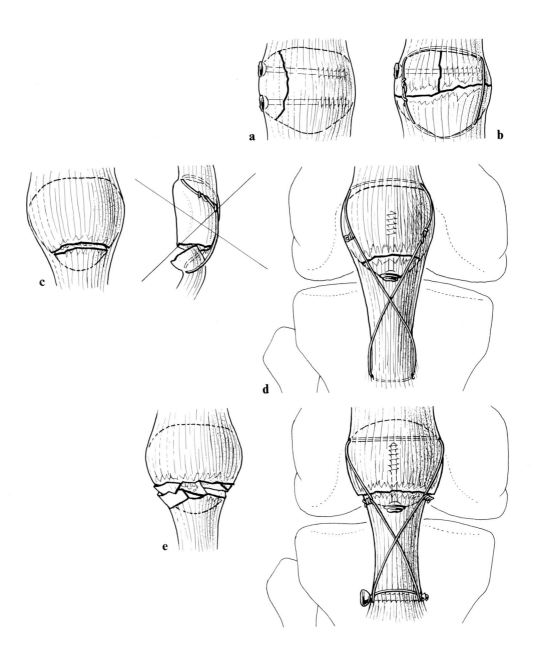

Fig. 134a–e. Internal fixation of the patella using the SFS

a Screw fixation of a longitudinal fracture

b Combination of screw fixation with tension-band wiring in a transverse fracture with a longitudinal component

c Tension-band wiring produces malposition of a small avulsed fragment at the distal pole

d Axial screw fixation combined with a figure-of-eight tension-band wire anchored in the tibial tuberosity

e Comminuted fracture of the distal pole of the patella. Partial patellectomy and fixation of the distal main fragment to the proximal fragment and a tension-band wire to the tibial tuberosity. The wire is prevented from tearing off the bone by the insertion of a transverse screw. If no distal fragments are available for screw fixation, the patellar liament is sutured directly to the proximal main fragment

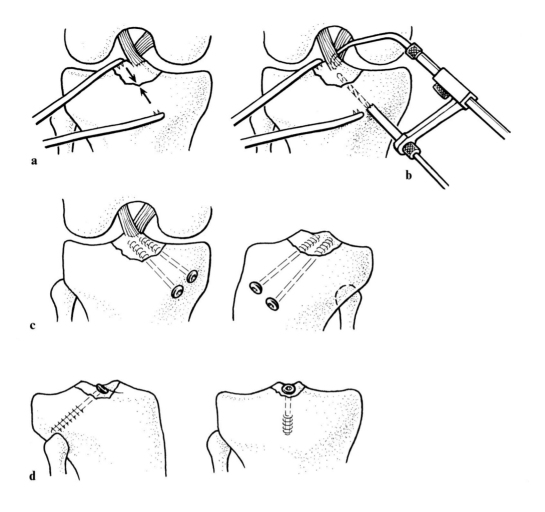

Fig. 135 a–d. Screw fixation of the intercondylar eminence

a Reduction and temporary fixation with a forceps

b Drilling of a 2.0-mm screw hole with the drill guide for the knee joint, from the medial aspect

c Two small cancellous screws are inserted in different planes and provided with washers

d So-called direct fixation of a small fragment with a screw: By retracting the patella laterally the screw is inserted from the proximal aspect through the fragment. By this means the fragment may be displaced to the dorsal side and produce loosening of the anterior cruciate ligament

Fig. 137 a, b. Screw fixation of a loose body in osteo- ▷
chondritis dissecans

a Fixation of an osteocartilaginous fragment, which is not detached completely

b Reduction and fixation of a displaced fragment after freshening of the bed and filling in with a cancellous bone graft

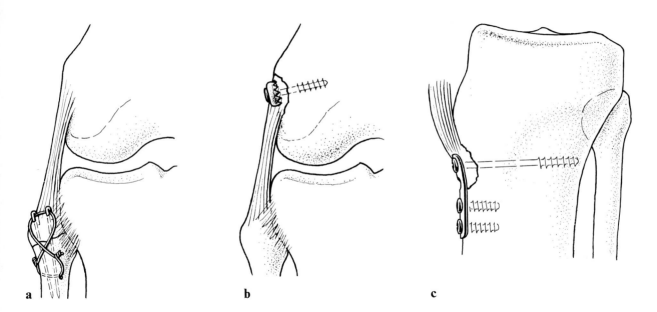

Fig. 136 a, b. Internal fixation of small avulsed fragments at the knee joint

a Avulsion fracture of the head of the fibula: fixation by parallel Kirschner wires combined with a figure of eight tension-band wire

b Avulsion of the fibular collateral ligament with a bony fragment: Screw fixation using a spiked polyacetal resin washer

c Avulsion of the tibial tuberosity: fixation with a tension-band wire or a small tension-band plate

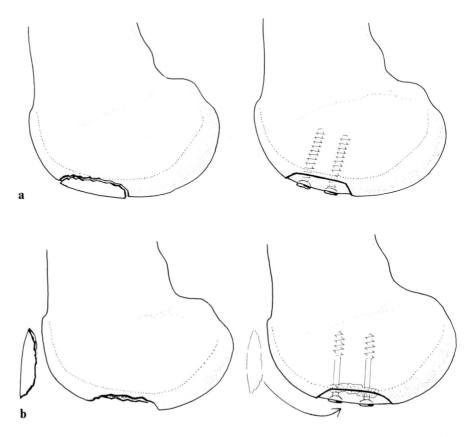

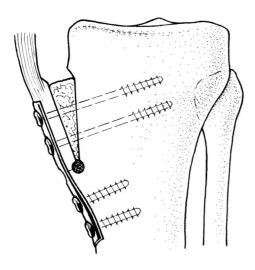

Fig. 138. Osteotomy of the tibial tuberosity

Anteromedial displacement of the tuberosity according to the Roux-Maquet-Bandi technique. The tuberosity remains in contact with the periosteum distally. A corticocancellous bone graft is interposed and fixed distally together with the tuberosity with a one-third tubular plate

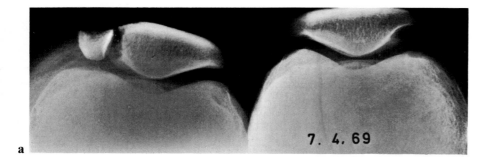

a

Fig. 139a–d. Clinical example: Screw fixation of a longitudinal fracture of patella

H., Claus, merchant aged 38. He had fallen, hitting his left knee on a stone

a Longitudinal fracture of the patella with a 90° tilt of the fragment. The fracture is only visible in the tangential view. There was much swelling of the joint

b The fracture was reduced on the 4th day and fixed with two 4.0-mm small cancellous screws. The postoperative course was uncomplicated. The joint was mobilized after the wound had healed. Then a plaster cast was applied for 4 weeks. Weight bearing was started immediately

c Removal of the screws after 1 year: the patient had no complaints and a full range of motion

d Review after 11 years. Still no symptoms and full function without arthrosis. The lateral X-ray view still shows the screw holes

238

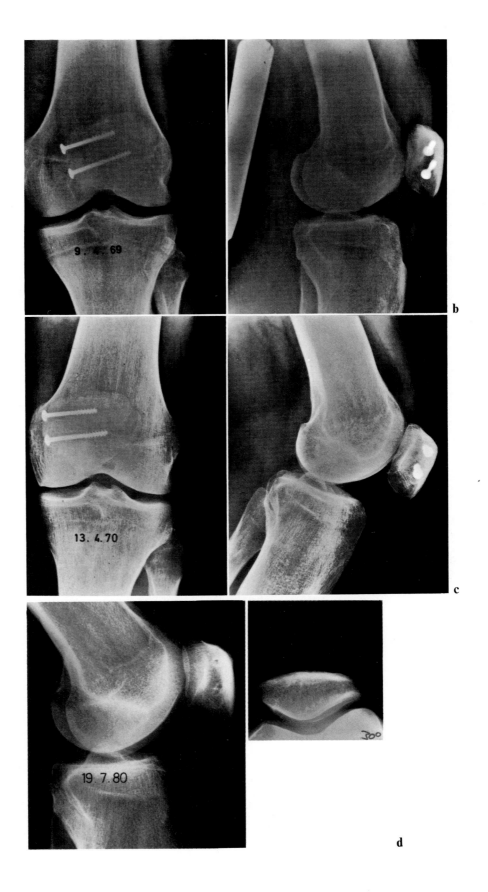

9 . 4 . 69

13. 4. 70

19. 7.80

b

c

d

239

Fig. 140 a–c. Clinical example: Fracture of the distal pole of the patella

D.S., Jose, a kitchen aid, aged 22 years. He had fallen on his left knee

a Transverse fracture of the lower pole of the left patella

b Internal fixation with two small cancellous screws and washers
Functional treatment without complications. Full weight bearing after 6 weeks, when he was back at his work

c Review and removal of the implants at 10 months: The joint was pain-free and had a full range of movement. No atrophy of the muscles. One of the small screws had broken at the junction of the thread with the shaft in the attempt to remove it, and it was left behind

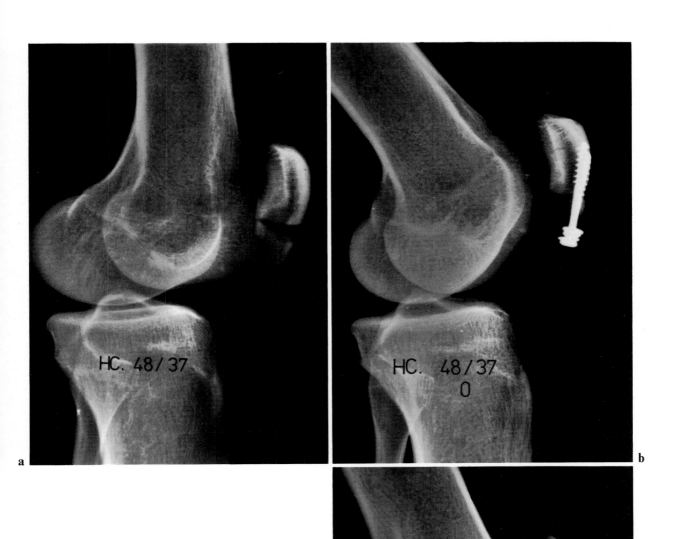

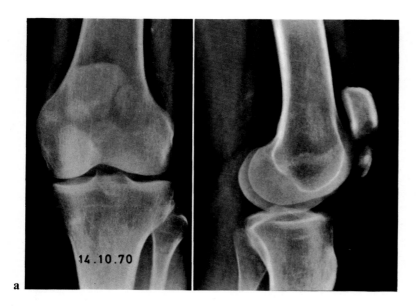

a

14.10.70

Fig. 141 a–d. Clinical example: Transverse fracture of the patella with a longitudinal component

M., Elisabeth, a housewife aged 57 years, had a road accident, sustaining concussion

a Comminuted fracture of the lower pole of the patella. The large proximal fragment shows a longitudinal fissure fracture

b A partial patellectomy was performed as an emergency procedure. The longitudinal fracture of the main fragment was fixed with screws and the patellar ligament reinserted into the proximal fragment. Reconstruction was protected by a figure-of-eight tension-band wire, anchored to the tibial tuberosity.
No complications in the postoperative course. The knee was immobilized with a plaster cast for 2

months. The implants were removed after 8 months

c At review after 16 months the patient was symptom-free and had full function of the joint, without arthrosis

d The patient is still free of pain 9 years after the fracture and she is able to go on long walking tours. She has slight atrophy of the calf muscles, but a full range of movement of the knee. The patella has nicely remodelled on the radiograph and there is no arthrosis

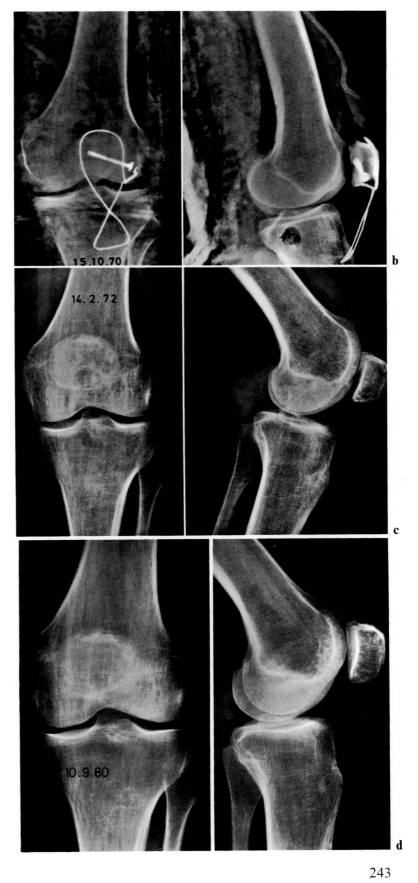

15.10.70

14. 2. 72

10.9.80

b

c

d

243

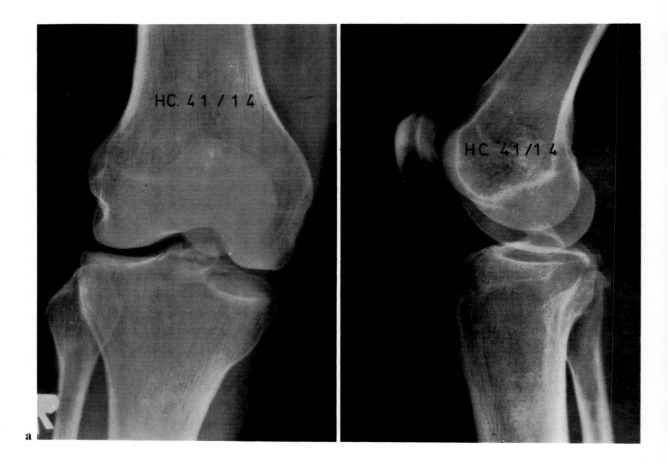

Fig. 142a–c. Clinical example: Avulsion fracture of the intercondylar spine of the tibia combined with rupture of the medial collateral ligament

B., Jutta, a woman doctor aged 44 years, who had a skiing accident

a Avulsion of the intercondylar spine of the tibia, anteromedial instability of the joint with rupture of the femoral insertion of the medial collateral ligament and with a partial rupture of the anterior cruciate ligament

b Repair was done as an emergency procedure by screw fixation of the intercondylar spine, fixation of the collateral ligament to the femur with a screw and a spiked washer, and suture of the cruciate ligament and the capsule.

The postoperative course was uneventful. Exercises for the quadriceps were started immediately. The patient was discharged with a plaster cast. At 10 weeks, mobilization and full weight bearing was started

c The implants were removed at 8 months. The joint was stable and pain-free and showed a full range of movement. There was slight atrophy of the muscles. Two small washers were overlooked during removal of the screws and left behind

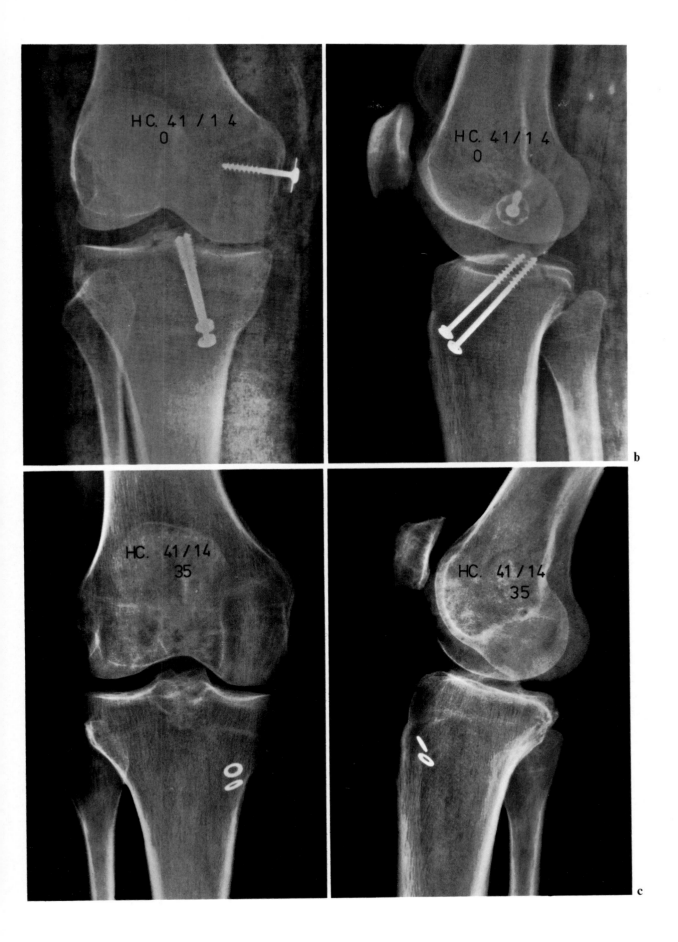

b

c

Fig. 143 a–c. Clinical example: Screw fixation of a loose body in the knee joint, resulting from osteochondritis dissecans

C., Constantino was an unskilled worker in the building trade, aged 25

a He had been kicking a football with a slightly twisted left knee which then became locked. Extension was limited to 30° and there was a slight effusion. A loose body was found to have been avulsed from the medial femoral condyle and was lying in the intercondylar notch. Arthrotomy was performed 2 days later. It was found that the loose body had been avulsed from an area of the medial condyle of the femur. It was fixed back in place with a small cancellous screw. He was immediately mobilized. A week later a plaster cast was applied and left in place for 6 weeks without any weight bearing. He was then mobilized without weight bearing for 10 weeks. He returned to full work $4^1/_2$ months after operation

b Review at 11 months: he was symptom-free and had function in this knee equal to that on the other side. X-ray shows that the loose body had been reincorporated

c Removal of the metal at 16 months. X-ray showed no sign of arthrosis

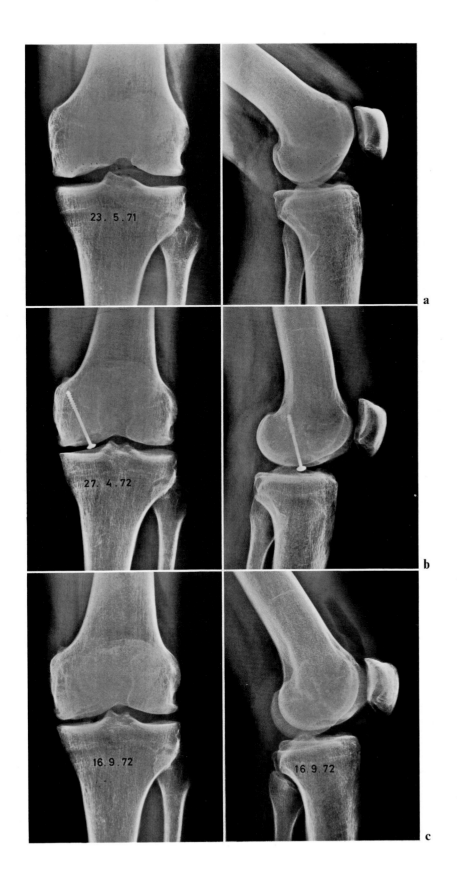

247

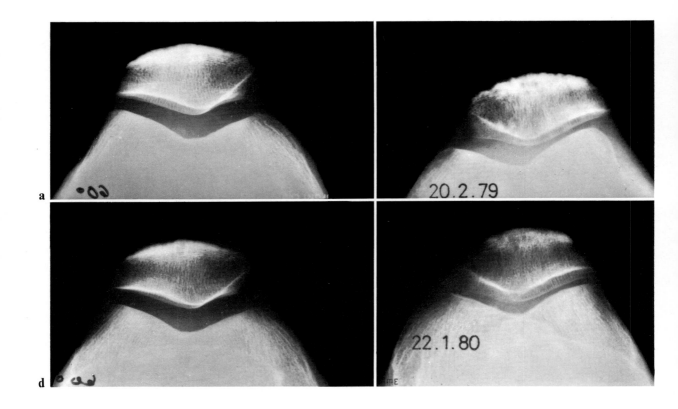

Fig. 144a–d. Clinical example: Osteotomy of the tibial tuberosity for advancement and medialization, and osteotomy of the femoral insertion of the medial collateral ligament

B., Caspar, 34-year-old railway official who incurred a torsion injury of the knee while skiing. From this time he suffered from a progressing chondromalacia of the patella with slight medial instability of the joint and symptoms of a tear of the meniscus. At operation 1¹/₂ years later he had smoothing down of the articular surface of the patella, section of the lateral and medial patellar retinacular ligament and a medial meniscectomy.

After operation the symptoms did not subside, instability of the joint progressed and he had trophic disorders

a A year later a pronounced lateralization of the osteoporotic patella was found, together with a syndrome of patellar overload.

6 weeks later the tibial tuberosity was osteomized for advancement and medialization. A wedge-shaped corticocancellous bone graft from the iliac crest was interposed and fixed by a one-third tubular plate and an additional screw. The femoral

insertion of the medial collateral ligament was osteotomized and reinserted proximally and fixed by another one-third tubular plate.

The postoperative course was slow and building up of the quadriceps difficult. At discharge the knee was immobilized with a plaster cast for 8 weeks. Mobilization and progressive weight bearing was started thereafter. Osteoporosis subsided slowly

b After 8 months the osteotomies are healed and the implants are removed

c Anterior displacement of the tibial tuberosity after removal of the implants

d Remodelling of the articular surface for the patella 11 months after operation compared to the preoperative X-ray.

1¹/₂ years after operation the function of the joint is full. Quadriceps muscle has nearly normal volume, the knee is stable and the patient is fit for sport

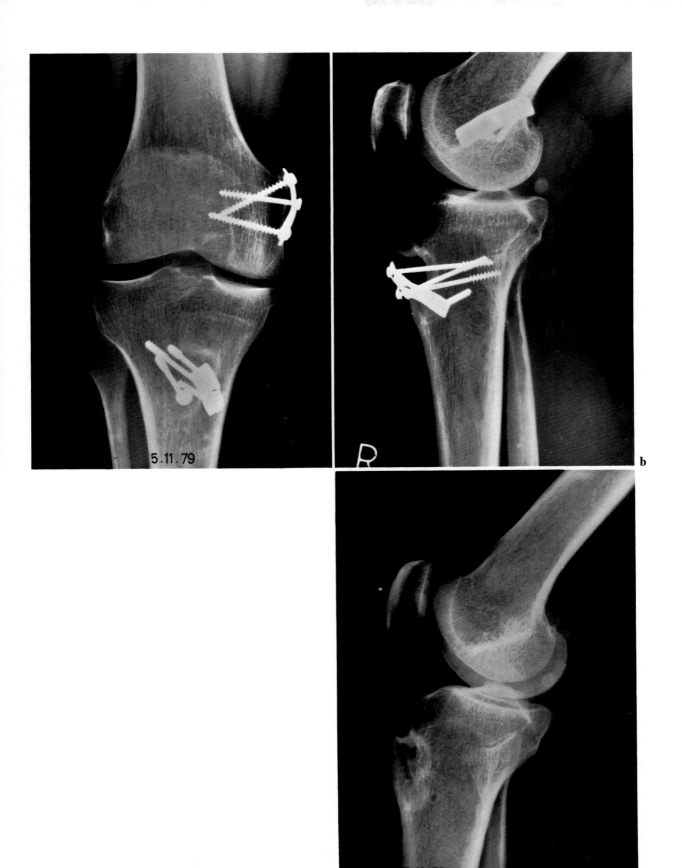

5.11.79

R

b

7.11.79

c

XV. The Shaft of the Tibia

In the very rare indications for internal fixation of the tibial shaft in children the DCP with 3.5-mm screws has proved best because of its strength and small size.

Internal fixation of the tibial shaft in adults normally involves implants of the standard size, but individual small screws may be used. The use of 3.5-mm cortex screws is recommended, since cancellous screws with the smooth shank are very difficult to remove. They are inserted according to the technique shown (Fig. 17.) The use of the drill sleeve is mandatory, as the slender 2.0-mm drill bit may break if it has to penetrate the hard cortical bone of the tibia twice. The same danger is avoided by inserting the 3.5-mm tap through the canal of the gliding hole. Special care is needed if the posterior cortex is very hard.

Small screws are used in the internal fixation of the tibial shaft in three situations:

a) Narrow Tips of Fragments

The 3.5-mm cortex screw is especially useful for the fixation of such tips. The danger of splitting the fragment is much less than if larger screws are used.

b) Detached Cortical Fragments

The accurate reduction and fixation of small cortical fragments is recommended in comminuted fractures. Reduction of the main elements of the fracture is facilitated, and the stability of the entire structure is increased. Stable fixation promotes revascularization of the fragments from the surrounding bone, since the fixation with small screws is less traumatic. Cortex lag screws of 3.5 mm are used in the shaft, while in the distal cancellous area 4.0-mm small cancellous screws are more suitable (Fig. 145).

c) Thin Butterfly Fragments

The same observations have led to the increasing use of small lag screws for the fixation of thin butterfly fragments. The flat screw heads do not splinter the cortex or damage the periosteum (Fig. 145).

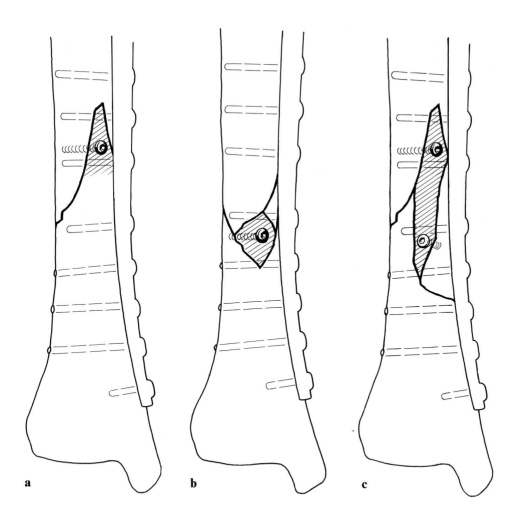

Fig. 145a–c. The use of small cortex lag screws for internal fixation of the tibia

a For the fixation of tips of narrow fragments

b For the fixation of detached cortex fragments

c For the fixation of thin butterfly fragments

XVI. The Ankle Joint

The use of the SFS in the ankle joint has become routine. This holds true for the different types of malleolar fracture and for articular fractures of the tibia and fractures of the talus. Most of these fractures have been indications for internal fixation from the inception of the ASIF group. Techniques have since been developed, founded on well established principles. Progress was based on a better understanding of the accompanying injury to soft tissues, by study of the problems of approach and by critical analysis of the long-term results.

The small implants have completely replaced both the medullary nail for the fibula and the large cancellous screw, and have superseded malleolar screws in most cases. Small plates occupy little space, spare the soft tissues and are easily contoured, and have proved increasingly successful.

The following account deals mainly with technical details rather than with indications.

A. Distal Articular Fractures of the Tibia

Fractures of the weight-bearing surface of the lower end of the tibia are referred to as fractures of the tibial pilon, a term derived from French. From an anatomical standpoint the fracture of Volkmann's triangle should be included. Nevertheless, we prefer to classify these avulsions of the dorsolateral joint surface under malleolar fractures.

Much has been written about the classification of these fractures and people have attempted to assess the technical difficulties and the prognosis from X-ray appearances. For surgical practice a simplified outlook seems appropriate. We distinguish three types of fractures, each with their own indications and techniques for internal fixation.

1. Multifragmentary Fractures

These fractures may vary from the simple wedge fracture to the comminuted one, but they never have a cancellous defect. Reduction is easier, stability of the reduced tibial joint surface is better and there is little damage to the blood supply. This type of fracture occurs chiefly in the adolescent skier and in a simple axial impaction.

A bilateral incision gives the best access. On the lateral side anterolateral tibial fragments, ruptures of ligaments and fractures of the fibula can be repaired, while on the medial side the ankle must be opened and fractures reduced under direct vision (Fig. 146).

Screw fixation alone may be enough but in multifragmentary cases medial support is recommended in the form of a DCP or clover-leaf plate.

2. Depressed Comminuted Fractures

The main feature of these fractures is a cancellous bone defect in the metaphysis. In recent years, many workers have studied the problems involved in their treatment. The fracture has certainly become more common and two different mechanisms must be distinguished:

– The Fracture in ski accidents (French: "pilon-ski") is closed, multifragmentary, and usually very complex. Bandi has described a combination of impaction, shearing and bending.

– The pure axial impaction (French: "pilon-choc") is usually due to a fall from a height or to an impact in a car accident. Many are open fractures, often occurring in old or psychiatric patients whose ability to co-operate is limited. The difficulties presented by the mental state of the patient and by the soft tissue injuries in these cases are quite different from those resulting from sports injuries and have special requirements as regards the type of operation as well as influencing the prognosis.

The operation for the injured skier follows regular lines, described below.

a) Definition and Signs

Operation can confirm the following components of the injury, listed in order of frequency rather than biomechanical significance (Fig. 147):

– A large *medial malleolar fragment* similar to that in an adduction fracture.

– A *defect in the cancellous bone* of the metaphysis.

– An *anterior impaction of the articular surface* with proximal displacement of the fragments.

– An *anterolateral fragment of the tibia,* consisting of Tillaux-Chaput's tubercle.

– A *type C malleolar fracture.* Because the anterior tibiofibular syndesmosis is intact, the lateral malleolus is attached to the anterolateral tibial fragment. If there is no fracture of the fibula, i.e. in about 10% of cases, either the anterior syndesmosis or the fibulotalar or fibulocalcaneal ligaments are ruptured as a consequence of impaction and/or displacement (Fig. 147b).

– A *transverse fracture of the posterior cortex.* The anterior impaction and the dorsal fracture are responsible for backward bowing.

To summarize, bony injuries encompass the whole circumference in most cases and the impaction of the joint surface produces complete instability of the distal tibia.

b) Planning for Operation

The consensus of opinion is that only operative treatment of this type of fracture can provide good results. The fundamental principles of this treatment have been published in 1968 (Ruedi et al. 1968) and have been widely accepted. The following procedure is recommended:

– Internal fixation of the fibula
– Reconstruction of the articular surface of the tibia
– Autogenous cancellous bone graft
– Internal fixation of the tibia with a medial buttress plate.

The above sequence can be varied somewhat: First the articular surface is reduced, and the remaining elements of the fracture are approached. The scattered fragments, which may resemble a jig-saw puzzle, must be reassembled and are fixed provisionally, after which the extent of the defect in the metaphysis becomes evident. The defect is filled in with autogenous cancellous bone graft to provide a solid block of bone for the lower tibia. Finally this block is connected to the tibial shaft by a medial plate. It acts not only as a buttress but helps in the beginning of the procedure to assemble the metaphyseal block.

There is some discussion about the choice of the appropriate implants. In the case of large fragments a DCP is best as the distal screws can be inserted parallel to the joint line. In circular fractures with anterior and posterior fragments the slender clover-leaf plate has proved most suitable, as it embraces the bone and can be easily made to fit the tibia. When anterior impaction is dominant, the spoon plate gives excellent support. The operative procedure must be altered in open fractures with major soft tissue damage. Here primary internal fixation of the fibula is useful to help in restoration of the full length of the tibia and to simplify later reconstruction. Primary procedures may be combined with traction on the os calcis or with external three point fixation of the tibia, talus and os calcis.

c) Pre-operative Preparations

The depressed, comminuted fractures are characterized by impaction of the articular surface of the tibia. This results in broadening of the epiphysis, shortening of the tibia and bone loss in the cancellous area of the metaphysis. Conventional X-ray films are often inadequate to demonstrate all the details of the injury. In every case X-rays must be of perfect quality and additional oblique views or tomograms are needed. The surgeon must study the X-rays carefully to anticipate difficulties and plan the operation beforehand.

In most of these fractures considerable swelling occurs, the extent of which is difficult to foresee immediately after the injury. Os calcis traction and elevation of the limb on a frame are recommended to avoid damage to the soft tissues, especially necrosis of the skin. This is continued until the swelling in the lower leg has diminished, usually after 3–4 days, at which time it is safe to operate.

d) Approach

To obtain excellent reconstruction, all the above-mentioned elements of the fracture must be exposed. Long bilateral incisions giving full access to the deep structures are indispensable.

Medial Incision (Fig. 148 a). This runs in a curve from the anterior border of the lower tibia, in front of the medial malleolus to the foot and provides wide exposure of the ankle joint immediately in front of the deltoid ligament. A view is thus obtained of the large medial malleolar fragment, the depressed anteromedial articular surface, and the adjacent depression of the epiphysis or defect of cancellous bone, as well as the medial aspect of the upper surface of the talus. In order to correct or prevent backward bowing, the dorsomedial border of the tibial fracture, which

lies just proximal to the groove for the tendon of the tibialis posterior, must be exposed.

Lateral Incision (Fig. 148 b). A lazy-S incision runs from the posterior border of the distal shaft of the tibia to the anterior edge of the lateral malleolus distally. The superficial branch of the peroneal nerve should be protected. Exposure must display the frequently complex fracture of the lateral malleolus and the anterolateral fragment of the tibia. The lateral aspect of the articular surface of the tibia and the upper surface of the talus must be just as fully exposed as the anterior tibiofibular syndesmosis and the fibulotalar ligament. If the latter has been ruptured it must be sutured.

The skin bridge between the two incisions must be at least 5 cm wide to maintain an adequate blood supply (Fig. 148 c).

e) Reduction

Internal fixation of the fibula is the first step; its correct length and position provide guidelines and partial support for the accurate reduction and reconstruction of the depressed surface of the tibia, which may be in valgus or varus deformity, backwardly bowed or rotationally displaced. A long one-third tubular plate with six to eight holes is usually applied (Fig. 149 a), providing rigid fixation of the comminuted ends. For details of this technique reference may be made to the section dealing with type C malleolar fractures.

Reduction and *reconstruction of the articular surface of the tibia* may be difficult. A medial or lateral approach can be used, but often both are needed to deal with the depressions of the joint and bony defects. The approach will depend upon the lesions that have been found. In order to expose anterior steps in the joint, the medial malleolar fragment must sometimes be temporarily retracted (Fig. 149 b–d). Provisional fixation is done with Kirschner wires to hold the joint fragments and to fix the epiphysis to the shaft (Fig. 150).

f) Autogenous Cancellous Bone Graft

When the articular surface has been restored attention is turned to the cancellous bony defect, which must be completely filled in with autogenous cancellous bone graft to prevent subsequent collapse (Fig. 150). This graft has a biological as well as a supporting function, and contributes to early fracture healing.

The usual donor sites in elderly patients, and whenever a large amount of graft is needed, are the iliac crest and inner surface of the ilium (Fig. 151 a). The operation for obtaining the cancellous bone should be a separate procedure, undertaken before the actual internal fixation is begun, to reduce the tourniquet time.

In young patients, and when only a small volume of graft is needed, enough cancellous bone can be obtained during the main procedure from the upper end of the tibia of the injured leg (Fig. 151 b). The advantages of this include the accessible donor site, the simple safe procedure and the saving of time. The blood supply is separate for the distal and the proximal tibia so the healing of the fracture is not disturbed, and as the leg is immobilized after operation there is no danger to the upper end of the tibia.

The technique is simple. A 4-cm incision is made over the medial aspect of the upper end of the tibia. The periosteum is incised and elevated, after which a window is chiselled in the cortex and cancellous bone obtained with a curette. More cancellous bone may be obtained from the same site during the operation if necessary. Enough bone can always be obtained from this site, and the volume can be measured at the end of the operation by filling the cavity with Ringer's solution. The wound is closed by suture of the periosteum and the skin without a drain.

The bone graft is packed into the defect through a natural or artificial window in the cortex of the anteromedial aspect of the tibia. It may be done after reduction or provisional stabilization with Kirschner wires, or after the provisional fixation of the plate and before the screws are inserted into the area of defect. The full extent of the defect must be firmly filled in and impacted.

g) Internal Fixation of the Tibia

We usually begin by screw fixation of the lateral fragment of the tibia. A clover-leaf plate is then contoured and applied medially. It may be necessary to cut off the posterior lug of the plate to prevent the groove for the tibialis posterior being narrowed.

Rigid fixation of a comminuted fracture can only be achieved if the screws can grip at all levels and in all directions, and therefore an epiphyseal block must first be established in the sagittal and transverse planes. The plate must first be fixed distally and special attention paid to the stability of the individual parts. Any malalignment which occurs should be corrected immediately. The plate is fixed temporarily to the shaft with forceps, after which individual fragments can be fixed with additional single screws. It is not necessary to fill every hole in the plate, but solid fixation of the large medial malleolar fragment is vital. At this point the temporary Kirschner wires are removed and the plate is screwed home to the main proximal fragment (Fig. 152).

The operation is completed by suturing the periosteum and closing the joint capsule. A suction drain is placed on either side. The closure of the soft tissues over the flat clover-leaf plate presents no difficulty as it occupies little space, and the patient can wear normal shoes afterwards.

h) Postoperative Treatment

The ankle joint should be held at a right angle with a plaster splint and no forced movements should be attempted until all the swelling has subsided. Hospital treatment of these patients must therefore last a few days more than in the simpler internal fixation of the tibia. No weight bearing should be attempted before the 16th week.

The clover-leaf plate is left in place until the 14th month. The large number of screws does not seem to be detrimental. The contact surfaces are limited, and we have not so far encountered corrosion between the screws and the plate.

3. Transitional Fractures

In transitional fractures the impaction of the articular surface is at the anteromedial aspect, which is a zone of low mechanical stress within the weight-bearing area of the joint. On the medial side there is always a fracture of the medial malleolus, usually of the adduction type, and laterally there may be ruptures of ligaments, which need to be reconstructed.

In these fractures also reduction and reconstruction of the fracture are important to prevent post-traumatic arthrosis and allow active postoperative movement. The bony defect is usually small and can be filled with a graft from the upper end of the tibia. Stabilization of the anterior impaction is provided by a small T-plate, or even by the L-plates used in operations on the hand and foot. The screws, which obtain a good grip on a posterior cancellous bone, give good stability to the plate. At the medial malleolus small cancellous screws are used together with washers (see adduction fractures of the malleolus, Fig. 178).

4. Secondary Operations

For pseudarthrosis or malunion, operative correction is sometimes needed at the lower end of the tibia. Malunion is due either to varus deformity, often combined with backward bowing or rotational deformity, to valgus position or to rotational deformity alone. Osteotomy of the fibula is not always necessary but double plate fixation may be used on the tibia. The small tissue-protecting plates which require little space are particularly appropriate here. The main plate must be applied medially where it can obtain a good purchase on the medial malleolus. The broad clover-leaf plate gives more rigidity than the long narrow semitubular plate. Axial compression is necessary to provide early consolidation.

a) Varus Deformity

Correction is indicated where malalignment exceeds 8°. Osteotomy of the fibula is not necessary but a small incision can be made laterally to fix a one-third tubular plate with two holes which is adequate for the coaptation of the distal and proximal fragments with one screw each. Thus rupture and splitting of the lateral cortex is avoided (Fig. 153a).

Reconstruction or opening of the pseudarthrosis and osteotomy are carried out medially (Fig. 153b). A wedge-shaped defect is produced and this is filled with cancellous bone graft. Axial alignment is checked with an X-ray. The medial buttress plate is applied and fixed distally (Fig. 153c), and if necessary compression can be applied from the upper end. A slight overcorrection of the malalignment may sometimes be advisable as the plate can then compress the graft, which promotes early healing (Fig. 153d).

b) Valgus Deformity

Correction is indicated where malalignment exceeds 14°. It is achieved by simple oblique osteotomy about 3 cm above the joint surface. Fixation is obtained with a medial plate and axial compression. Osteotomy of the fibula is not usually necessary (Fig. 154).

c) Rotational Deformity

This is often combined with varus or valgus deformity. Combined osteotomy of the tibia and fibula is needed for correction. The tibia is fixed with either a clover-leaf plate or two one-third tubular plates (Fig. 155).

d) Postoperative Treatment

The rigidity achieved in this type of osteotomy allows postoperative active movement without any external support in almost every case. Joint movement is quickly regained during the healing process of the bone and this improves the blood supply. The bone is usually consolidated enough to allow weight bearing within 8–12 weeks.

5. Clinical X-ray Examples
(Figs. 156–159)

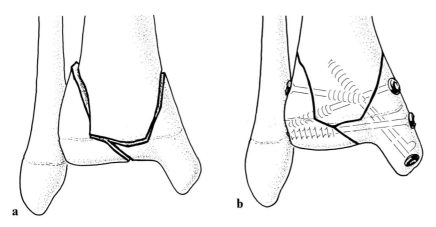

Fig. 146 a, b. Comminuted fractures of the lower tibial epiphysis

Internal fixation with cancellous screws via a bilateral approach

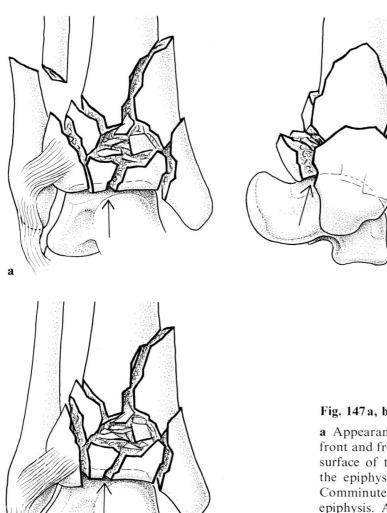

Fig. 147 a, b. Impacted comminuted fracture

a Appearance of the fracture, viewed from the front and from the side: Impaction of the articular surface of the tibia together with broadening of the epiphysis. Large medial malleolar fragment. Comminuted zone of the cancellous bone of the epiphysis. Anterior joint fragment. Anterolateral fragment of the tibia. Fracture of the fibula. Posterior fracture with backward angulation

b When the fibula is intact, impaction leads to rupture of the anterolateral ligaments

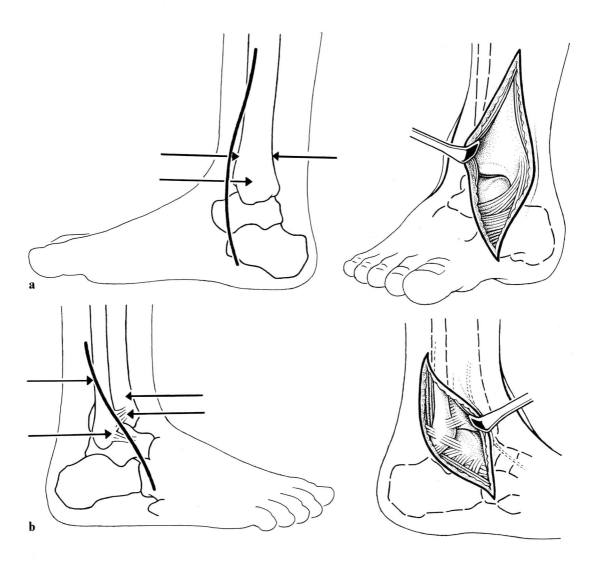

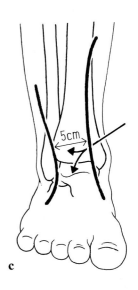

Fig. 148 a–c. Incisions and approaches

a A medial incision allows exposure of the ankle joint. The arrows mark the critical points to be observed in this approach

b A lateral incision to expose the ankle joint. The arrows mark the critical points for this approach

c Anterior view of both incisions. The minimal distance between the two incisions is 5 cm. The arrow marks the exposure of the anterior part of the ankle joint obtained by the combined approaches

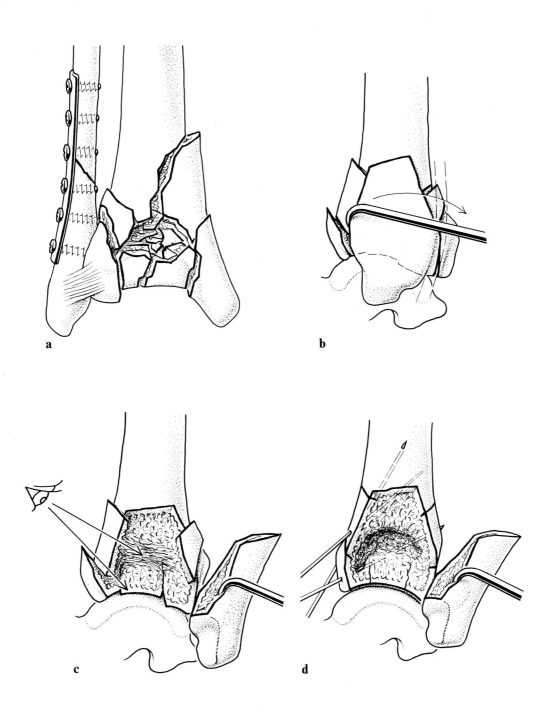

a

b

c

d

Fig. 149 a–d. Reduction of the fracture

a The first step is the fixation of the fibula by a one-third tubular plate

b–d Reduction and reconstruction of the articular surface using the anteromedial approach. A large medial malleolar fragment is temporarily retracted. Provisional fixation with Kirschner wires. A wide gap develops at the site of impaction

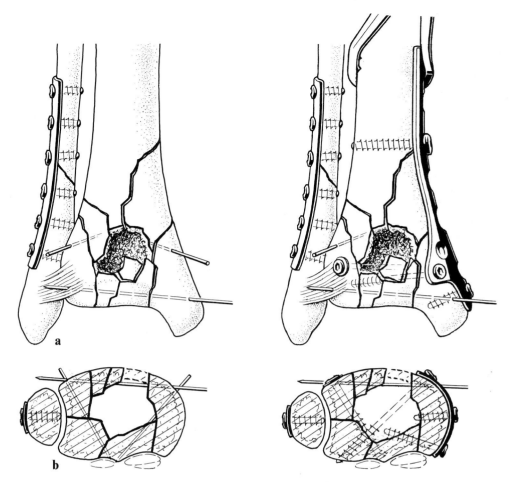

Fig. 150 a, b. Provisional medial stabilization and autogenous cancellous bone graft

a Anterior view and section through the reduced and temporarily fixed fracture. The defect in the cancellous bone is shown

b The clover leaf plate is provisionally fixed. Cancellous bone graft is filled in through a natural or chiselled window in the cortex

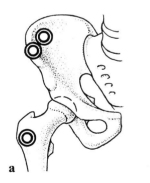

Fig. 151 a, b. Donor sites for the cancellous bone

a The anterior superior spine and the iliac crest as well as the greater trochanter are selected in elderly patients, and if a large amount of bone is needed. The graft is obtained in a separate preliminary operation

b If the amount of graft is insufficient or if an unexpected amount is required, cancellous bone may be obtained from the upper end of the tibia. Through a small longitudinal incision the graft is taken, using a sharp spoon. This site is preferable in younger patients and if only a small amount of graft is required

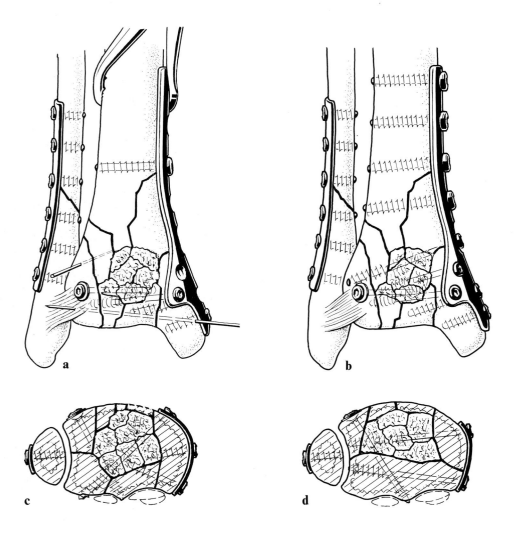

Fig. 152 a–d. Internal fixation of the tibia

a, b After filling in of the cancellous bone defect the plate is fixed with screws and the Kirschner wires are removed

c Section through the epiphyseal area of the fracture: the whole width of the clover-leaf plate is in contact. The screws obtain a powerful, circumferential grip

d Section through the epiphyseal area of the fracture: the posterior end of the plate has been cut off. The plate is therefore shorter on the anterior surface and circumferential support is reduced

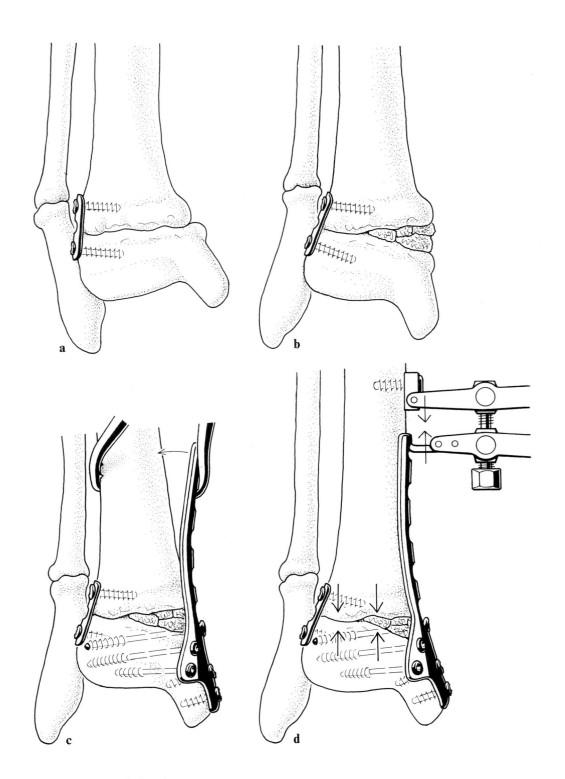

Fig. 153a–d. Correction of a varus deformity

a Lateral fixation with a short plate preventing distraction of the fragments

b Medial osteotomy and over-correction with cancellous bone in the gap

c Positioning and distal fixation of the clover-leaf plate

d Plate is placed under tension until the over-correction is removed. The graft is then under compression

263

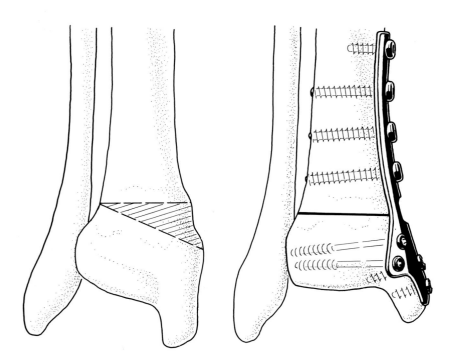

Fig. 154. Correction of a valgus deformity with a clover-leaf plate

In some instances the interposition of an antero-lateral wedge-shaped graft is required to prevent shortening. Osteotomy of the fibula may be necessary

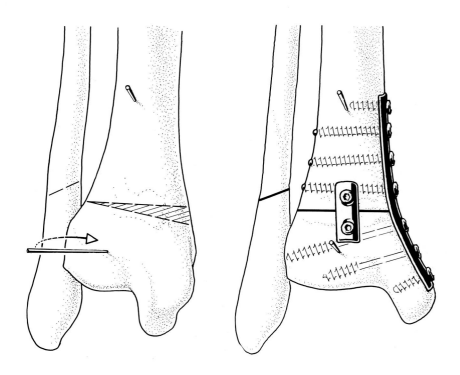

Fig. 155. Correction of a rotational deformity with two one-third tubular plates

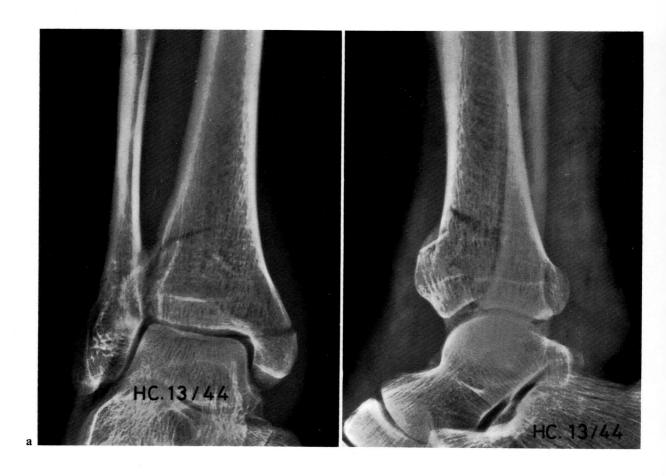

Fig. 156a–c. Clinical example: Fractures of the lower end of the tibia without cancellous defect

G., Franz, 47-year-old mechanic who had a skiing accident

a Multifragmentary fracture of the lower end of the tibia with slight anterior impaction, without cancellous bone defect

b Internal fixation with five small lag screws as an emergency procedure.

Uneventful postoperative course. Full weight bearing after 12 weeks. He was back at work after 4 months, Removal of the implants at 8 months

c Review at 7 years. The patient is free of pain, with a linear scar. He has full range of movements in the ankle joint. He has no atrophy of the muscles and X-ray shows no signs of arthrosis

266

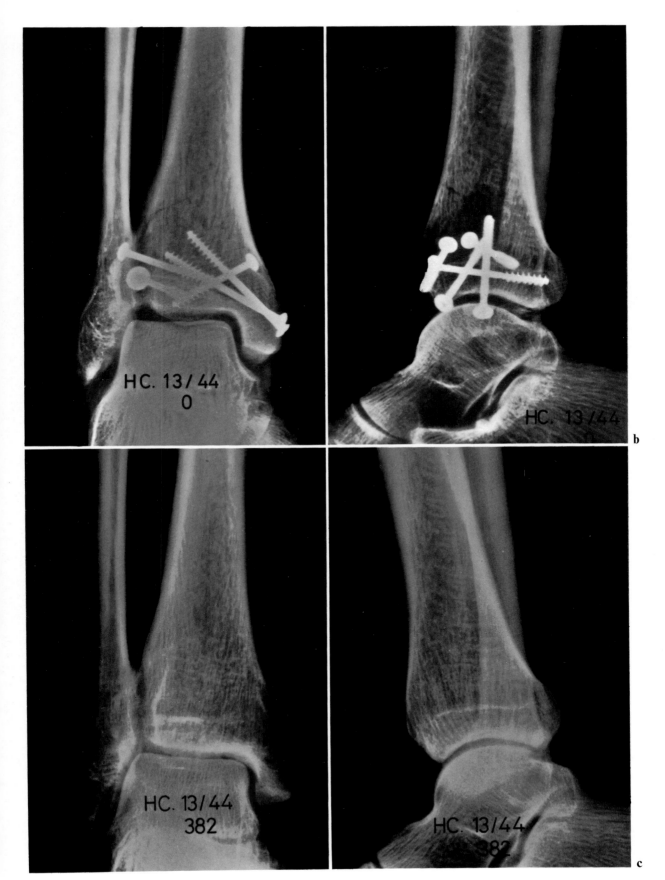

HC. 13/44
0

HC. 13/44

b

HC. 13/44
382

HC. 13/44
382

c

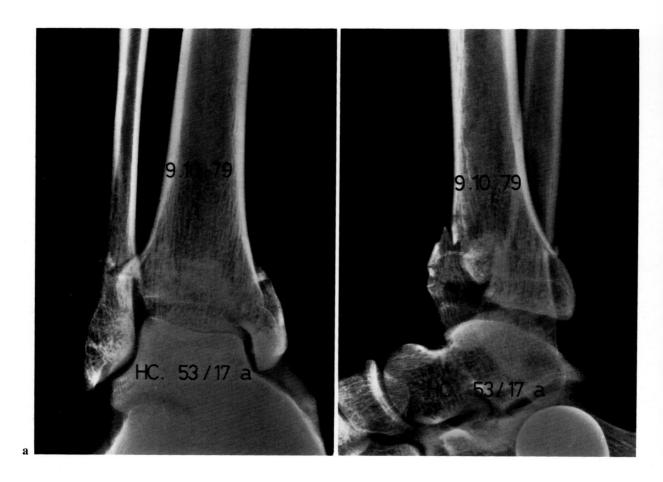

a

Fig. 157a–c. Clinical example: Fracture of the lower tibia with anterior impaction in a polytrauma patient

J.E., Klara, 25-year-old unskilled immigrant worker who had a crash with a motorcycle while driving a car. He suffered from concussion and bilateral fracture of the tibial heads

a Fracture of the lower end of the tibia with impaction of the anterior articular surface.
Because of the bad condition of the soft tissues, treatment in traction was instituted first

b Internal fixation was done on the ninth day. The fractures of both tibial heads and of the lower end of the right tibia were fixed by plates. A small T-plate for the radius was fixed to the anterior surface of the tibia since the dorsal cortex was

intact. There was a large piece of cartilage sheared off the talus.

The postoperative course was uncomplicated. Mobilization was difficult because of the injuries to both legs. At 8 weeks walking was started in the pool. At 6 months he was partially back at work and at 8 months he had full capacity for work

c Review at 9 months: He is free of pain and can walk for an unlimited distance. The ankle joint is somewhat thickened and extension and flexion are reduced by 10° each. There is no atrophy of the muscles. The X-ray shows narrowing of the tibiotalar joint space as an early sign of arthrosis

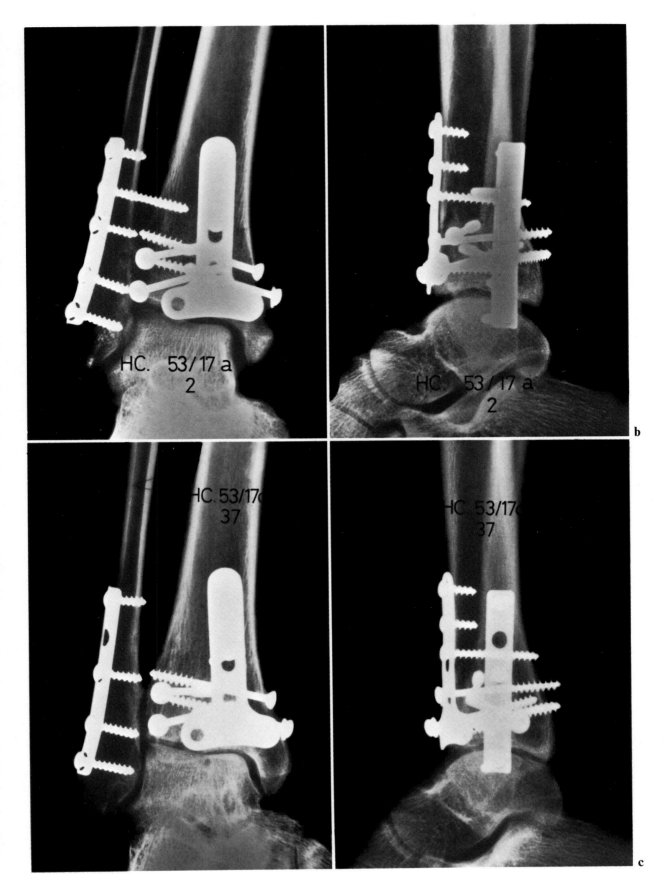

HC. 53/17 a
2

HC. 53/17 a
2

b

HC. 53/17c
37

HC. 53/17c
37

c

Fig. 158a–d. Clinical example: Fracture of the lower end of the tibia

B., Heidi, 41-year-old housewife who had a skiing accident

a There is a complex fracture of the lower end of the tibia which involves the shaft. Primary treatment was with elevation of the limb and traction

b After the oedema had subsided, internal fixation was undertaken on the second day. Internal fixation of the fibula using a one-third tubular plate with five holes. A long clover-leaf plate was used medially with additional screws. Cancellous bone graft was obtained from the iliac crest.
Uneventful course. The patient was discharged with a removable plaster splint. Weight bearing was started at 4 months and was full at 5 months

c, d see page 272f

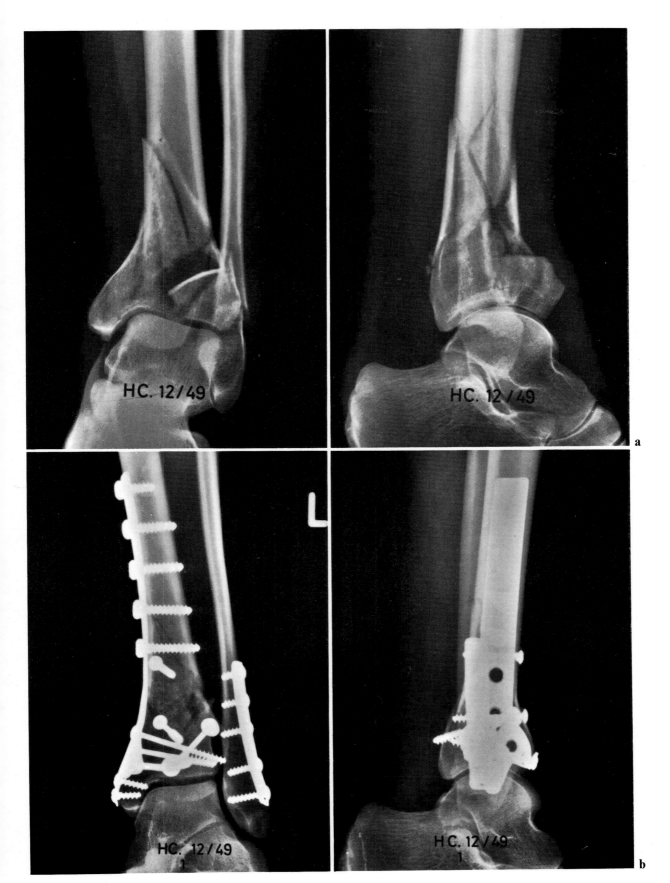

HC. 12/49

HC. 12/49

HC. 12/49
1

HC. 12/49
1

a

b

271

Fig. 158c, d.

c At 5 months the lateral implants have been removed: Structure of the bone in the grafted area is still uneven.

The remaining implants have been removed at $1^1/_2$ years: the patient is pain-free and has a full range of movement of his joint and no atrophy of the muscles. The fracture is healed.

d At 7 years the patient claims slight but constant discomfort in starting walking and in weight bearing, but is fully fit for sports. The X-ray shows moderate arthrosis of the joint

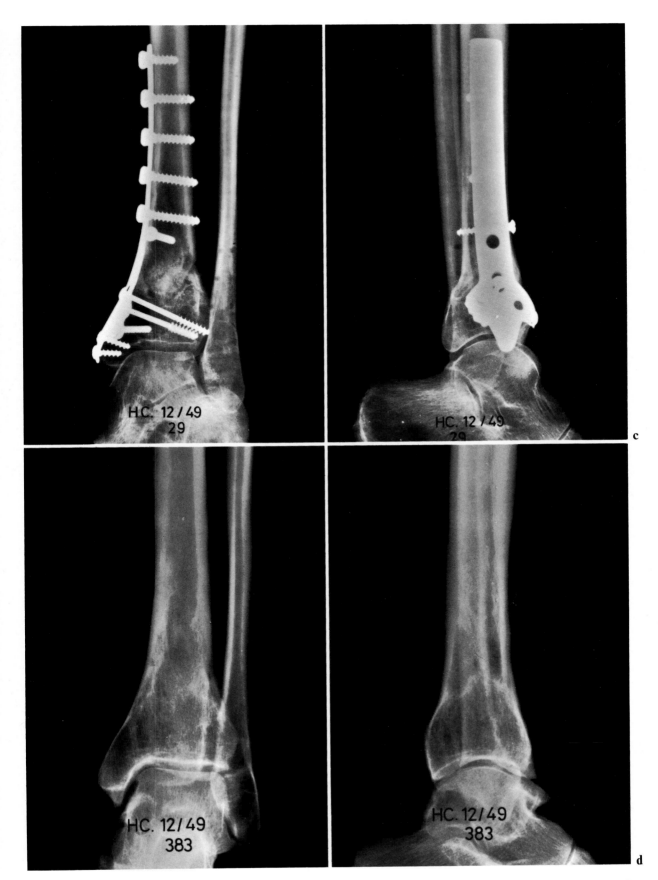

HC. 12 / 49
29

HC. 12 / 49
29

c

HC. 12 / 49
383

HC. 12/49
383

d

273

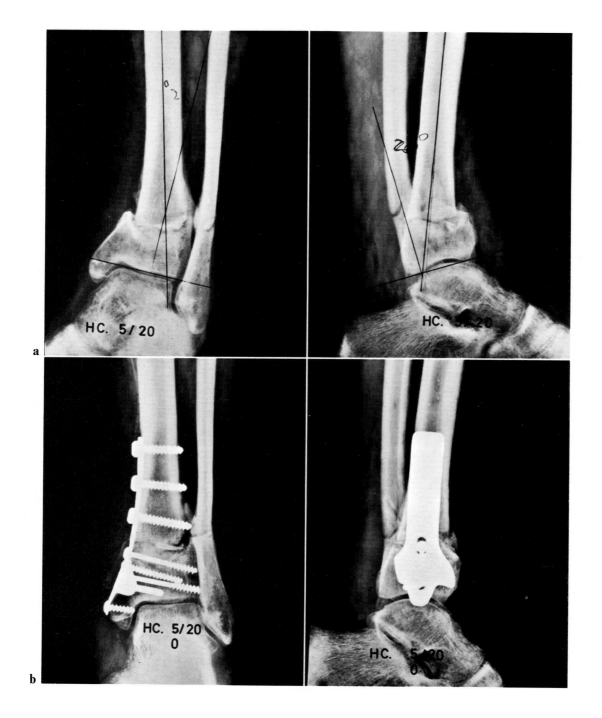

Fig. 159 a–c. Clinical example: Osteotomy for axis correction in non-union of the distal tibia

H., Brigitte, a 16-year-old pupil at a commercial school who had a skiing accident. Supramalleolar fracture of the lower leg. Primary treatment by extension, followed by a plaster cast resulted in increased deformity. The patient was referred to us three months after the accident

a Firm pseudarthrosis of the lower leg with a varus deformity of 20° and backward angulation of 20°

b Osteotomy by a medial approach. Interposition of a cancellous bone graft from the iliac crest and internal fixation by a clover-leaf plate at the medial side. Plaster-free postoperative treatment. Full movement and consolidation at 8 weeks. Full weight bearing at 10 weeks

274

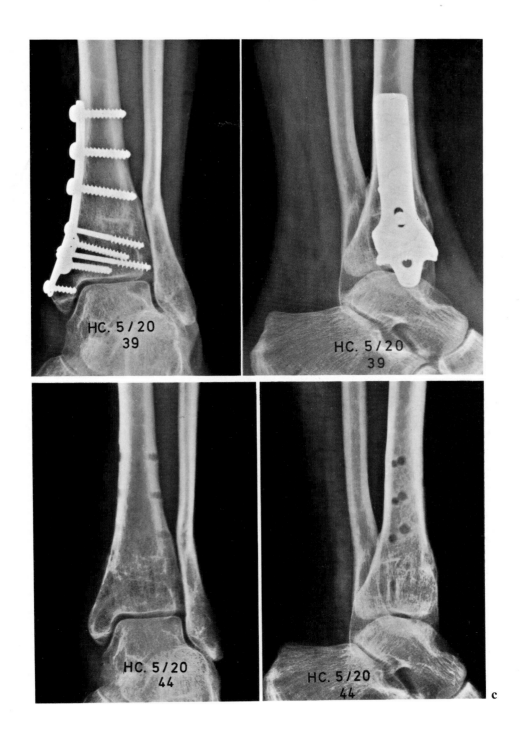

c

c Review and removal of the implants at 10 months: no pain, full function of the joint. The angle of the joint is reconstructed. There is no arthrosis.

At 9 years the patient, who lives at a distance, asserts that she is free from pain. The X-rays which were sent to us are not suitable for reproduction. The fracture is already scarcely visible; the joint is in good condition

B. Malleolar Fractures

1. Classification and Indication

Malleolar fractures are among the most common injuries to the human skeleton. They are characterized by a wide variety of lesions and have been the continuous subject of aetiological, clinical and therapeutic studies. Developments in recent years have led to the increasing use of operative treatment. The credit for this is chiefly due to H. Willenegger and B.G. Weber who have developed a clear and useful classification of the fracture types based on Danis' and Bonnin's studies. This scheme has rapidly gained acceptance and the surgical as well as the technical principles derived therefrom are now commonly applied. A second edition of Weber's "Verletzungen des oberen Sprunggelenkes" has been published.

Attention now focuses on the pathology of the tibiofibular syndesmosis and the following classification deals with the fracture-dislocation of the ankle joint (Fig. 160):

Type A: Fracture of the fibula either at the level of, or distal to the tibiotalar joint.

Type B: Fracture of the fibula at the level of the syndesmosis.

Type C: Fracture of the fibula proximal to the syndesmosis, which is always associated with rupture of the syndesmosis.

In type A the tibiofibular syndesmosis remains intact, in type B it is often ruptured, while in type C it is invariably torn and must be repaired.

The chief aim of operation is to reconstruct the fibula exactly and stably, and this must be done if active postoperative treatment is to be carried out.

Stability of the malleolar mortice is decisive. It is always unsatisfactory if the fibula is not securely fixed into the tibial notch by its ligaments. The importance of the anterior tibiofibular ligament is usually overestimated. The state of the complete ligament apparatus must be taken into account. It consists of the syn-desmosis, which is made up of connective tissue, the anterior ligament, the strong posterior ligament or its equivalent, the posterior Volkmann's triangle, and the interosseous membrane. The interosseous membrane deserves more attention as it may be ruptured well above the fracture level and be responsible for lasting instability of the ankle mortice after internal fixation.

We shall now discuss the range of application of the small implants. Not all malleolar fractures can be repaired with them. In some cases tension-band wiring is better, or in severe osteoporosis a fan of Kirschner wires may be inserted. Suture reinforcement of the ligaments is discussed, as they are closely relevant to the SFS. It is convenient to separate treatment into the internal fixation of the lateral and medial side and reconstruction of a ligament.

2. Lateral Internal Fixation and Suture of the Ligaments

Lateral internal fixation is required in fractures of the lower fibula associated with spiral fractures of the tibia; in the various type C malleolar fractures; in type A and B malleolar fractures; in fractures of the posterior triangular fragment of the tibia (Volkmann); and in fractures of the anterior tibial triangle (Tillaux-Chaput).

a) Anatomy and Topography of the Lower Fibula

The shape and structure of the lower fibula must be considered when using the SFS for fixation. The lateral side is suitable for a plate, as there are no muscular insertions. Level with its articular surface, the fibula widens out considerably and has a double bend which requires special attention. Small plates must be contoured into this S-shape (Fig. 161a). In this region the bony structure changes from hard cortical to softer cancellous bone (Fig. 161b). As the latter gives a weaker grip, 3.5-mm cortex screws or 4.0-mm cancellous screws should be used as they both have sufficiently wide threads. There is a lateral prominence 2–3 cm above the ankle joint which widens proximally (Fig. 161 b) and accounts for the lateral surface rotating increasingly in a dorsal direction. Plates must be twisted to fit this surface to avoid any rotational deformity (Fig. 161).

At this level the fibula is more posterior to the tibia so that screws must be aimed more forward towards the tibia. This may be helpful when a screw is needed to transfix the fibula at right angles to the tibia, and using the 2.0-mm bit the cortex can be penetrated without producing a crack (Figs. 161 e, 166).

b) Fractures of the Lower Fibula Associated with Other Fractures of the Lower Leg

Most of these fractures are of the "vassal" type. Internal fixation of the tibia results in spontaneous reduction of the fibula which then needs no further treatment (Fig. 28). This, however, is not always the case, and in about 7% of fractures of the shaft of the tibia additional operative fixation of the lower fibula is indicated. This may occur in two situations:

Irreducible axial deformity of the lower fibular fragment may occur after internal fixation of the tibia. Open reduction of the fibula is then needed to prevent any disturbance of the mobility of the ankle mortice (Fig. 162). A short longitudinal incision made directly over the fracture usually gives sufficient access. Oblique fractures are reduced and then fixed with small cortex screws. In the case of an indented transverse fracture or in the presence of small fragments, a short one-third tubular plate may sometimes be applied (Fig. 162 b).

Instability of the ankle mortice after internal fixation. Here the fibular fracture is associated with rupture of the anterior tibio-fibular syndesmosis. The looseness of the ankle joint cannot be diagnosed with certainty before the tibial fixation; afterwards the mortice must be carefully examined, either clinically or with the image intensifier, which is rather more reliable. If there is no movement, the fibula can be fixed with a long one-third tubular plate and the ligaments repaired following the procedure used in type C fractures (Fig. 163).

c) Internal Fixation of the Fibula in Type C Fractures

The fracture is proximal to the syndesmosis, which is always ruptured. Fixation is usually with neutralization plates. The one-third tubular plate has almost completely replaced medullary nailing of the fibula as the latter offers very little resistance to rotation and can sometimes damage the bone badly. Three special conditions are now discussed in detail:

Comminuted Type C Fractures

The fibula must be restored to its normal length, axial alignment and rotation, and this can often be difficult. In addition to the special forceps, temporary cerclage wiring may occasionally be necessary for reduction. Long one-third tubular plates with 6–8 holes are suitable for use here. To prevent rotational deformity the plates must be bent and twisted so that they exactly fit the shape of the lower fibula (Fig. 163 a). Small defects of cortical bone, which are often present, heal early and do not require cancellous grafting.

The next step is to repair the syndesmosis (see below), after which the stability of the mortice is checked. Any looseness in the transverse direction is tested with a hook or spreading forceps and the drawer sign is manually tested in the anterior and posterior direction (Fig. 164). When the stability is inadequate it is best to fix even a small posterior Volkmann triangle fragment. Only when this has been done and instability remains should the fibula be screwed to the tibia, as this is a non-physiological procedure.

Screwing the Fibula to the Tibia

A screw is passed 3–5 cm above the ankle joint proximal to the syndesmosis. It is inserted from behind forwards and should run parallel to the ankle joint surface (Figs. 165, 166). It should only stabilize the syndesmosis and not compress it. A cortex screw is therefore chosen, not a cancellous or a malleolar screw. It should fit the fibula and not have a gliding hole. The screw must gain a grip in three cortices, the lateral and medial cortex of the fibula and the lateral cortex of the tibia. This provides an elastic fixation which does not interfere with the movements of the ankle mortice.

A transfixion screw can be passed through a hole in the plate, which is already in place. If there is still instability after internal fixation of the fibula and suture of the ligaments, a screw is removed from the plate at the appropriate level, a drill hole is made through the hole in the plate and the lateral cortex of the tibia with a 1.8-mm Kirschner wire. This is better than using the drill bit as this may bend or break if its broad point does not meet the lateral cortex at right angles (Fig. 166 b). The hole made with the Kirschner wire is easily found with a 2.0-mm drill bit and can be widened. A 3.5-mm thread is tapped and a 24–28 mm long screw inserted. This transverse screw can also be inserted away from the plate (Fig. 167). The angle of insertion must be 30° forward to make the drill bit meet the tibial cortex at right angles to its dorsolateral margin (Fig. 166 a). After the screw has been placed it must be confirmed that there is free movement of the ankle joint, especially in dorsiflexion.

It has been found that early removal of the transverse screw is not necessary. As there is no compressing effect, the ankle can move freely and calcification or ossification in the syndesmosis does not occur. If the screw is stressed by rotation of the fibula at an early stage, a small area of bone resorption may be seen on X-ray. The screw may also break during mobilization without interfering with the postoperative treatment, in which case the tip of the screw can be left behind, buried in the tibia.

High Type C Fibular Fractures

Here special operations are required.

Direct Fixation. Rigid internal fixation of the shaft of the fibula can be obtained either by screw fixation or by a neutralization plate. After repair of the ligaments and internal fixation, stability of the ankle mortice must be checked again. When this is adequate the transverse screw can be omitted but it must always be inserted if there is insufficient stability.

Indirect Fixation. Direct internal fixation of the fibula is possible up to the middle of the shaft but above this it becomes difficult, as the fibula is embedded deeply in muscles and exposure may jeopardise the peroneal nerve. The fracture should then be indirectly fixed as follows:

– A small drill hole is made in the lateral cortex of the distal fibula. A hook is inserted into this hole and the fibula pulled downwards until it exactly fits into the notch of the tibia at its full length and in proper rotation. Assessing the correct position of the fibula needs some experience.

– Temporary transfixion of the fibula to the tibia near the joint, using a transverse 1.8-mm Kirschner wire.

– The correct position of the fibula can be checked by comparing a centred X-ray film with a pre-operative one of the normal ankle. The length of the fibula can be confirmed, and the reduction checked, using an X-ray or the image intensifier.

– Final fixation of the fibula may be done with one or two transverse screws above the syndesmosis, according to the above-described technique of the "three point fixation" (Fig. 165 d).

In this procedure one must pay attention to the following details:

– Suture of ligaments must be carried out before bony stabilization. The ease of suture of the anterior ligament to its proper place is a useful indication of the correct position of the fibula. Additional transosseous sutures are usually required to obtain perfect stability.

– Transfixion must always be carried out with 3.5-mm cortex screws according to the "three point fixation" technique. It is not necessary to drill the tibia right through to the medial cortex, as the lateral cortex alone provides adequate fixation. Use of the

4.5-mm cortex screw has been discontinued, as it is too rigid and the screw heads project too far.

Maisonneuve's fracture

In this unusual type C fracture, the break is at the neck of the fibula near the knee joint, and is often missed. A Maisonneuve mechanism may also cause dislocation of the head of the fibula without fracture, when the ligaments alone are ruptured. Diagnosis must be made clinically, as pathological movement of the fibular head can be seen and felt. In these cases the entire interosseous membrane has been ruptured. Fixation of the fibula is carried out as described above.

d) Internal Fixation of the Fibula in Type B Fractures

Here the fibula is fractured level with the syndesmosis, which is usually ruptured. Long oblique or spiral fractures are fixed with cortex or small cancellous screws. In short or comminuted fractures, a well contoured one-third tubular plate is appropriate (Fig. 168). If the fracture plane is suitable, it is useful to apply the plate posteriorly to give a better fixation (Fig. 168 d). The incision of the peroneal tendon sheath, which is necessary for this procedure, does not have any ill effects.

In comminuted fractures and in osteoporosis, stabilization can be achieved by a number of intersecting Kirschner wires, to which a tension-band wire loop may be added. The transfixion of the fibula and tibia by these pins is not detrimental; good stability of the ankle mortice must be guaranteed by some means (Fig. 168 e).

e) Internal Fixation of the Fibula in Type A Fractures

The fibula is fractured below the level of the ankle joint and the syndesmosis is intact. Fractures are usually transverse or short oblique; such fractures can rarely be fixed by screws alone. In some cases a neutralization plate or a small T-plate may be used, but normally these fractures are treated with a combination of Kirschner wires and a figure-of-eight tension-band wire loop (Fig. 168 f). If there is an isolated fracture of the medial malleolus there may be ruptures of the distal ligaments (anterior fibulotalar and fibulocalcaneal) at this site, in which case they must be repaired to maintain stability of the ankle joint.

f) Repair of the Ligaments at the Ankle Joint

The importance of the different ligaments in maintaining the stability of the ankle joint is usually underestimated. The following injuries may occur.

Anterior tibiofibular ligament:
- Avulsion of the ligament from the tibia with or without a small bone fragment (tubercle of Tillaux-Chaput).
- Intermediate rupture of the ligament itself, which is often Z-shaped.
- Avulsion from the fibula with or without a cortical bone fragment.

Posterior tibiofibular ligament:
- This is not exposed during internal fixation and is probably most often avulsed from the tibia.

Interosseous Membrane:
- Avulsion from the tibia predominates.

Fibulotalar and Fibulocalcaneal Ligament:
- Avulsion is usually from the fibula.
- Avulsion from the talus
- Intermediate rupture of the body of the ligament.
- Avulsion from the os calcis which is usually V-shaped anteriorly.

Deltoid Ligament:
- Avulsion from the tibia (frequent).
- Z-shaped rupture
- Avulsion from the talus (rare).

When operative repair of these ruptures is advocated, one is often met with the argument that torn ligaments cannot be properly sutured. In such situations the suture is in fact only an adaptation. For mechanical stability, reinforcement is required by transosseous suture.

The following procedures have proved to be necessary in suturing ligaments:

- Avulsion of ligaments with bony fragments of sufficient dimension are fixed with screws. The small spiked polyacetal resin washer is very useful here (Fig. 169 b).
- Avulsions of the periosteum are repaired by transosseous suture on one side. Drill holes are made with Kirschner wires, a drill bit or the small finger chuck. They can be opened with a towel clip passed backwards and forwards to allow a curved needle to carry a suture through (Fig. 169 d, e).
- At the fibula, sutures can be anchored round implants like plates, wire loops or Kirschner wires (Fig. 169 g).
- Ruptures of the body of the ligament must be reinforced with a heavy suture passed through the bone on each side (Fig. 169 f).
- For many years we have used only inert absorbable suture material of calibres 1 and 2. There is no disturbance of wound healing and the material holds well enough until connective tissue has regenerated. Because the material is elastic the minor movements within the syndesmosis are not interfered with.
- After this reinforced suture of a ligament, movement of the joint is possible if there is no inflammation of the wound. Movements should not be forced and when the wound has healed a plaster slab or circular plaster cast should be applied and left until the connective tissue has settled down, which is at about 6 weeks. The general postoperative management depends on the fracture healing.

g) Volkmann's Posterior Triangle Fragment of the Tibia

This "third malleolus" fracture may occur in two forms, which are mechanically and anatomically different (Fig. 170).

The Shorn-off Fracture. Here there is a larger fragment including part of the posterolateral articular surface, the area of the ankle joint which carries the highest load. Anatomical reduction is indispensable if post-traumatic arthrosis is to be avoided. It used to be said that only large fragments needed reduction and fixation, but nowadays we feel that all articular fragments should be replaced. Interpretation of the radiographs may be difficult, especially when there is a fracture-dislocation. Minor impaction may be seen at the edges of posterior triangle fragments, so that in doubtful cases it is better to decide on internal fixation.

The Avulsion Fracture. Here the posterior tibiofibular ligament avulses a fragment from the tibia. The fragment is small and takes no part in the joint surface. The only indication for internal fixation of this fragment is instability of the mortice which does not disappear with internal fixation of the fibula and the reinforced suture of the anterior tibiofibular ligament. In this case fixation of the posterior fragment stabilizes the fibula, and is more physiological than passing a tibiofibular transfixion screw.

Two different techniques are available for fixing the posterior malleolar fragment.

Indirect Screw Fixation

The fragment is exposed and reduced from a dorsomedial approach (Fig. 174), but the screw fixation is done from the front of the tibia, as follows:

After internal fixation of the fibula and suture of the lateral ligaments a long, curved incision is made in front of or behind the medial malleolus (Fig. 171 d). If there is a fracture of the medial malleolus, this is fixed or the suture of the deltoid ligament prepared.

The tendon sheath of tibialis posterior is opened longitudinally. The approach is along the surface of the tibia, retracting the tendons, nerves and vessels dorsally with a Hohmann retractor. The posterior fragment is exposed, the medial edge of which is close to the medial malleolus. The periosteum at the proximal margin of the fragment is incised to confirm the reduction. The fragment can be reduced accurately with a hook and is temporarily fixed with reduction forceps, which can embrace the whole tibia. From the anteromedial aspect of the tibia a 1.8-mm Kirschner guide wire is inserted. In the same direction as this but in different planes two small cancellous screws may now be inserted. In small fragments where the screw would penetrate too far, preventing interfragmentary compression, the thread may be shortened by cutting it with a special forceps (Fig. 172a, b).

If there is doubt about the accuracy of the reduction, an X-ray should be taken before the screw fixation is carried out. It is not possible to check the reduction satisfactorily with the image intensifier.

Direct Screw Fixation

This technique (Fig. 172c) provides much better interfragmentary compression, but involves a difficult exposure. The patient has to be positioned preoperatively (Fig. 171). Screw fixation may be achieved by a dorsolateral or dorsomedial approach. The latter procedure is preferred if the articular surface of the tibia is impacted at the posterior circumference and needs reduction.

Dorsolateral Approach. The patient lies on his side or back with the knee joint flexed (Fig. 171c). The surgeon is seated working from the upper side and must be free behind, so the patient's arm must be elevated. The supine position is best if the medial malleolus has also to be fixed, as this is difficult in the lateral position. The prone position is not used because of its risks of anaesthesia complications.

A curved incision, similar to but somewhat longer than that for internal fixation of the fibula, is made (Fig. 171e). The incision is made primarily behind the lateral malleolus. The posterior fragment is approached between the tendons of flexor hallucis and peroneal muscle. The fragment is exposed by incising the periosteum at the proximal edge and it can be reduced and temporarily fixed with a Kirschner wire. Short cancellous screws with washers are used to fix the fragment. Drilling must be conducted carefully to avoid penetrating the ankle joint, as this may easily happen with the joint in the inclined position after flexing the knee. The direction of the screws must therefore be downwards from behind or upwards from the front (Fig. 173d).

h) The Anterolateral Triangle of the Tibia (Tillaux-Chaput)

An anterolateral fragment of the tibia may be missed on the X-ray but oblique views may be helpful. The size of the fragment varies from a very small avulsed chip at the insertion of the syndesmosis to a larger wedge-shaped fragment. Stabilization is imperative because the fracture line runs into the syndesmosis and influences the integrity of the ankle mortice, and because the anterior tibiofibular ligament is inserted into the fragment. Internal fixation is usually carried out using a small cancellous screw with spiked metallic or polyacetal resin washer (Fig. 169b).

The approach to the anterior margin of the lateral malleolus must preserve the fine cutaneous branch of the superficial fibular nerve, which varies in position.

i) Dislocation of the Peroneal Tendons

Traumatic anterior displacement of these tendons has become more common in recent years. It may be an isolated lesion or occur in combination with other injuries of the ankle joint like malleolar fractures, rupture of the Achilles' tendon or ruptures of ligaments. Swelling may obscure the lesion but it should be repaired. The injury occurs in two forms (Fig. 175).

– Rupture of the retinaculum with avulsion of the periosteum from the fibula. Displaced tendons lie below the avulsed periosteum, which is continuous with the retinaculum. After reduction of the tendons the ligament can be fixed at the posterior edge of the fibula using a screw with a spiked polyacetal resin washer and additional sutures of the periosteum.

– Direct rupture of the retinaculum at the edge of the fibula: Direct suture of the ligament is impossible because of swelling. The retinaculum is retracted dorsally and reconstructed with a free tendon graft from the

281

plantaris longus, or with a periosteal flap with its base at the tip of the fibula. Recurrence is rare.

In a long-standing displacement of the peroneal tendons, Kelly's osteotomy may be carried out. A disc of bone is chiselled off the lateral malleolus, displaced dorsally and fixed with screws; thus a block is provided which prevents further displacement of the tendons (Fig. 175c). Reconstruction may also be carried out with a free tendon graft from the plantaris longus or with a strip of Achilles' tendon, which remains attached to the tendon distally.

3. Fixation of the Medial Malleolus

Biomechanically, fractures of the lateral malleolus are much more important than those of the medial side of the ankle joint. Because of this, technical difficulties in reduction of the medial side of the ankle joint have been somewhat neglected. These fractures must also be accurately reduced and rigidly fixed. The special shape of the medial malleolus, consisting of a double curve, calls for careful consideration. Particular attention must be paid to the intermediate area, to impactions of the anterior edge of the articular surface and to posterior fractures within the canal for the tendons.

In isolated medial fractures one has to consider that there may be a lateral ligamentous injury. This usually consists of rupture of the anterior fibulotalar ligament or the fibulocalcaneal ligament, which do not show up on X-ray. Since fixation of the medial malleolus does not achieve thorough stability of the ankle mortice, repair of the lateral ligaments at the lower end of the fibula is mandatory.

a) Malleolar Fracture Associated with Fracture of the Tibial Shaft

Ankle joint involvement in spiral fractures of the tibia is quite common, and in our experience occurs in 10% of cases. The fracture usually involves the medial malleolus at its edge, and these fissures may not be seen in standard X-rays, only being discovered in the course of internal fixation. They are often unstable and, if displaced, must be accurately reduced. Experience has shown that reduction of the more proximal main fracture is made easier by first reducing and fixing the articular part of the fracture. This is especially true in posterior fractures.

Approach and Internal Fixation. The classical incision for fracture of the tibia is extended at its distal end above the anterior border of the medial malleolus. The saphenous vein is divided between ligatures, taking care not to disturb the saphenous nerve. The ankle joint is opened just in front of the deltoid ligament and the haemarthrosis aspirated, after which the incision in the capsule is widened laterally until the fracture line is exposed and the fracture can be reduced.

The fragment may be screwed through the tibial plate, if the level of the fracture calls for a distally placed lower end of the plate. When a DCP is used, a screw may be inserted parallel to the joint surface, i.e. obliquely through the plate, to fix the malleolus (Fig. 176a).

Usually the distal fracture is fixed by separate small cancellous screws with washers (Fig. 176b).

b) Oblique Fracture of the Medial Malleolus

This fracture is an ideal indication for internal fixation with two small cancellous screws. In a large fragment the procedure follows stabilization rule 1 (Fig. 26). The fragment is temporarily fixed with Kirschner guide wires. Two small cancellous screws are inserted in different planes to secure interfragmentary compression.

Comminuted fractures may be fixed with Kirschner wires and tension-band loops (Fig. 177).

If the soft tissues are in poor condition a separate screw introduced through a stab incision may be useful.

c) Small Avulsion Fracture

This may be only part of the injury, and the deltoid ligament may be ruptured anteriorly or posteriorly. Internal fixation is achieved either with a screw or a tension-band wire loop, depending on the size of the fragment (Fig. 177d). Ruptured ligaments should be repaired.

d) Posterior Fractures

Boat-shaped fragments may extend well backwards and involve the articular surface. They border a shorn-off posterior triangular fragment of the tibia. Incision of the tendon sheath and backward retraction of the tibialis posterior tendon is required to expose and reduce such a fragment. The fragment is temporarily fixed with Kirschner wires and then screwed so that the screw heads lie at the edge of the tendon canal to prevent any rubbing. It is not necessary to suture the tendon sheath.

e) Adduction Fractures

Adduction fractures are those in which the fracture surface extends to the medial proximal cortex of the tibia. They are fixed with small cancellous screws and washers, the screws being roughly parallel to the joint surface in different planes (Fig. 178).

Special attention must be paid to any impaction of the anteromedial joint surface of the tibia, which may be small but rather dense, and may hinder reduction of the fragments. There may also be wider impactions, approaching those found in comminuted distal tibial fractures. Before reduction, these impacted areas must be carefully identified. Any bony defect remaining after reduction should be filled in with cancellous bone graft. If only a small graft is needed it can be obtained from a non-weight-bearing part of the adjoining tibial metaphysis, and this may be termed "a local shift of cancellous bone" (Fig. 178b). Screw fixation thus compresses the recon-

structed articular surface and prevents further breakage.

4. Secondary Operations

a) Delayed Internal Fixation

Malalignment which cannot be corrected by conservative treatment or which occurs later may need operation. If it is still mobile and soft callus can be removed, internal fixation can be carried out in the same way as in a primary operation. This may be possible weeks or even months after the injury.

b) Pseudarthrosis

This is rare after primary operation for malleolar fractures but occurs more commonly after conservative treatment, chiefly in the medial rather than the lateral malleolus. Treatment is by compression with small cancellous screws and washers, with the addition of an autogenous bone graft in cases of osteoporosis.

c) Osteotomy

Shortening of the lateral malleolus after inadequate treatment is the most common indication for osteotomy in the ankle joint. Weber and Willenegger especially have emphasised the techniques and advantages of these corrections. A lengthening osteotomy of the fibula can easily be fixed with a one-third tubular plate. Distraction can be obtained with the reversed articulated compression device and the plate fixed to one side of the osteotomy, or with an external fixator. The resulting defect is filled in with a block of cancellous bone or with a corticocancellous graft (Fig. 34). Reconstruction of the anterior tibiofibular ligament may be achieved using strips of skin.

5. Clinical X-ray Examples
(Figs. 180–188)

C. Fractures of the Talus

1. Internal Fixation

We distinguish between peripheral and central fractures of the talus. Internal fixation is indicated in avulsion fractures of the lateral and posterior process of the talus to restore joint stability. The same holds true for larger flake fragments of the dome of the talus. Internal fixation is obtained with screws (Fig. 179 a).

Central fractures of the talus at its neck or dome are prone to necrosis. If the fragments are displaced, reduction and internal fixation must be carried out immediately. A medial approach is used and small cancellous screws inserted in different planes (Fig. 179 b). Bony defects are filled with cancellous bone. The vital part of the postoperative treatment is relief from weight bearing, enforced with the use of a walking caliper for many months.

2. Clinical X-ray Examples
(Figs. 189–190)

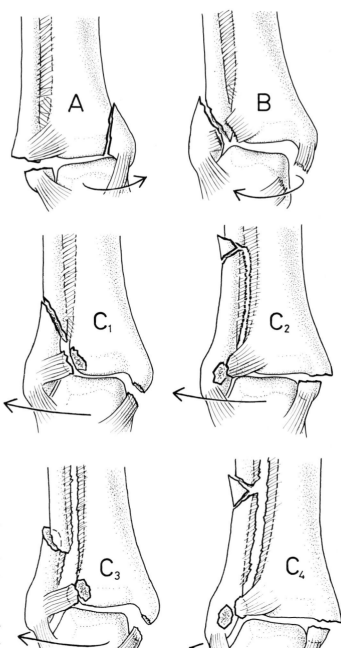

Fig. 160. Classification of malleolar fractures (see also *Manual of Internal Fixation,* 1979, p. 289)

Type A Transverse fracture of the fibula, either at the level of, or distal to, the joint. Possible shear fracture of the medial malleolus

Type B Spiral fracture, level with the syndesmosis, together with rupture of the anterior tibiofibular ligament. Rupture of the deltoid ligament or avulsion fracture of the medial malleolus

Type C Fracture of the fibula above the syndesmosis. A rupture of the tibiofibular ligament is always present. There may be an avulsion of the posterior margin of the tibia. A medial avulsion fracture or a rupture of the deltoid ligament is common.

One distinguishes: Cl, a low type C fracture type; and C2, a high type C fracture, as well as the proximal fibular fracture of Maisonneuve. If the interosseous membrane is ruptured above the fracture site there is a pronounced instability of the Maisonneuve fracture (C 3 and C 4)

Fig. 161 a–e. Anatomy of the lower fibula

a Lower fibula seen from the front with an accurately contoured one-third tubular plate, and a lateral view

b Cross-sections of the lower fibula at different levels: Changes of the bony structure. Lateral spur marked with arrow

c Topographical relations between the fibula and tibia. Dorsal position of the fibula in relation to the tibia. Posterior inclination of the lateral surface of the fibula in the area above the malleolus

d The slope of the lateral fibular surface requires a twist to be applied to the one-third tubular plate

e Cross-sections at different levels to show the situation of the one-third tubular plate. Plate screws above the malleolus are also inserted in a direction towards the tibia and this allows one to be used for transfixation

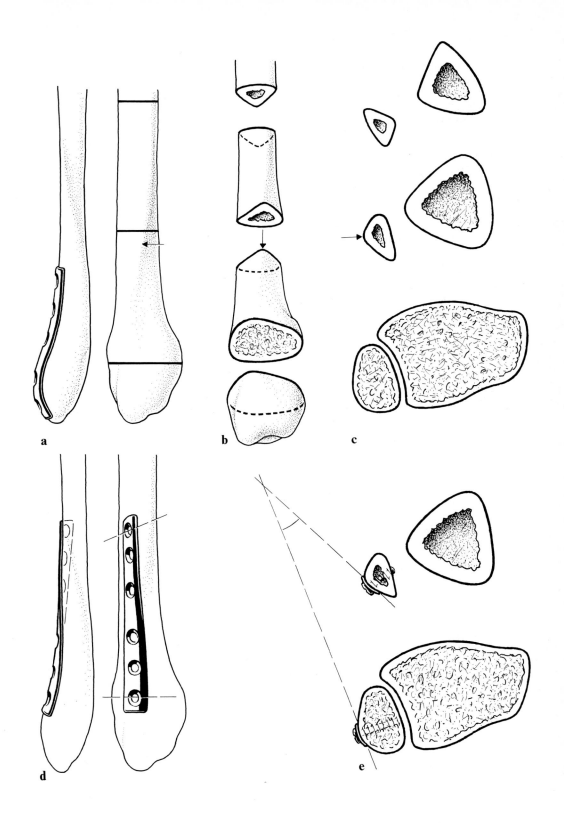

a

b

c

d

e

287

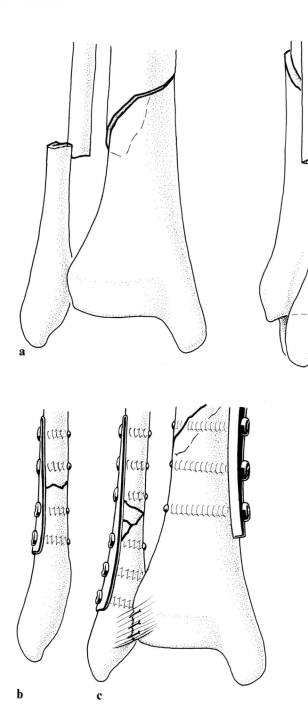

Fig. 162 a–c. Associated fracture of the lower fibula with fracture of the lower leg

a Persistent displacement of the lower fibula in internal fixation of the tibia. It disturbs the physiology of the ankle mortice and is usually combined with a rupture of the anterior tibiofibular ligament

b Internal fixation of a transverse fracture: Open reduction through a separate incision and fixation with a short one-third tubular plate

c In a complex fracture with rupture of the tibiofibular ligament: a long one-third tubular plate is used and the ligaments are sutured

Fig. 163a–c. Internal fixation of the fibula in type C fracture

a Comminuted fracture: long one-third tubular plate and repair of the syndesmosis including the interosseous membrane

b High type C fracture: one-third tubular plate and repair of the syndesmosis or screw fixation of a small anterolateral fragment of the tibia

c In a case with a small fragment or a comminuted area: screw fixation using a spiked polyacetal resin washer

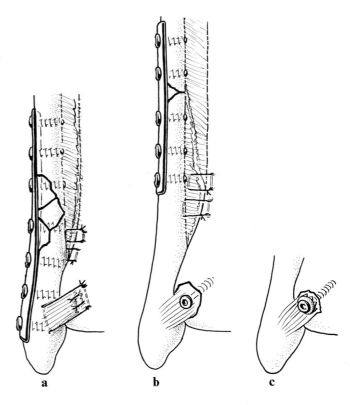

a   b   c

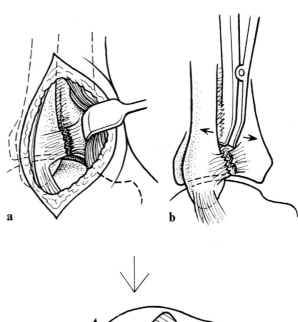

a   b

Fig. 164a–c. Checking of stability of the ankle mortice in a malleolar or Maisonneuve fracture

a Exposure of the anterior tibiofibular ligament and the distal part of the interosseous membrane by dissection of the fascia and anterior retraction of the extensor tendons

b Insertion of the spreading forceps between the tibia and the fibula: the fibular mortice, the posterior tibiofibular ligament or a posterolateral fragment of the tibial margin may be exposed

c The pathological movements of the fibula are demonstrated in a case of rupture of the tibiofibular ligaments and the interosseous membrane, in a cross-section superposing different levels: diastasis between the tibia and the fibula, anterior drawer movement which is limited by anterior margin of the fibular notch, posterior drawer movement (large arrow)

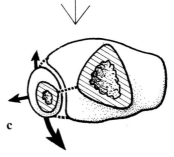

c

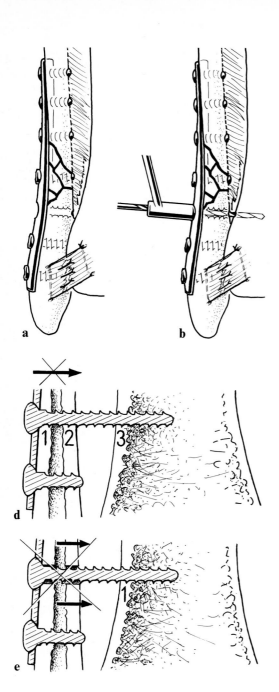

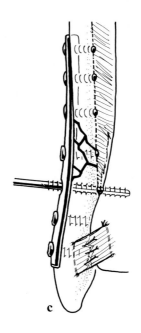

Fig. 165a–e. Transfixion of the fibula and tibia

Carried out in a case of persistent instability of the joint after completion of internal fixation and repair of the ligaments

Principle of stabilization without compression

a Removal of one plate screw 3–4 cm above the ankle joint

b Drill hole in the fibula is extended to the lateral tibial cortex with a 2.0-mm drill bit. The thread is preserved in the fibula

c The thread is tapped in the lateral tibial cortex

Cross-section in the frontal plane

d Since the transfixion screw is anchored in three cortices (1–2–3), compression is avoided

e Incorrect procedure: If the hole in the fibula is converted into a gliding hole, the transfixing screw is anchored in only one layer of cortical bone, that is the lateral tibia, and this results in compression between the tibia and fibula if the screw is tightened

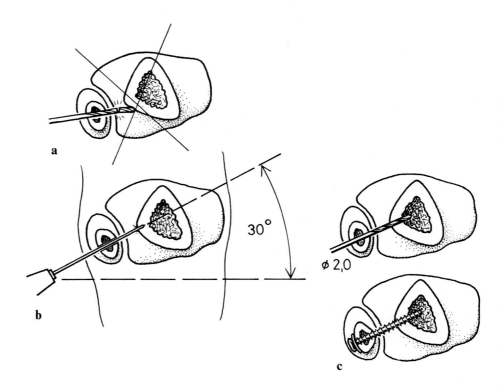

Fig. 166a–c. The procedure in the cross-section

a The drill hole is made in the fibula at an angle of 30° from the laterodorsal aspect to the medial side. The 2.0-mm drill bit is used. Direct drilling to the tibial cortex increases the danger of the drill bit slipping away and breaking at the posterior aspect of the tibia

b Recommended procedure: a pointed 1.8-mm Kirschner wire is introduced through the fibular

hole and drilled into the tibia as a pathfinder for the 2.0-mm drill bit. This prevents it slipping away to the dorsal side

c The 2.0-mm drill bit is introduced into the hole which was prepared by the Kirschner wire in the lateral tibial cortex and then the screw is placed according to the above technique (three cortices)

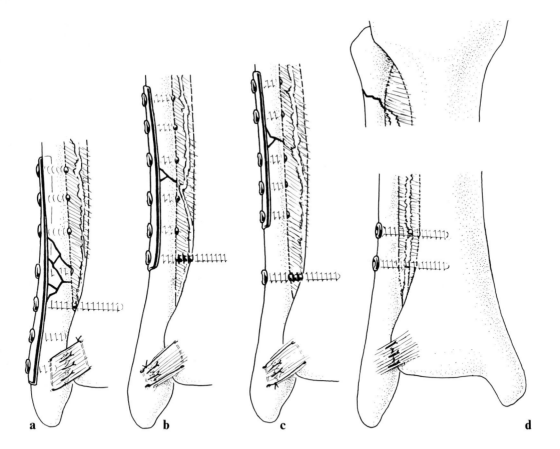

Fig. 167a–d. Different types of transfixation

a Supramalleolar comminuted fractures: transfixation by the lowest plate screw but two

b High fracture of the fibula: transfixation via the lower end of the plate

c Transfixion with a screw inserted independently from the plate when the latter is placed at a higher level

d Positioning screws in a Maisonneuve's fracture. The fibula is reduced into the fibular notch of the tibia and temporarily fixed with Kirschner wires. The anterior tibiofibular ligament is sutured. Two parallel 3.5-mm screws are usually inserted for better stability. They bite in three cortices each

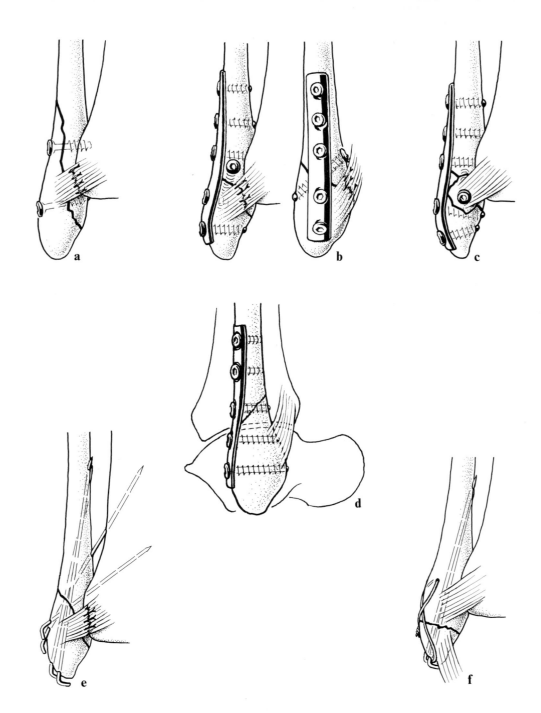

Fig. 168a–f. Internal fixation of the fibula in type A and B fractures

a Screw fixation of a long spiral or oblique type B fracture and repair of the anterior syndesmosis

b Screw fixation and neutralization plate placed on the lateral aspect, as well as suture of the ligaments

c Neutralization plate and screw fixation of an avulsion fracture of the anterior fibular cortex at the insertion of the anterior tibiofibular ligament

d Dorsal position of the plate with central lag screw in an oblique fracture

e Procedure in a case of severe osteoporosis: stabilization by multiple Kirschner wires and oblique transfixation may be combined with a tension-band wire loop

f Tension-band wiring of a type A fracture

Fig. 169 a–g. The technique of ligament repair in the ankle

a Usual adapting suture of a rupture of the substance of the ligament

b Ideal solution from the mechanical standpoint: reinsertion of a bony avulsion of the ligament with a screw and a spiked polyacetal resin washer

c Preparing oblique drill holes for an intraosseous suture with the 3.5-mm drill bit and drill sleeve

d Repair of the deltoid ligament: a supporting suture is placed in the anterior part of the ligament and anchored within the bone at one side. The remaining tear is adapted with conventional sutures

e Supporting sutures passed through the bone at one side (anterior tibiofibular ligament and anterior fibulo-talar ligament). Conventional suture of the remaining tear

f Mattress suture, which is passed through the bone on both sides

g Anchoring the supporting, transosseous sutures round the implant used for internal fixation of the distal fibula

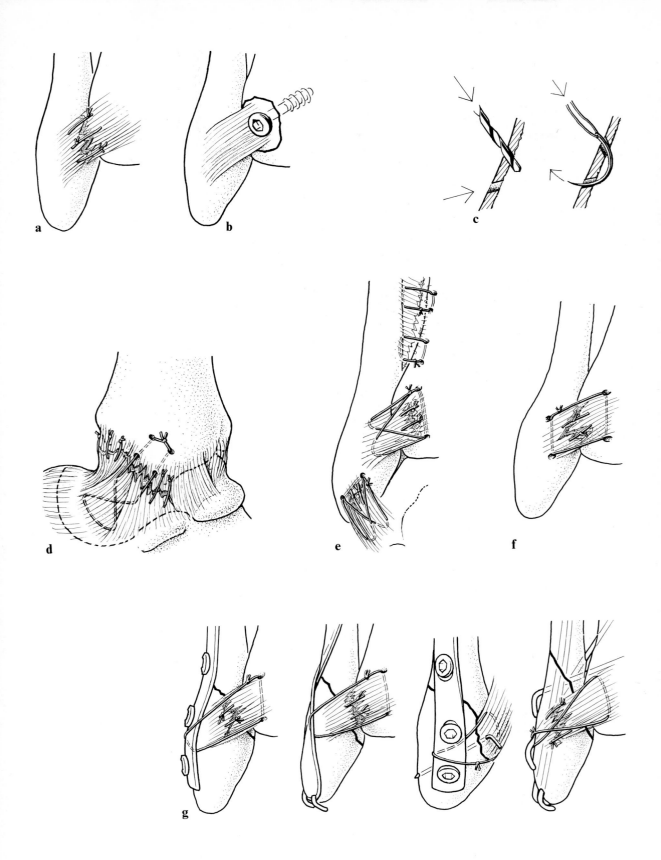

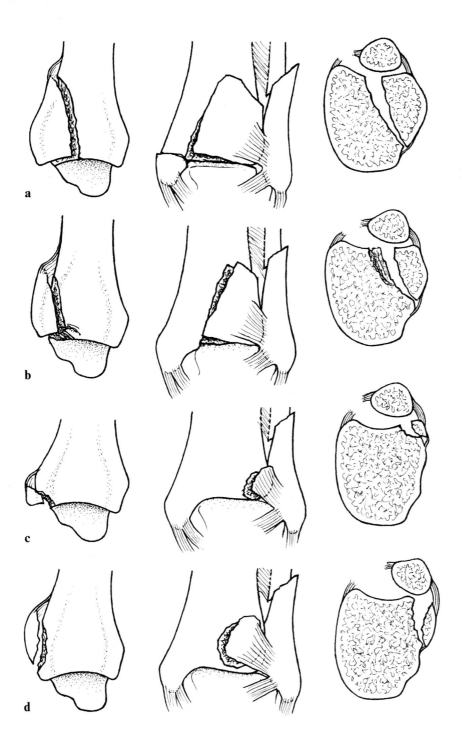

Fig. 170 a–d. Posterolateral triangle of the tibia (Volkmann): classification

a Large posterolateral triangle involving a large part of the articular surface of the tibia

b A small triangle with impaction of the anterior articular surface of the tibia

c A small posterior triangle with only slight involvement of the tibial articular surface

d Avulsion fracture of the insertion of the posterior tibiofibular ligament without involvement of the tibial joint surface

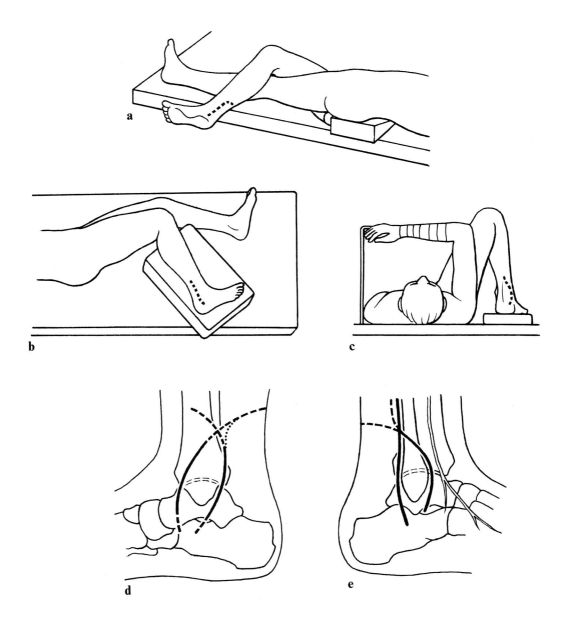

Fig. 171a–e. Positioning and incisions for simultaneous internal fixation of the malleoli and a posterolateral triangle

a Change of position from initial supine position for approach from the mediodorsal side: a sandbag is placed under the opposite buttock and the lower leg is flexed at the knee and crossed over

b Lateral position with the knee flexed for the dorsolateral approach of the lower fibula and the posterolateral triangle. Internal fixation of the medial malleolus is not possible in this position

c Position of the lower leg for dorsolateral approach to the posterolateral triangle. Note the position of the ipsilateral arm

d Typical incisions for the internal fixation of the medial malleolus and the possibilities for extension to expose the posterolateral triangle from the medial side

e Typical incisions for the internal fixation of the lateral malleolus and the extensions to expose the posterolateral triangle from the dorsolateral side

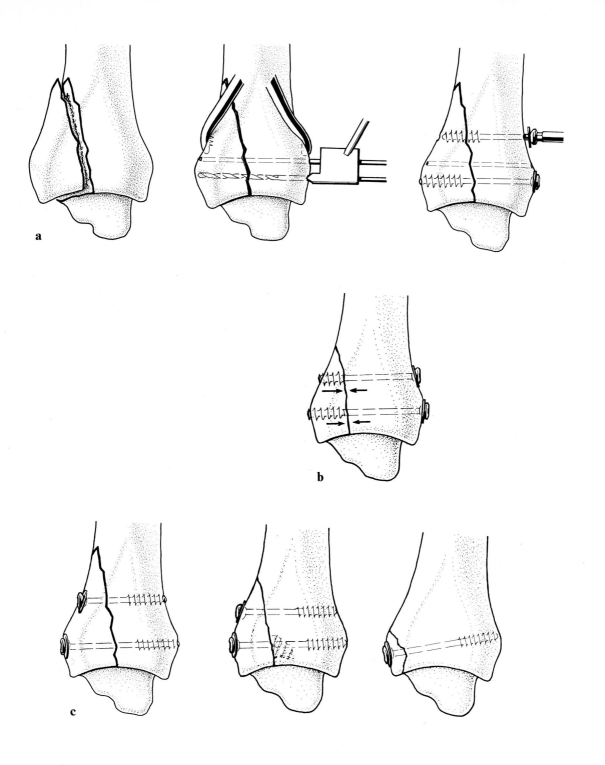

Fig. 172 a–c. The principles of internal fixation of the posterolateral triangle (Volkmann)

a Indirect screw fixation from the front: the reduction is temporarily fixed with a reduction forceps and a guiding Kirschner wire. Drilling through the triple drill guide

b Indirect screw fixation of a small posterolateral triangle: the threads of the screws have been shortened with the cutting forceps

c Direct screw fixation from the back

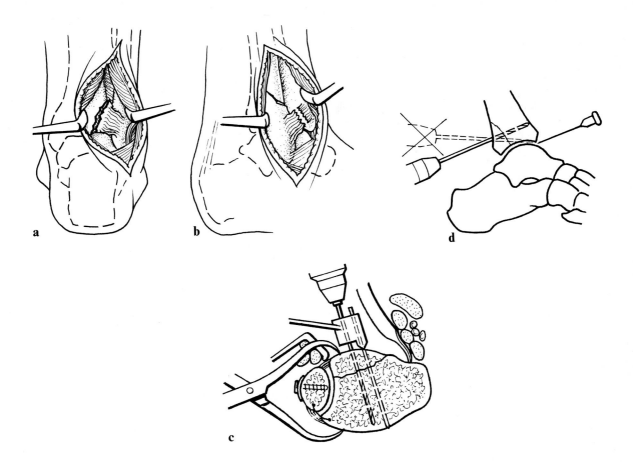

Fig. 173a–f. Direct screw fixation of a posterolateral triangle through the dorsolateral approach

a Exposure of the posterolateral triangle by lateral retraction of the peroneus tendons

b Exposure of the fracture of the fibula and the rupture of the anterior tibiofibular ligament

c Cross-section of screw fixation: fixation of the triangle with reduction forceps. Lateral retraction of the peroneus tendons. The Achilles' and the flexor tendons are retracted medially with a Hohmann retractor. Temporary fixation with a Kirschner wire. Drilling with a 2.0-mm bit through the triple drill guide

d Correct and incorrect position of the drill bit. To avoid the ankle joint, drilling must be done from the dorsal-distal to the ventral-proximal aspect. The joint space is marked by a hypodermic needle, which is inserted from the ventral side

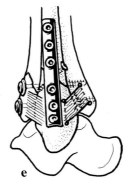

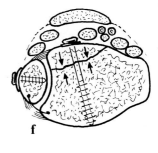

e Lateral view of the completed repair: lag screw and neutralization plate for the fibular fracture, transosseous mattress suture of the anterior tibiofibular ligament, direct screw fixation of the posterolateral triangle

f The completed repair in cross-section

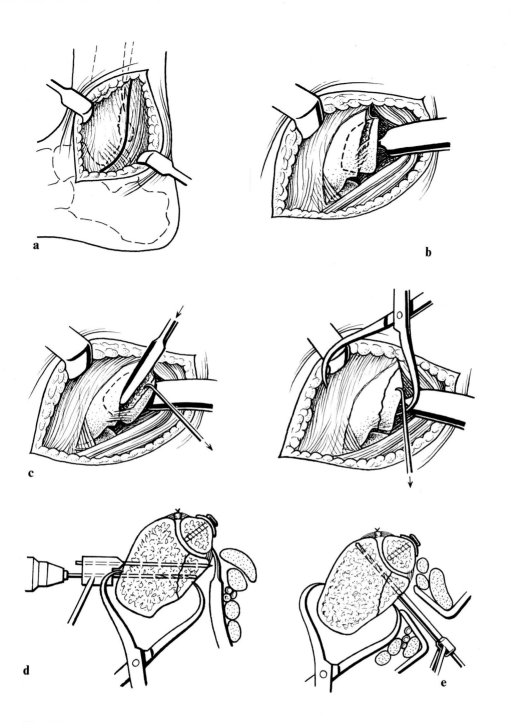

Fig. 174a–e. Screw fixation of the posterolateral tibial triangle by the mediodorsal approach

a Incision of the tibialis posterior sheath

b Dorsal retraction with Hohmann retractor of the tibialis and the flexor tendons as well as of the neurovascular bundle. Exposure of the triangle

c Reduction of a depressed articular fragment with an elevator. The triangle is then pulled distally with the help of a hook. Provisional fixation with reduction forceps

d Cross-section: Indirect screw fixation guided by a Kirschner wire and the triple drill guide from the anteromedial aspect

e Second procedure: Direct screw fixation. Positioning and incision according to Fig. 171a. Reduction according to a–d. The screw is inserted between the Achilles' and the flexor tendons or the neurovascular bundle

Fig. 175a–c. Repair of the dislocation of the peroneal tendons

a Classification of the primary dislocation: rupture of the retinacular ligament at the tip of the fibula, avulsion of the periosteum with the ligament intact, avulsion fracture from the fibula

b Fixation of the retinacular ligament or an avulsed fragment with a small cortex screw and spiked polyacetal resin washer

c Dorsoventral osteotomy of the fibula to produce a gutter (Kelly's operation). Fixation of the disc with two small cancellous screws

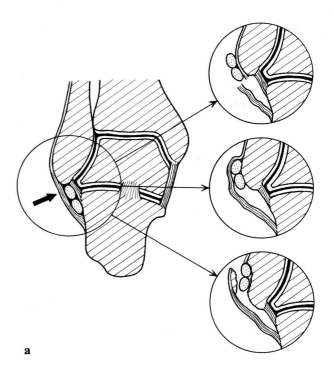

a

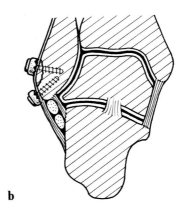

b

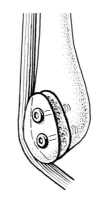

c

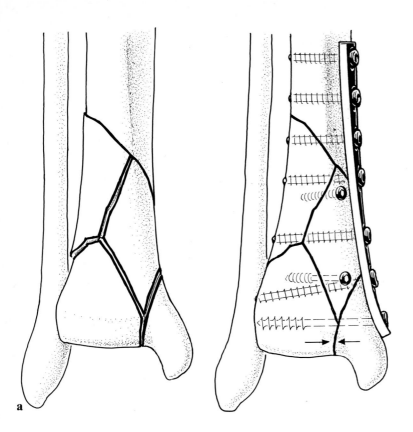

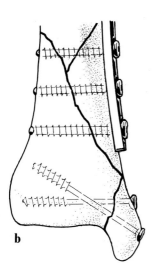

Fig. 176a, b. Internal fixation of a fracture of the medial malleolus combined with a fracture of the tibial shaft

a The DCP, fixed with 4.5-mm cortex screws and a 6.5-mm cancellous screw, holds the articular fragment as well. The fracture line of the medial malleolus is compressed by the distal cancellous screw, which is inserted parallel to the joint

b The main fracture of the tibial shaft and the distal malleolar fracture are stabilized independently (small cancellous screws in the malleolar fracture)

Fig. 177a–e. Various methods of internal fixation of the medial malleolus

a Screw fixation of a large anterior fragment

b Multiple fragments are reduced by screws and Kirschner wires

c Reduction of comminuted fracture by tension-band wiring

d Tension-band wiring in a small avulsed fragment

e Screw fixation of a posteromedial fragment. Screws are inserted between the grooves for the tibialis posterior and the toe flexors

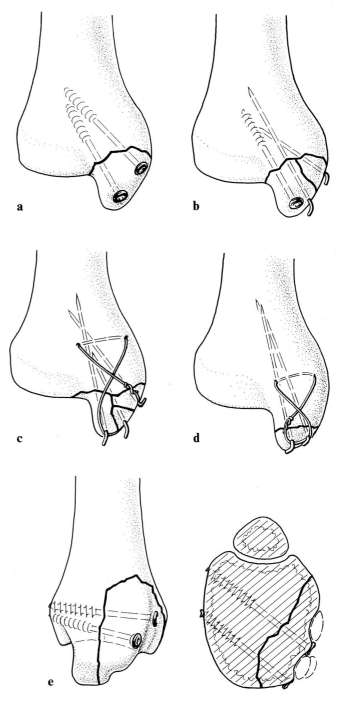

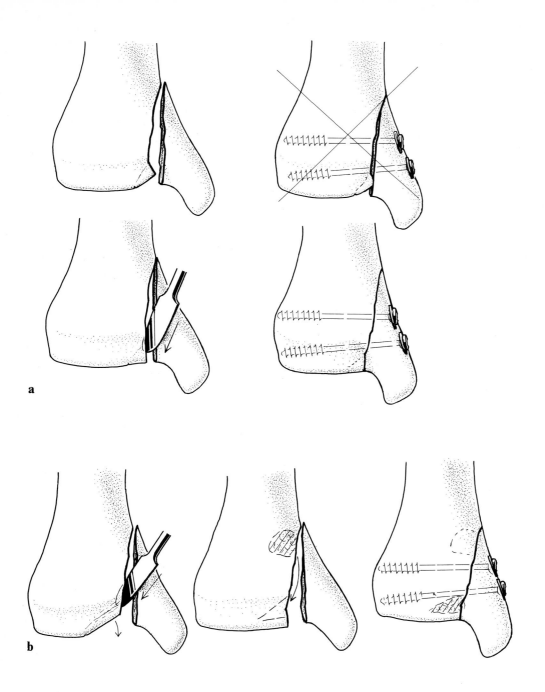

Fig. 178a, b. Adduction fractures

a The small impacted area at the medial articular border of the tibia impedes exact reduction. The impacted area must be lifted up with an elevator

b In the presence of larger impacted areas, the defect is filled with cancellous bone taken from the adjoining tibial epiphysis

Fig. 179 a, b. Internal fixation of fractures of the talus

a Screw fixation of peripheral fractures of the talus: Shearing off of an articular fragment and avulsion fracture of the lateral process with its ligamentous insertions

b Screw fixation from the anteromedial side of a fracture of the neck of the talus. A bony defect must be filled with an autogenous cancellous bone graft

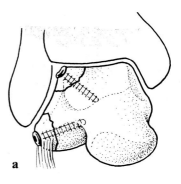

a

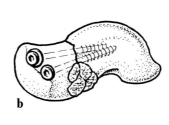

b

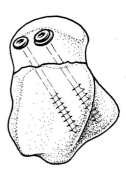

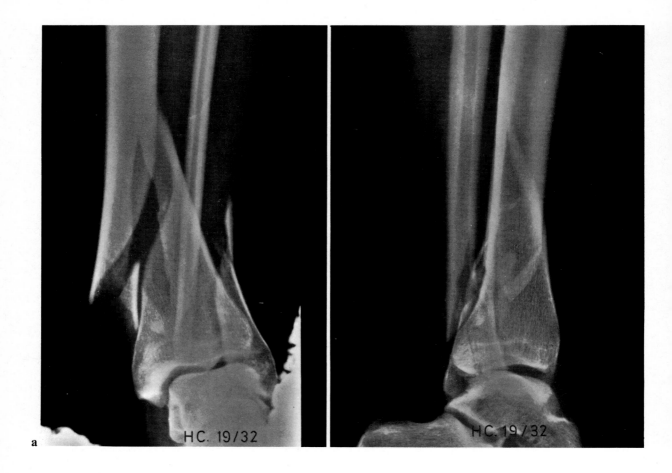

a   HC. 19/32   HC. 19/32

Fig. 180a–c. Clinical example: Additional internal fixation of the fibula in a fracture of the lower leg, screw fixation of small fragments of the tibia with small cortex screws

B., Christiane, 45-year-old housewife who had a skiing accident

a Grossly displaced fracture of the lower leg with wedge fragments of the tibia and fibula

b Internal fixation as an emergency procedure: Fixation of the tibia with a DCP reaching close to the ankle joint. The dorsal wedge-shaped fragment is fixed by a 3.5-mm cortex screw. The fibula remains unstable within the mortice. Therefore the

fibula is fixed using a one-third tubular plate with six holes and two separate 3.5-mm lag screws. Uneventful course with functional treatment. Full weight bearing after 4 months

c Review and removal of the implants at 14 months. No pain, full range of movements, slight atrophy of the muscles, primary healing of the fractures

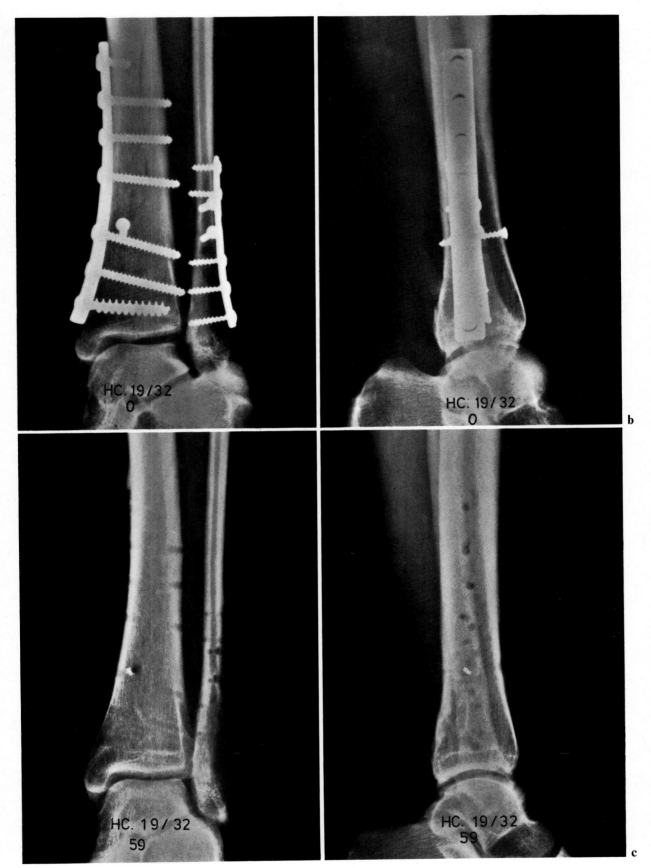

HC. 19 / 32
O

HC: 19 / 32
O

HC. 19 / 32
59

HC. 19 / 32
59

b

c

307

Fig. 181a–e. Clinical example: High type C fracture of the fibula with posterolateral tibial triangle of Volkmann. Internal fixation with a plate, indirect screw fixation of the triangle by anteromedial approach

H., Betty, 68-year-old housewife who had a fall on a staircase

a A high type C fibular fracture. Large posterolateral triangle of Volkmann. Rupture of the anterior tibiofibular ligament. Oblique fracture of the medial malleolus

b Emergency operation: Fixation of the fibula using a one-third tubular plate with six holes. Suture of the ruptured ligament. Fixation of the medial malleolus with two small cancellous screws. Indirect fixation of the posterolateral triangle with two small cancellous screws from the front.
Uncomplicated postoperative course. Mobilization but protection with a removable plaster splint. At discharge a plaster cast is worn for 10 weeks, then a walking cast, followed by free mobilization. At 12 weeks full weight bearing

c–e see page 310f

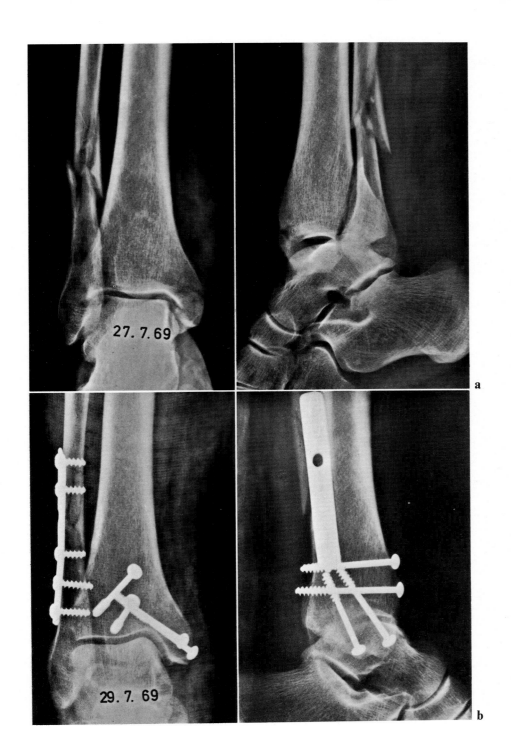

27. 7. 69

29. 7. 69

a

b

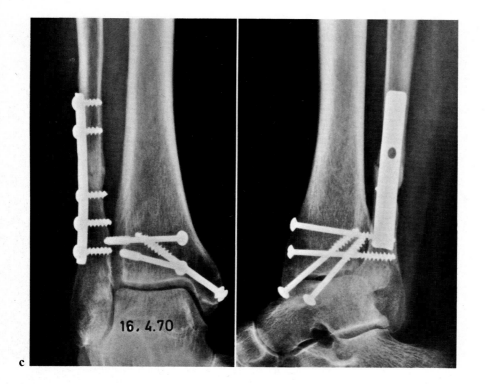

c

Fig. 181 c–e.

c Review and removal of the metal at 9 months. A zone of instability at the fibula is missed

d Review after 1¹/₂ years. The patient is pain-free and has full function of the joint. There is callus formation at the fibular fracture with slight short-

ening, causing slight arthrotic signs at the syndesmosis

e Review at 11 years. No disturbance; the ankle is somewhat thickened, but has full function. There is no atrophy of muscles. In the X-ray no progression of arthrosis during the last 8 years

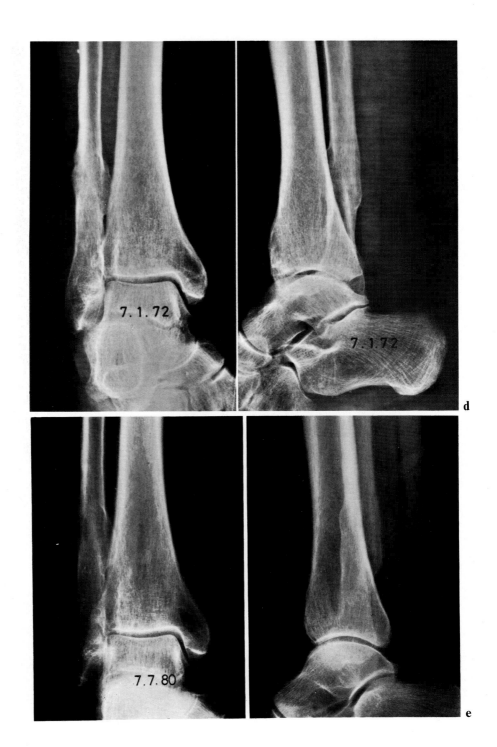

7. 1. 72

7. 1. 72

7.7.80

d

e

311

Fig. 182 a–d. Clinical example: Malleolar type C fracture with tibiofibular transfixion

K., Lotti, 37-year-old housewife who had a skiing accident

a Spiral type C fracture of the fibula with a small posterolateral tibial triangle of Volkmann and rupture of the medial ligaments

b Internal fixation the same day. On the lateral side the main fragments have been fixed by lag screws and a neutralization plate with five holes has been added. Repair of the anterior tibio-fibular ligament. Since instability of the fibula persisted, the second plate screw from above was replaced by a long transfixing screw. The threads within the fibula have been preserved.

At the medial side the deltoid ligament avulsed from the tibia was repaired.

Uneventful course. Immediate mobilization but protection by a removable plaster splint. Discharge with a plaster cast left in place for 10 weeks. Full weight bearing after 12 weeks

c, d. see page 314f

312

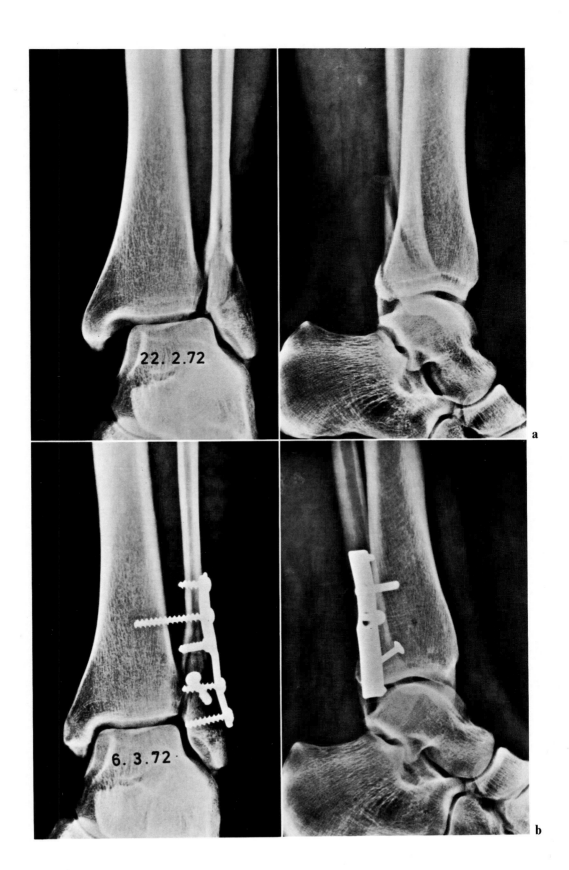

22. 2.72

6. 3.72

Fig. 182c, d

c Review and removal of the implants after 33 weeks: no pain, full range of movements, no atrophy of the muscles. The fracture is healed and there is no arthrosis

d Review after 8 years: the patient is free of pain and has no arthrosis

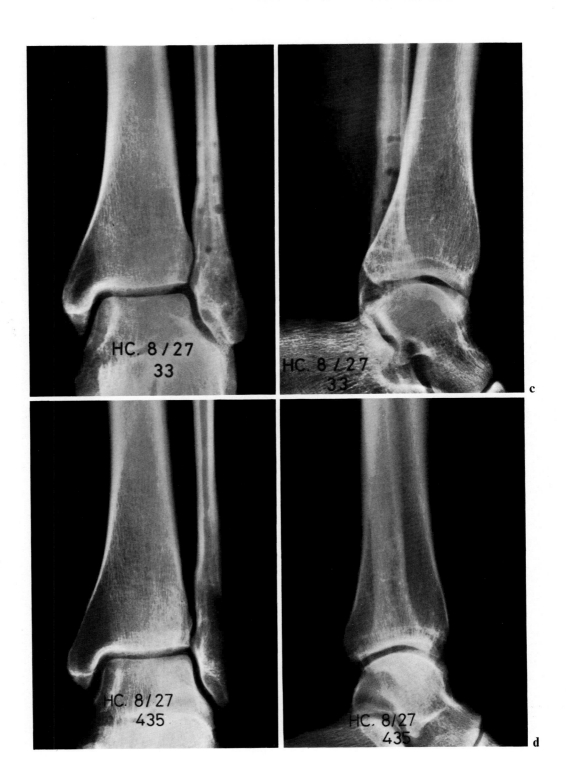

HC. 8 / 27
33

HC. 8 / 27
33

c

HC. 8 / 27
435

HC. 8/27
435

d

315

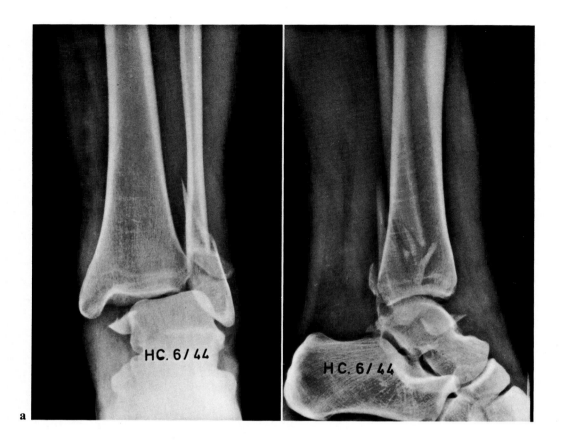

a

Fig. 183 a–c. Clinical example: Malleolar type C fracture with a small medial avulsion fracture, plate and tension-band wire fixation

H., Heidi, 18-year-old apprentice who had a skiing accident

a Comminuted type C fracture of the fibula. Small avulsion fracture at the medial malleolus. Small posterolateral triangle of Volkmann

b Emergency internal fixation: Lag screw fixation of the wedge-shaped fragment of the fibula, one-third tubular plate with six holes for neutralization. Repair of the anterior tibiofibular ligament. At the medial side the fragment is fixed with two Kirschner wires and a figure-of-eight tension-band wire. Suture of the joint capsule.

No postoperative complications. The joint is mobilized out of a protecting splint. A plaster cast is applied on discharge for 10 weeks. Implants are removed elsewhere after 8 months

c Review after $8^{1}/_{2}$ years: The patient is symptom-free, has a full range of movements and no atrophy of the muscles. The X-ray demonstrates slight irregularity of the bone structure of the tibia in the area of the syndesmosis

316

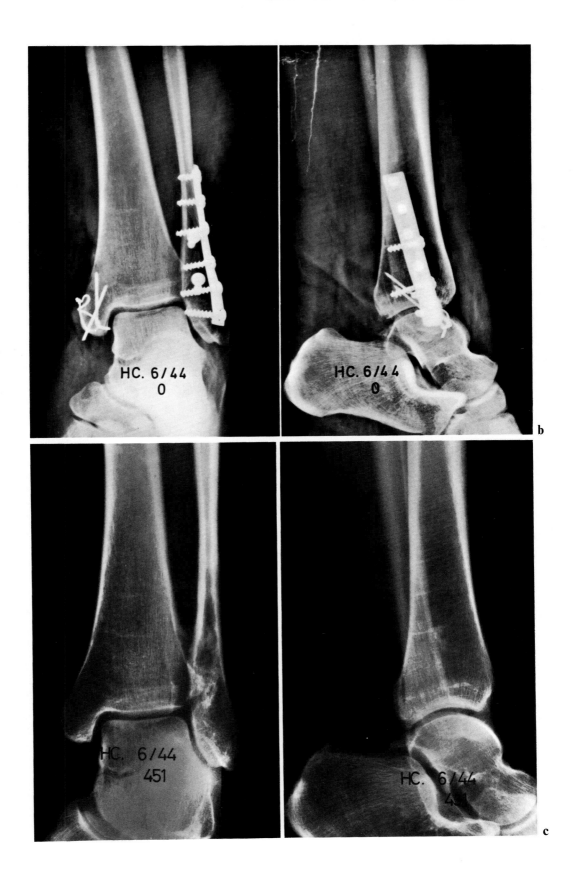

HC. 6/44
0

HC. 6/44
0

b

HC. 6/44
451

HC. 6/44
451

c

317

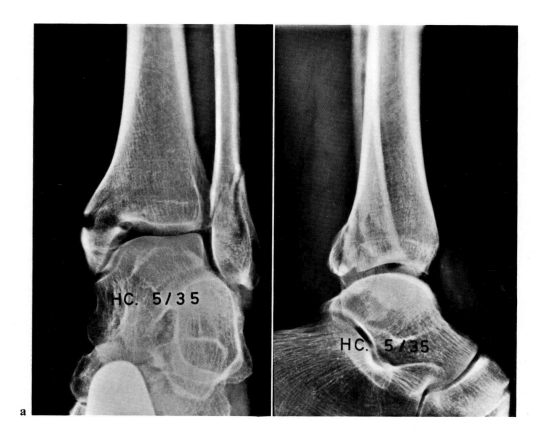

a

Fig. 184a–c. Clinical example: Bimalleolar type B fracture with a medial comminuted area

W., Ilse, a 51-year-old school teacher who had a skiing accident

a Oblique type B fracture of the fibula. Comminuted fracture of the medial malleolus with a dorsal extension

b Emergency internal fixation. At the lateral side, lag screw fixation of the fibula together with a neutralization plate. Repair of the syndesmosis by suture of a small avulsed fragment with a flexible wire. At the medial side a combination of screws, Kirschner wires and tension-band wire was used.

Uneventful postoperative course. Plaster cast. The implants have been removed after one year in a foreign country

c Review after 9¹/₂ years: The patient is pain-free and fit for sport. The movement of the subtalar joint is slightly limited. There is no atrophy of the muscles. One of the medial Kirschner wires was left behind, there is no arthrosis

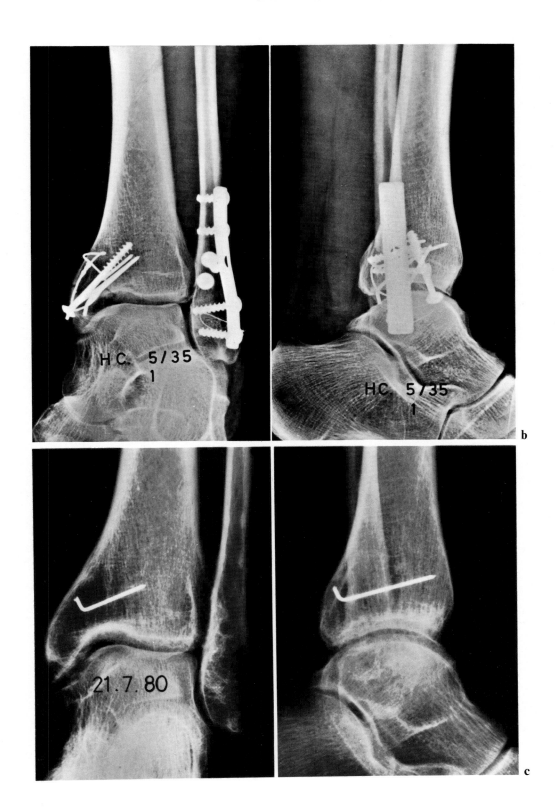

Fig. 185 a–c. Clinical example: Adduction fracture with impaction of the joint surface

K., Brigitte, a 28-year-old housewife who had a skiing accident

a Adduction fracture of the medial malleolus with an articular fragment impacted upwards and an undisplaced type A avulsion fracture of the lateral malleolus

b Emergency internal fixation: Medially the joint surface is reconstructed by reduction of the impacted fragment. Fixation by combining screws and Kirschner wires. Laterally a simple Kirschner wire is inserted as stability has been restored by the medial internal fixation.
Uncomplicated course. A primary plaster slab was replaced later by a plaster cast. Full weight bearing at 12 weeks

c Review and removal of metal after 8 months: No symptoms, full mobility, normal appearance of the articular surface.
The patient 9 years later had no symptoms and full range of movements

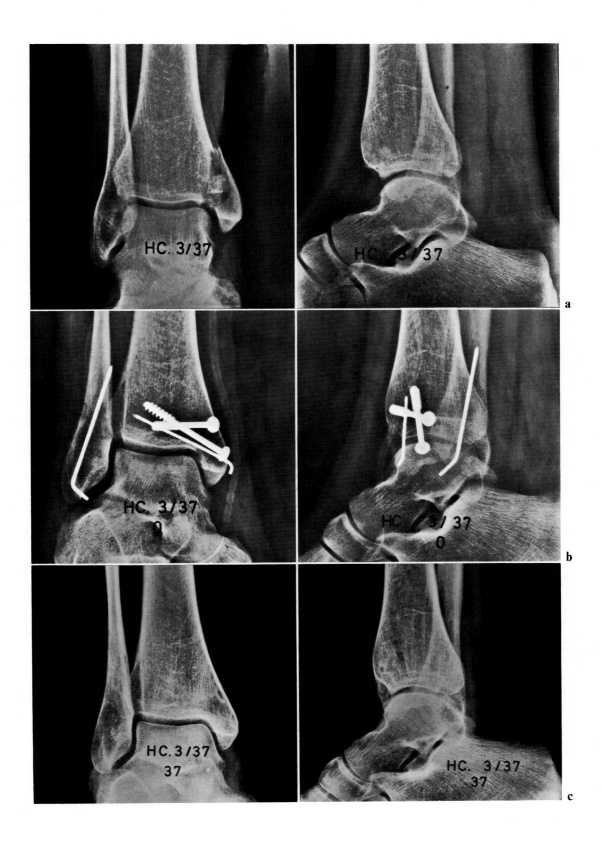

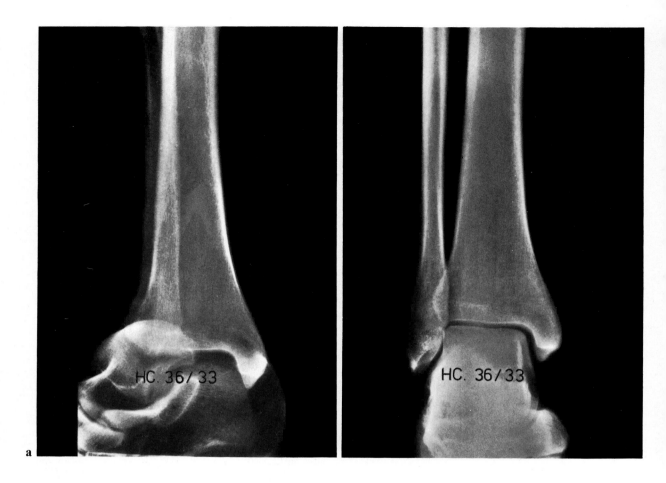

HC. 36/33

HC. 36/33

a

Fig. 186a–c. Clinical example: Fixation of a Maisonneuve fracture with 3.5-mm cortex screws

R., Edith, a 34-year-old housewife who had a skiing accident

a Fracture-dislocation of the ankle joint of the Maisonneuve type with rupture of the deltoid ligament. Spiral fracture of the fibula at the upper end of the shaft. After the immediate reduction of the dislocation no pathology was seen in the joint

b Operation as an emergency: Rupture of the tibiofibular ligaments as well as the anterior and posterior fibulotalar ligaments. Repair of the ligaments medially and laterally. Reduction of the fibula into the mortice. Indirect stabilization by two transfixion screws inserted transversely above the syndesmosis and each gripping three cortices.

No postoperative complications. After initial mobilization a plaster cast was applied for 6 weeks. Full weight bearing after 12 weeks. The implants have been removed elsewhere

c Review at $3^1/_2$ years: the patient is free of symptoms, she is skiing and playing tennis and her ankle moves fully. There is a slight limitation of subtalar joint movement but no atrophy of the muslces. The X-ray shows a regular joint surface without arthrosis. A small osteophyte can be seen at the anterior margin of the tibia

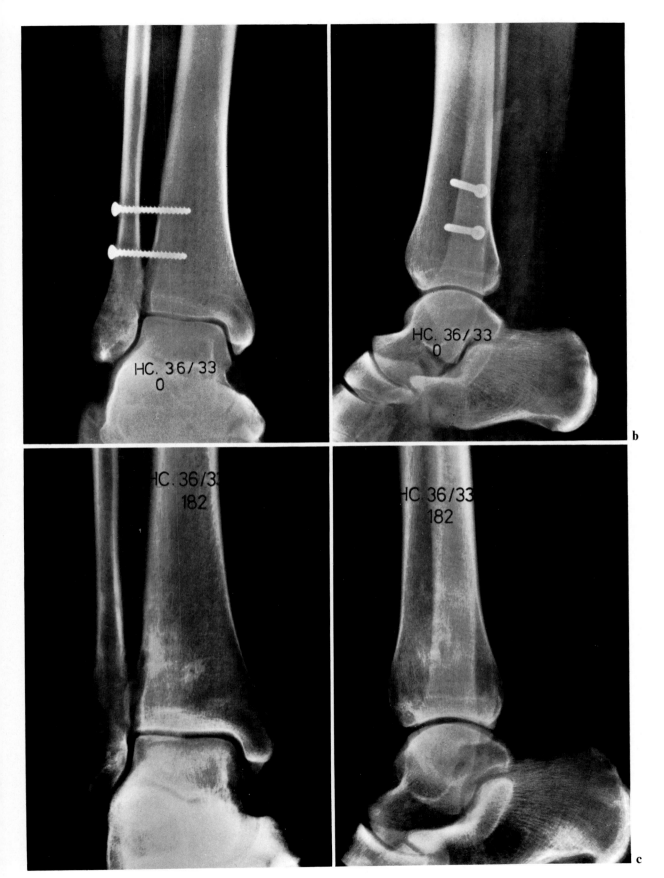

HC. 36/33
0

HC. 36/33
0

b

HC. 36/33
182

HC. 36/33
182

c

323

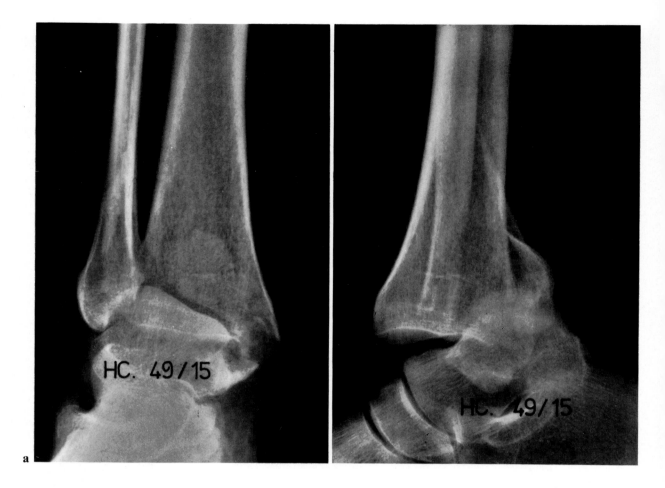

Fig. 187a–c. Clinical example: Direct screw fixation from the dorsolateral aspect of a small posterolateral triangle of Volkmann in a trimalleolar fracture

Sch., Paulina, a 58-year-old nun who was rather unathletic, fell on a walking tour in the mountains. She had mild diabetes

a Trimalleolar fracture-dislocation of the right ankle type B with a small posterolateral Volkmann triangle

b Emergency internal fixation: fixation of the fibula with an oblique lag screw and a one-third tubular plate with six holes for neutralization. Transosseous suture of the anterior tibiofibular ligament. The lateral incision was extended in a proximodorsal direction for internal fixation of the posterolateral triangle with two small cancellous screws

and washers. The medial malleolus was fixed with a small cancellous screw and a Kirschner wire.

Wound healing was uncomplicated. After initial active exercises, a plaster cast was applied for 6 weeks, followed by mobilization without weight bearing. From the 10th week she was treated in the walking pool and weight bearing was started at 12 weeks. Recovery was disturbed by some trophic disorders

c Review and removal of the implants at 10 months: The movements of the ankle and subtalar joints are slightly limited but osteoporosis is diminishing

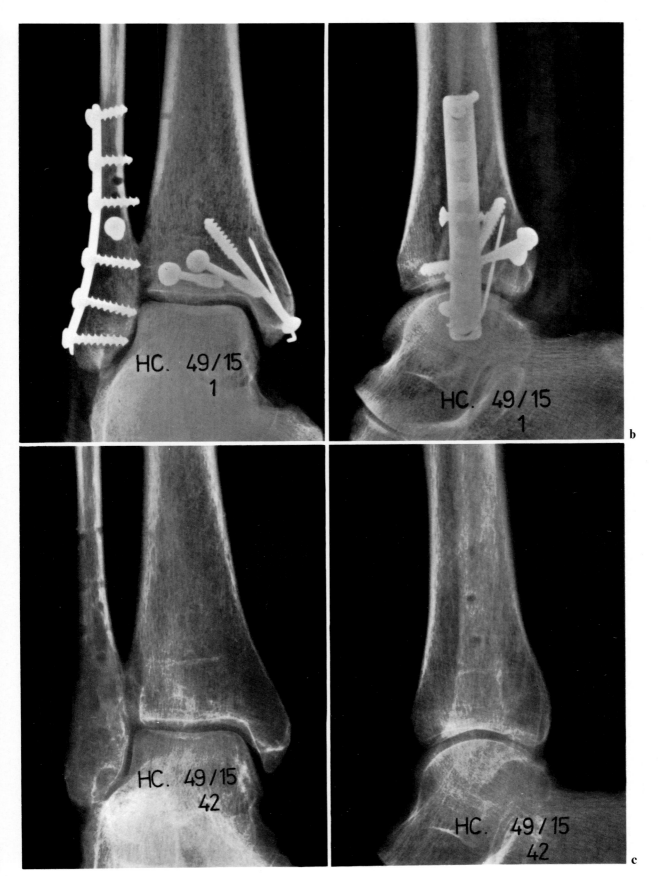

HC. 49/15
1

HC. 49/15
1

b

HC. 49/15
42

HC. 49/15
42

c

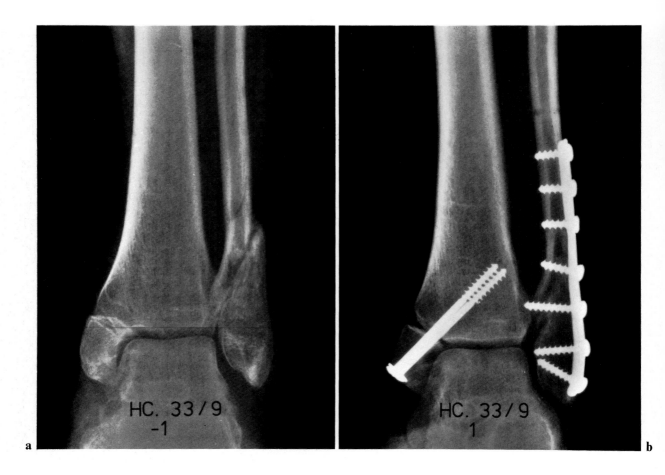

a

HC. 33/9
-1

HC. 33/9
1

b

Fig. 188a–f. Clinical example: Non-union of the malleoli

C., Nesa, a 48-year-old housewife who was hit by a car from behind. She suffered a bimalleolar fracture and a wound on the back of the lower leg. She was treated elsewhere with a plaster cast for 8 weeks

a Four months after the accident: non-union of the lateral malleolus with shortening of 6 mm and non-union of the medial malleolus with corresponding valgus deformity

b Internal fixation at 4 months. Lengthening of the fibula and internal fixation using a one-third tubular plate with seven holes. Fixation of the medial malleolus with two small cancellous screws and washers.
No postoperative complications. After initial active exercises a plaster cast is applied for 8 weeks

c Healing of the non-union of the fibula but persistance of the pseudarthrosis of the medial malleolus

d Reoperation 16 months after injury. Removal of the metal from the lateral side. One of the small cancellous screws in the medial malleolus is replaced by a large 6.5-mm cancellous screw and a washer

e Healing of the medial pseudarthrosis

f Review 4 years after injury: The patient is slightly disturbed by the screwhead at the medial malleolus. There is wasting of the calf muscles of 0.5 cm. Full range of movements. Some thickening of the ankle, no arthrosis. The patient is anxious about removal of the screws

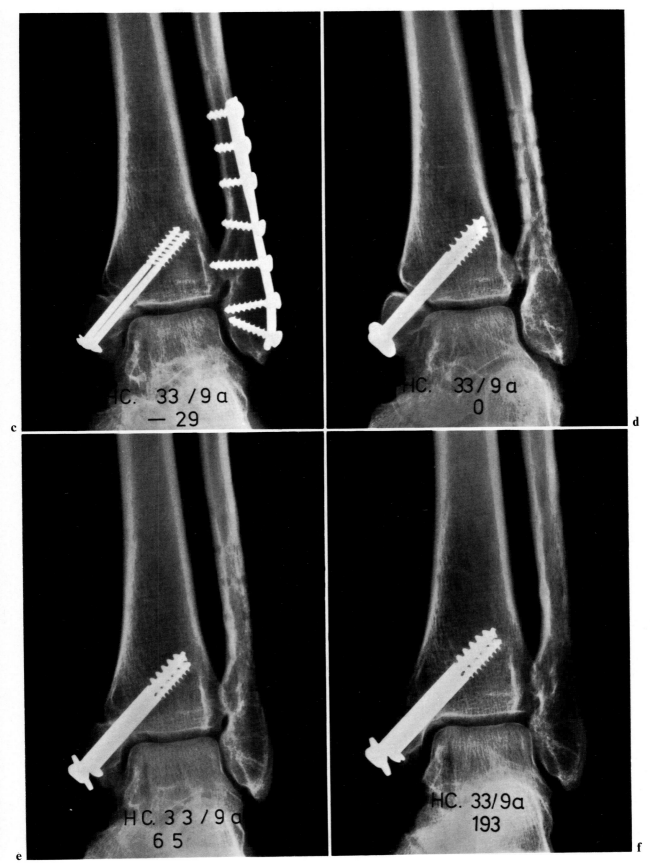

c

H.C.   33 / 9 a
— 29

d

H.C.   33 / 9 a
0

e

H.C. 3 3 / 9 a
6 5

f

H.C. 33/9 a
193

327

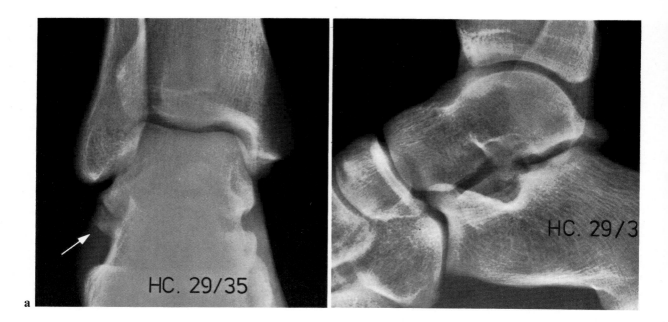

Fig. 189 a–c. Clinical example: Avulsion fracture of the lateral process of the talus

C., Silvio, a 21-year-old draughtsman who had a skiing accident. There was tenderness and swelling distal to the lateral malleolus

a The avulsion fracture of the lateral process of the talus is hardly seen (arrow). It indicates a rupture of the lateral ligaments

c Emergency internal fixation. Evacuation of the haemarthrosis. Reduction of the fragment and fixation by a 2.0-mm screw and an improvised washer. Repair of the ligaments.

Uncomplicated course. Discharge with a protective plaster slab. Weight bearing after 10 weeks. Removal of the screw at 9 months

c Review at $4^{1}/_{2}$ years after injury: the patient is symptom free, has full function and no atrophy of the muscles. The X-ray shows no arthrosis, but a little calcification at the back of the talus

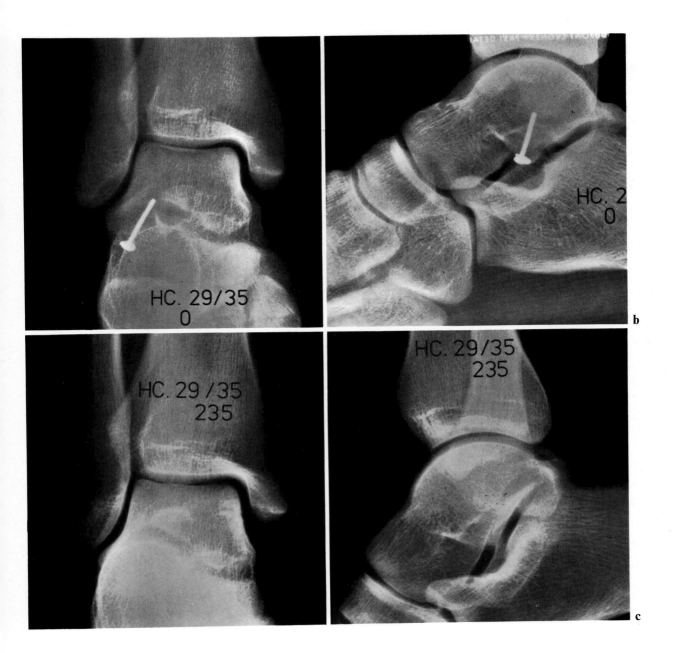

Fig. 190 a–c. Clinical example: Screw fixation of a fracture-dislocation of the talus

Sp., Daniel, an 18-year-old apprentice who had a fall while skiing

a Fracture-dislocation of the neck of the talus. Closed reduction is impossible

b Emergency internal fixation via a medial approach. Accurate open reduction, temporary fixation by two Kirschner wires and replacement of one of them by a small cancellous screw for interfragmentary compression, the second wire being left behind.
Uneventful course. Plaster cast for 4 weeks followed by a walking caliper for 12 months

c Review after $9^1/_2$ years: symptom-free, no muscular atrophy, normal radiologically

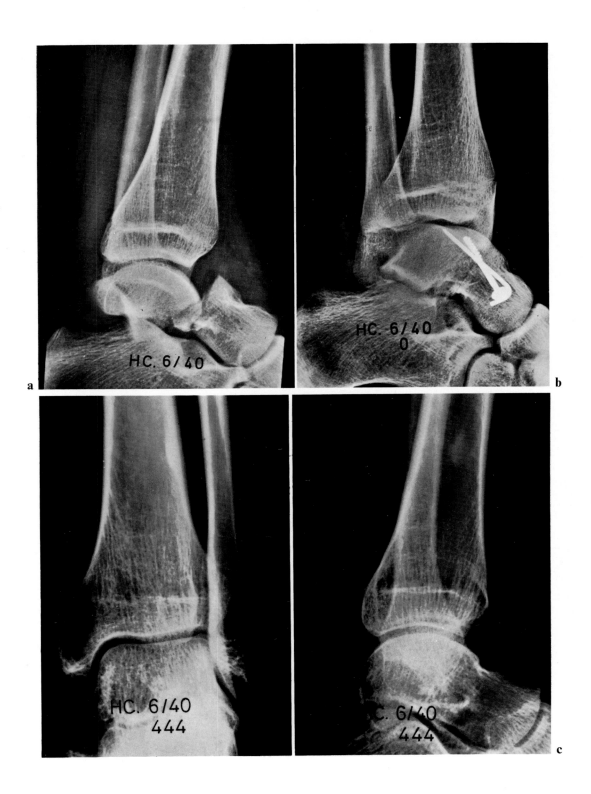

a

b

HC. 6/40

HC. 6/40
0

HC. 6/40
444

C. 6/40
444

c

XVII. The Foot

1. Calcaneum

Avulsion fractures of the anterior process of the calcaneum, where the fibulocalcaneal and interosseous ligaments are inserted, are treated by screw fixation.

The rare "duck beak" fractures, which are avulsion fractures of the Achilles tendon at the tuberosity of the calcaneum, are fixed by tension wires, usually in combination with Kirschner wires or cancellous screws.

For the central depressed fracture, Bezes has recently recommended internal fixation by a lateral approach. After loosening the tendon sheath of the peroneal muscles, the impaction is reduced under vision and the angle of the calcaneum restored. The resulting bone defect is filled in with cancellous bone graft. One-third tubular plates are applied, with the screws inserted into the tuberosity of the calcaneum, the reduced sustentaculum tali and the anterior aspect of the body. If necessary the plate may also be anchored to the cuboid (Fig. 191).

2. Tarsal Scaphoid

In dislocations there may be fractures of the tuberosity, which is the point of insertion of the tibialis anterior tendon. These are fixed by screws or by tension-band wiring. Displaced fractures of the body of the scaphoid are rigidly fixed with screws.

3. Cuboid

Depressed fractures of the cuboid occur in dislocations of the midtarsal joints. After re-duction, defects have to be filled in with cancellous bone graft and fixation obtained with lateral buttress plates (one-third tubular or small T-plates), which may be anchored to the calcaneum.

4. Metatarsus and Toes

a) Indications

It is widely accepted nowadays that rigid internal fixation of marginal fractures of the forefoot is more effective than traditional treatment. Its aim is the exact anatomical reconstruction of the plantar arch and particularly the functional postoperative treatment without any external support. This is the only method that can minimize trophic changes within this poorly vascularized area. Internal fixation in the metatarsus is more difficult than in the hand because implants have to be applied to the dorsum of the bone, which is not the side under tension. Sometimes plates can be placed on the lateral side of the bone; this improves their stabilizing effect but cannot achieve a real tension-band action. Early load bearing, which is the rule in the hand, must be avoided. In the presence of multiple injuries, we often find vassal fractures which require little internal fixation.

b) Approaches

Dorsolateral incisions similar to those in the hand are made for the first and fifth metatarsals and the big toe. They must never extend far enough downwards to reach the margin of the plantar surface of the foot, lest walking be interfered with or scarring lead to irritation when shoes are worn. A Z-shaped or longitudinal incision gives the best approach for fractures of the necks of the second to fourth metatarsals (Fig. 192).

c) Shaft Fractures

Fractures of the shaft of the first metatarsal occur frequently in the middle third. They are flexion fractures and stabilization is obtained with a one-third tubular plate or a small T-plate. The plate must be well contoured and because the bones are quite wide the proximal screws must be longer (Fig. 193a). Attention must be paid to small plantar wedge-shaped fragments or comminuted areas as they can delay healing. Cancellous bone grafting is often indicated (Fig. 193b).

Fractures of the proximal phalanx of the big toe are usually displaced and unstable because of the tensile force of the tendons. There is no doubt about the indication for internal fixation here and to get sufficient stability the small T or L-plates are preferred to simple screw fixation.

Displaced fractures of the terminal phalanx of the big toe are rare, but when they occur screw fixation may be indicated.

d) Joint Fractures

These must be reconstructed as exactly as possible. Avulsions of the ligaments are fixed with screws. Dislocation of the tarsometatarsal joint is treated by closed reduction and afterwards stabilized with transarticular Kirschner wires. Comminuted fractures of the tarsometatarsal and metatarsophalangeal joints of the big toe should be reduced anatomically. Defects are filled in with cancellous bone, and stabilization achieved with plates, which may sometimes be screwed to the neighbouring bone to act as a temporary arthrodesis.

e) Middle Three Metatarsals

Fractures seldom need internal fixation with plates or screws, but as the transverse arch must be maintained, exact reduction is imperative (Fig. 194). Axial medullary wiring carried out at the same time as open reduction has proved to be the best method. Thick Kirschner wires pointed at both ends are inserted from the fracture site with the help of the small chuck and passed distally through the distal fragment and the sole of the foot. The chuck is then changed to the other end, and the wire is introduced through the reduced fracture to the medullary canal of the proximal fragment, as far as the base of the metatarsal. The end of the wire at the sole is not buried below the skin but only bent. After closure of the wound the fracture is first protected by a padded plaster slab, which is later completed into a full plaster. The wires are removed after 5–6 weeks and a walking cast applied for another 2–3 weeks.

f) Fifth Metatarsal

Spiral and oblique fractures of the neck of this bone commonly occur, sometimes combined with a vassal fracture of the fourth metatarsal. Healing in this area tends to be poor for circulatory reasons and because of mechanical instability inside a plaster. Internal fixation is therefore often indicated, even in slight displacement. It is carried out with small T- or L-plates.

Apophyseal fractures of the fifth metatarsal are very common. The injury may occur in one of two ways:
– Avulsion fracture is produced by the sudden pull of the peroneus brevis muscle, which is inserted at this point. This occurs in supination trauma, and results in a small displaced fragment.
– Fracture may be produced by excessive weight bearing on the outer side of the foot in supination, or by a direct blow. Here the fracture is larger and there may be several fragments.

Conservative treatment with a plaster cast often results in pseudarthrosis. In our opinion, such fractures should be reduced by primary internal fixation. The choice of a small tension-band wire or screw fixation depends on the size of the fragment. The ligaments at the tip of the fibula must be checked before operation as they may have been ruptured in a supination injury; any ruptures should be repaired at the same time (Fig. 195).

5. Secondary Operations on the Forefoot

a) Pseudarthrosis

Delayed union and real pseudarthrosis are fairly common in the forefoot. They usually occur in the weight-bearing areas such as the proximal phalanx of the big toe and the fifth metatarsal. Because of the poor circulation in this area, metal fixation alone is insufficient and a cancellous bone graft should be taken from the iliac crest. The implants to be used are the same as with the corresponding fractures.

As some of the bones are short, a neighbouring joint may be involved in the internal fixation, in the sense of a temporary arthrodesis. This does not produce lasting disturbance of the joint.

b) Arthrodesis

In comminuted joint fractures secondary arthrodesis may be required. Resection of the first metatarsophalangeal joint should be avoided, but post-traumatic arthrosis of this joint may be successfully treated by a silastic prosthesis. Retrograde screw fixation is suitable for stabilizing the interphalangeal joint of the big toe (Fig. 38).

6. Clinical X-ray Examples
(Figs. 196–206)

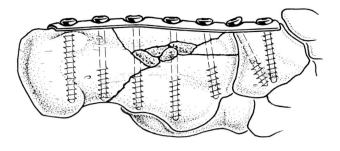

Fig. 191. Internal fixation of a comminuted fracture of the calcaneum

A one-third tubular plate is contoured to the lateral surface of the calcaneum. After reduction of the fracture the screws can be easily placed in those parts of the bone which experience shows can remain intact: the body, the sustentaculum tali and the anterior process. If comminution extends to the distal area, the plate may also engage the cuboid bone

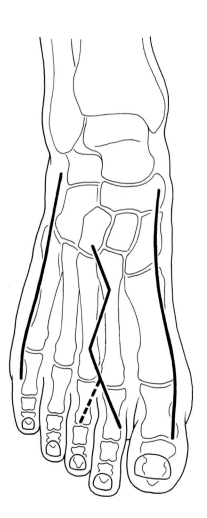

Fig. 192. Incisions for internal fixation of the forefoot

Fig. 193a, b. Typical internal fixations of the fore-foot with plates

a A one-third tubular plate must be placed as lateral as possible on the first metatarsal bone. L- and T-plate on the fifth metatarsal and the proximal phalanx of the big toe

b Small cancellous bone graft for a comminuted area at the base of the first metatarsal

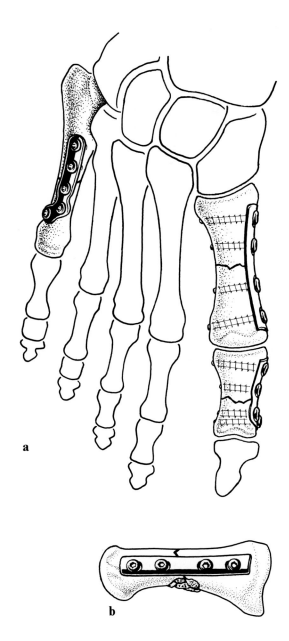

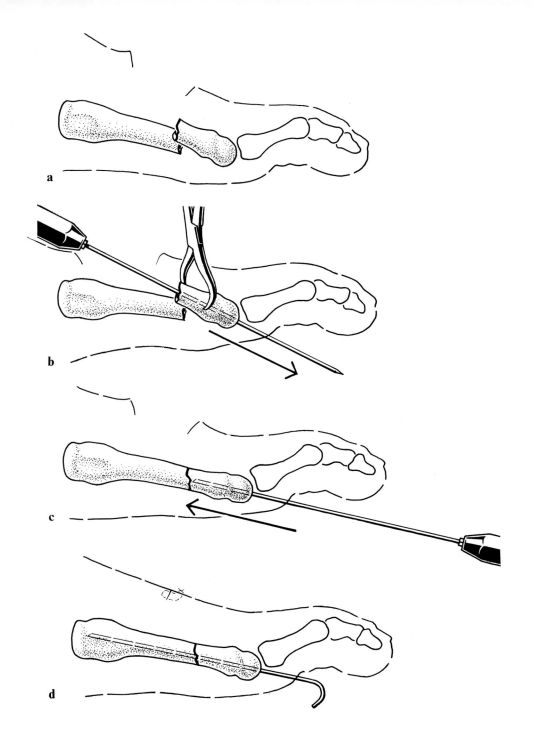

Fig. 194a–d. Open intramedullary wiring in fractures of the second–fourth metatarsals

a Initial situation and approach

b Insertion of the Kirschner wire dorsally from proximal to distal through the distal fragment and out through the plantar surface

c Open reduction of the fracture and drilling of the wire backwards into the proximal fragment

d The end of the wire is not buried under the skin

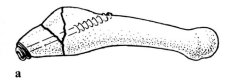

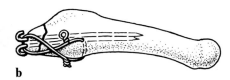

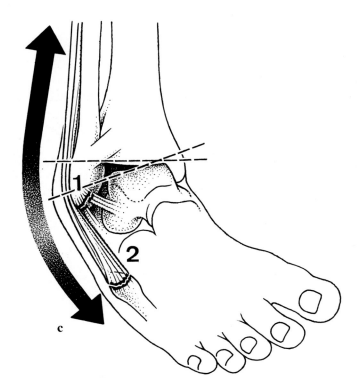

Fig. 195a–c. Fracture of the base of the fifth metatarsal

a Screw fixation of a larger fragment

b A small avulsed fragment is fixed by a tension-band wire procedure

c Inversion of the foot often results in an avulsion fracture of the base of the fifth metatarsal combined with rupture of the fibulotalar and the fibulocalcaneal ligaments

Fig. 196a–c. Clinical example: Avulsion fracture of the anterolateral calcaneum

B., Hans-Ulrich, a 21-year-old commercial employee who had a fall while skiing

a Avulsion fracture at the anterolateral margin of the calcaneum with slight dislocation of Chopart's intertarsal joint. Small avulsion from the lateral process of the talus

b Emergency operation: Fixation with two small cancellous screws. A small comminuted zone is below the avulsed fragment.
No complications. Discharge with plaster cast, left for 12 weeks. Removal of the screws after one year elsewhere

c Review at $5^1/_2$ years: no symptoms, full function, some pigmentation of the scar. The X-ray still shows sclerosis of the anterior process of the talus. No arthrosis. After removal of the metal the fracture is healed on the radiograph

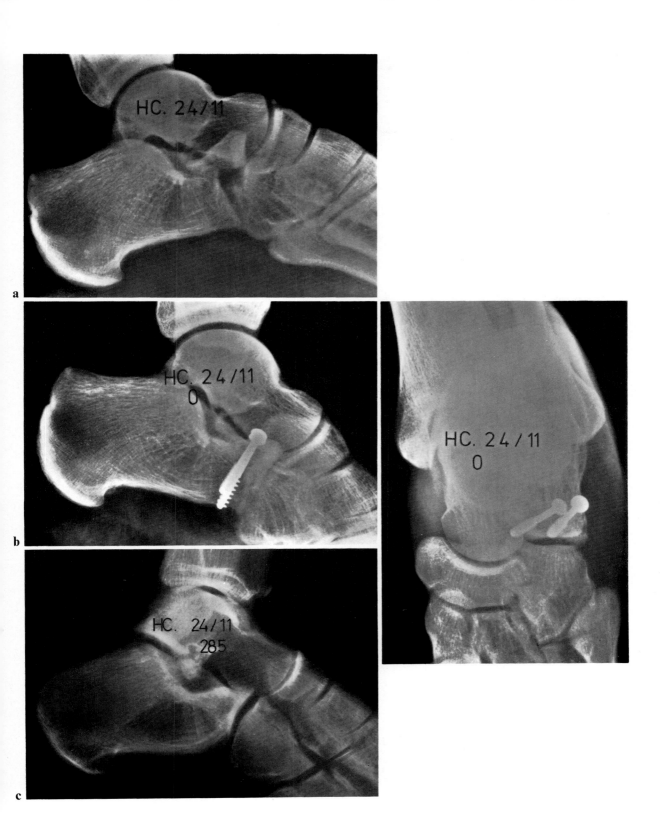

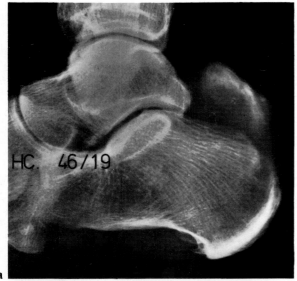

a

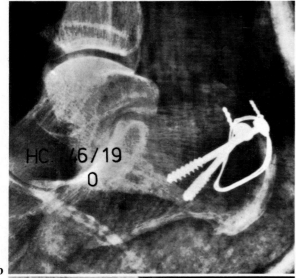

b

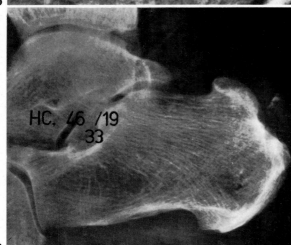

c

Fig. 197a–c. Clinical example: Fixation of an avulsion fracture of the Achilles' tendon with tension-band wiring

G., Eva-Maria, a 42-year-old housewife who had a skiing accident

a Avulsion of the Achilles' tendon from the calcaneum

b Emergency internal fixation with two small cancellous screws, washers and a double tension-band wire.
No postoperative complications. Primary wound healing. Plaster cast at discharge with plantar flexion of the foot. Walking plaster cast at the end of 3rd week up to 7 weeks

c The patient, who lives abroad, claims 13 months after operation that she has completely recovered and is fit for sports. The implants were removed after 8 months. The X-ray film after 33 weeks demonstrates a healed fracture

Fig. 198a–d. Clinical example: Dislocation of Chopart's intertarsal joint ▷

F., Verena, an 18-year-old apprentice in the hotel industry, who had a fall while playing badminton. Reduction and plaster cast by the family doctor. Admission to hospital on the 9th day

a Dislocation at Chopart's joint with impaction fracture of the scaphoid and cuboid bone

b Closed reduction as an emergency procedure under general anaesthesia with relaxation, with percutaneous Kirschner wire fixation between the scaphoid and the talus. The X-ray now shows an avulsion fracture and a defect of the cuboid bone more clearly. Because of the poor condition of the soft tissues further treatment is postponed

c, d. see page 344f

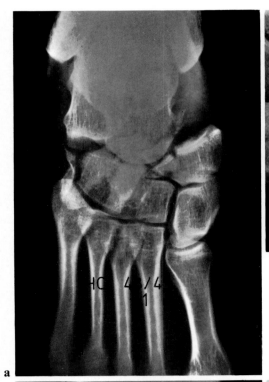
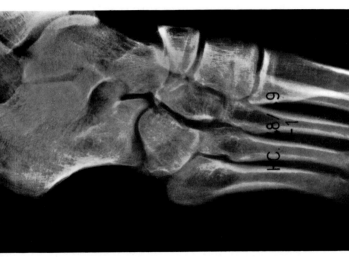

a

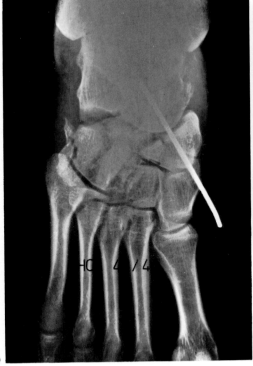
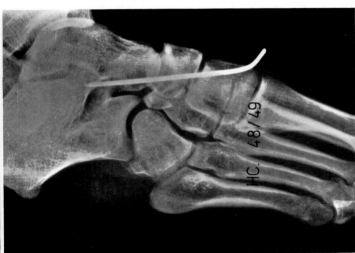

b

Fig. 198c, d

c One week later, the lateral internal fixation is done. Reduction of the cuboid bone, filling of the defect with a cancellous bone graft from the iliac crest. Neutralization T-plate fixed in the intact distal part of the cuboid and in the calcaneum. The medial Kirschner wire is buried beneath the skin. No complications. Functional treatment. At discharge a plaster slab is applied. The Kirschner wire is removed after 4 weeks because of local irritation. After 10 weeks the patient is back to school and full weight bearing is started

d Review and removal of the metal after 8 months: No symptoms, full ability to walk, good function with only a slight limitation of supination, no muscular atrophy. The X-ray shows a healed fracture with a congruent joint surface without arthrosis

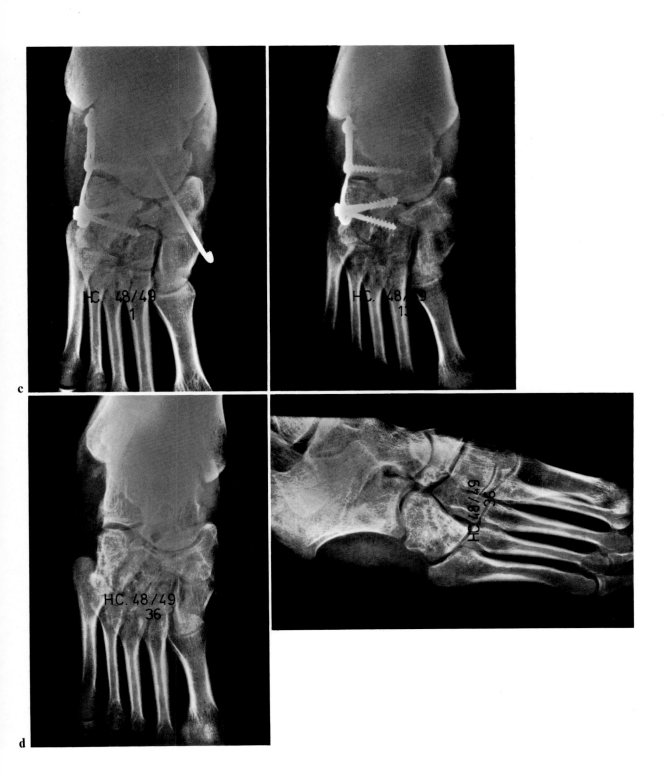

c

d

345

Fig. 199a–e. Clinical example: Internal fixation with plates of transverse fractures of the first and fifth metatarsals

C., Michele, 32-year-old building labourer. His foot had been squeezed in the shovel of an excavator

a Transverse fractures of the first and fifth metatarsals. Severe local swelling. The limb was elevated

b Internal fixation after 11 days: L-plate on the fifth metatarsal and one-third tubular plate on the first metatarsal. The comminuted area at the base of the first metatarsal is disregarded. The proximal screw of the plate is too short, the second in the comminuted area.
No postoperative complications. Functional treatment without plaster. Full weight bearing at 4 months. The patient is back at work after 6 months

c, d. see 348 f

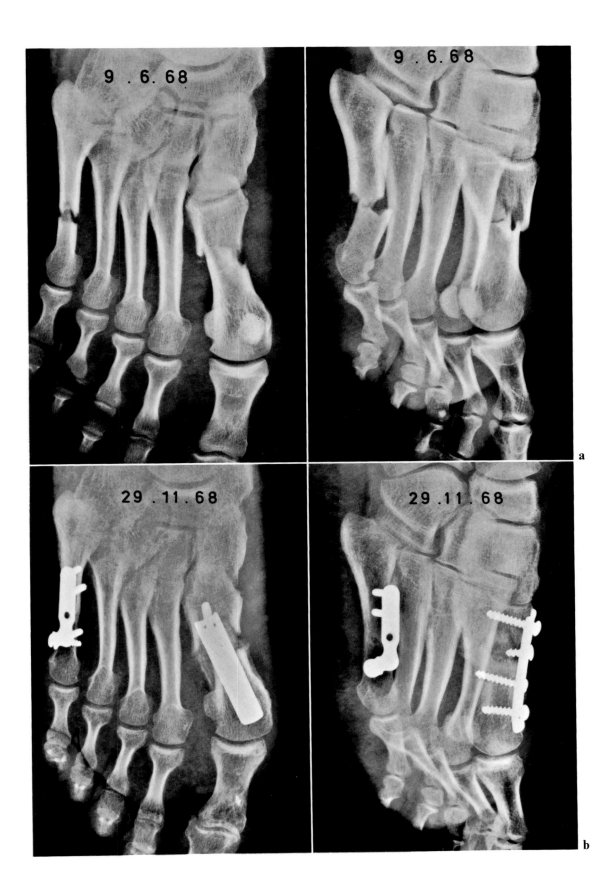

Fig. 199c–e

c Primary healing of the fracture of the fifth metatarsal. Considerable callus formation at the fracture of the first metatarsal because of instability; loosening of the proximal screw

d Review and removal of the implants at 8 months: symptom-free, full working capacity. Full mobility. Uneven structure of the bone at the base of the first metatarsal.

e 12.7.80 Review at 12 years: No pain and full working capacity as a building labourer. Linear scars. Full mobility of the joints. No muscular atrophy. The fractures are healed. The space of the tarsometatarsal joint is somewhat narrower

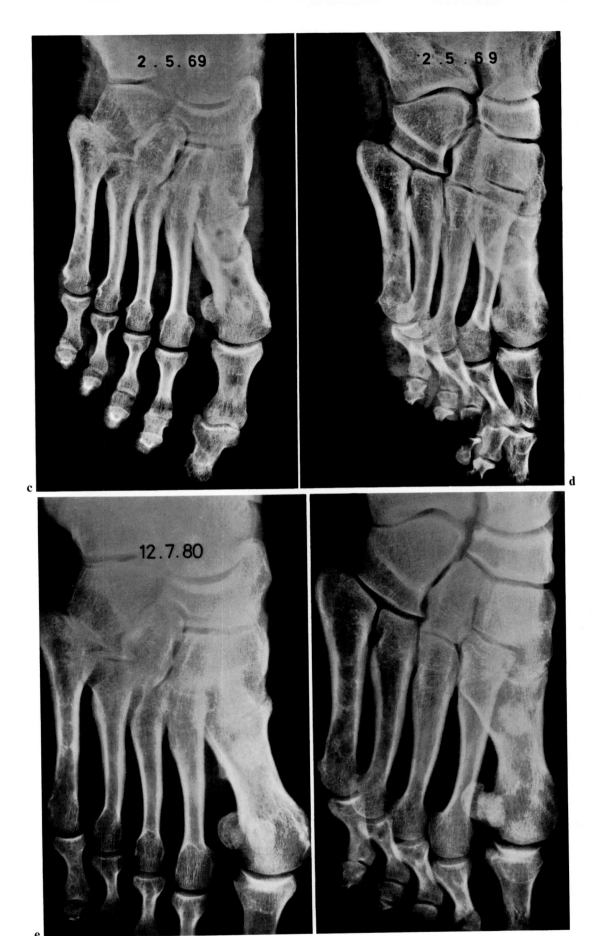

Fig. 200a–c. Clinical example: Fracture of the base of the first metatarsal

M.D., a 28-year-old electrician who had fallen from scaffolding

a Comminuted, proximal, articular fracture of the first metatarsal together with a fracture of the neck of the second metatarsal (vassal fracture)

b Operation after 2 weeks: Primary arthrodesis of the 1st tarsometatarsal joint with a one-third tubular plate and cancellous bone graft. Medullary wiring of the second metatarsal.
Removal of the medullary wire at the end of 4 weeks. Walking caliper used for 3 months. Working capacity of 50% at the end of 7 months

c X-ray at 13 months, just before removal of the implants. The fracture and arthrodesis are healed.
Review at 15 months: no symptoms, full working capacity. Reduction of extension and inversion of the foot by 30%

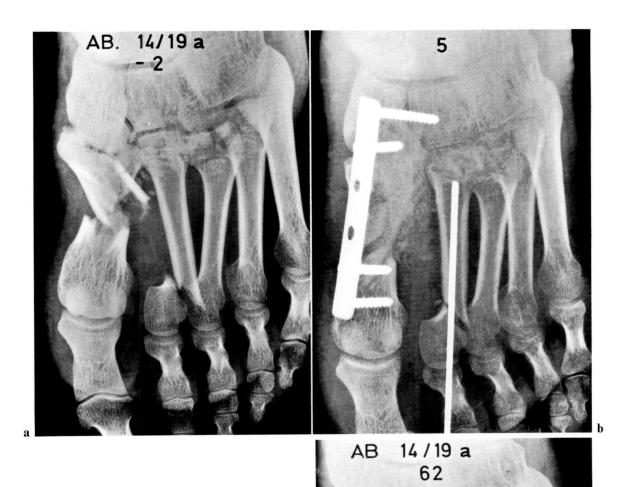

a

b

c

351

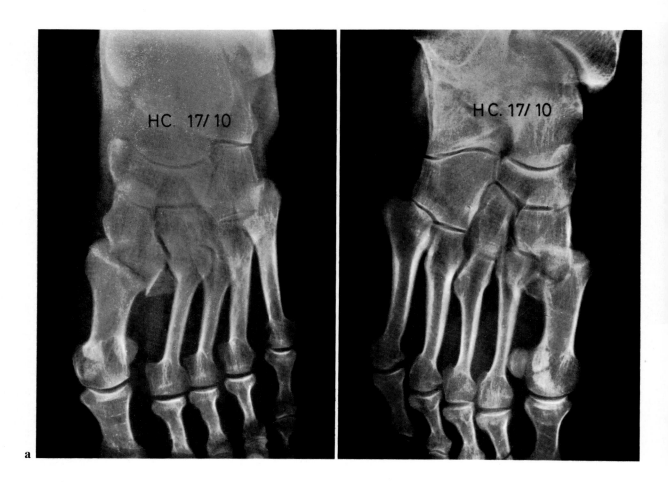

a

Fig. 201 a–c. Clinical example: Fracture-dislocation of the base of the first metatarsal

H., Hermine, a 60-year-old woman factory worker who had a fall at work. Conservative treatment by the family doctor. She was referred to the hospital after 6 days

a Fracture-dislocation of the base of the first metatarsal

b Internal fixation. Stabilization of the base of the first metatarsal with a radius T-plate engaging the medial cuneiforme as well.

Primary wound healing without complications. Discharge with a walking plaster cast because of neurological disorders unconnected with the accident. Removal of the implants at the end of 7 months

c Final review at 13 months: quite symptom-free, fracture healed, no significant arthrosis of the tarsometatarsal joint

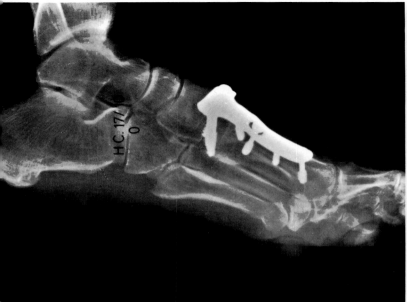

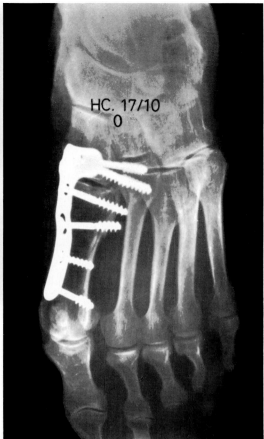

b

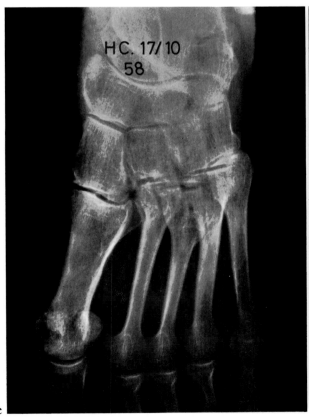

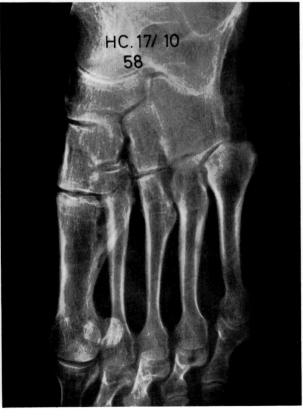

c

Fig. 202a–d. Clinical example: Delayed internal fixation of a comminuted fracture of the base of the fifth metatarsal

P., Agnes, a 53-year-old woman factory worker. Her left foot was squeezed between a fork-lift truck and a wall. Significant contusion of the skin. The X-ray shows a comminuted fracture of the base of the fifth metatarsal. Elevation of the limb at home, plaster slab, antibiotics for a perforating wound. Admission to hospital after 19 days. Failure of a first closed reduction

a The skin is bluish and oedematous, severe displacement of the comminuted fracture

b Internal fixation after 5 weeks, with a finger T-plate and a cancellous bone graft from the iliac crest.
Functional treatment without plaster. Primary wound healing. A removable splint was applied at discharge. Uncomplicated healing of the wound and the fracture. Full weight bearing with a walking plaster cast after 7 weeks. Full weight bearing without plaster after 18 weeks. Full working capacity after 34 weeks

c, d see page 356 f

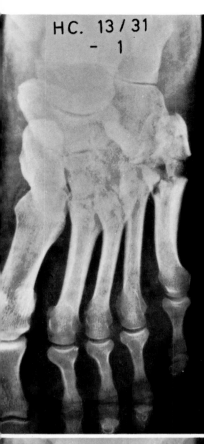

HC. 13 / 31
- 1

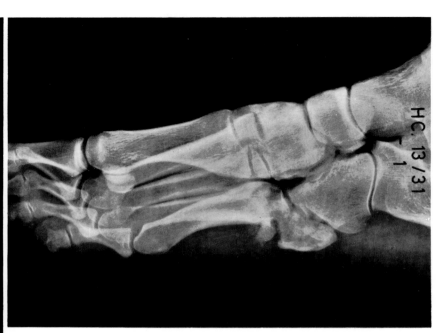

HC. 13 / 31
- 1

a

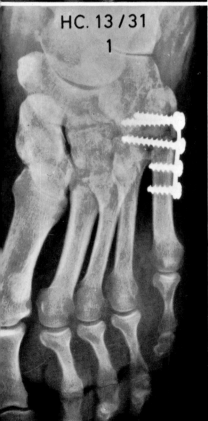

HC. 13 / 31
1

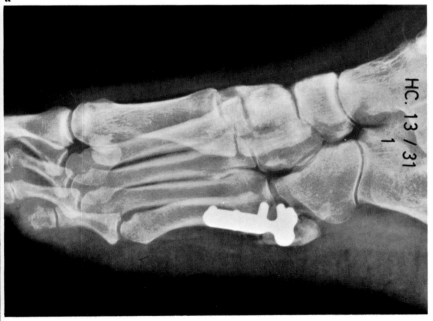

HC. 13 / 31
1

b

Fig. 202c, d

c Removal of the metal, the fracture being united, at $4^1/_2$ months

d Review after $7^1/_2$ years: The patient is symptom-free and is fully fit to work and to walk. Full range of movement, no atrophy of the muscles. X-ray demonstrates restoration of the base of the fifth metatarsal

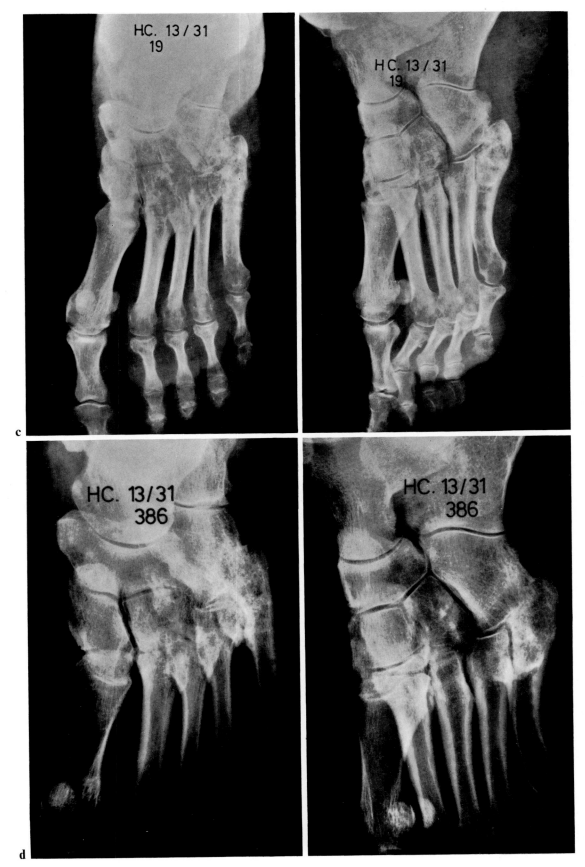

c

d

357

Fig. 203a–c. Clinical example: Bicondylar fracture of the proximal phalanx of the big toe

M., Esther, a 27-year-old unskilled woman worker. She had a fall on a staircase

a Bicondylar fracture of the proximal phalanx of the left big toe. Some local swelling

b Internal fixation with a mini T-plate the next day.
Uneventful course. Functional postoperative treatment. A walking plaster cast was applied at discharge for 6 weeks. Full weight bearing at the end of 6 weeks. She was back at work at 10 weeks

c Review and removal of the implants at 9 months: No complaints. Limited function of the interphalangeal joint of the toe. The fracture is healed, no arthrosis

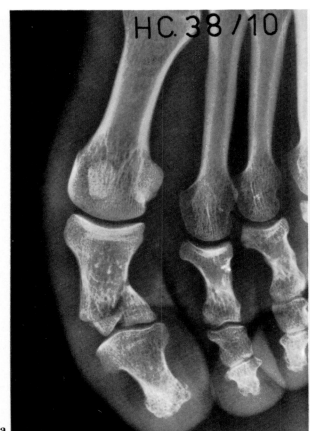

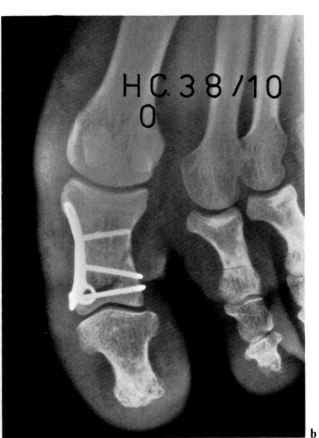

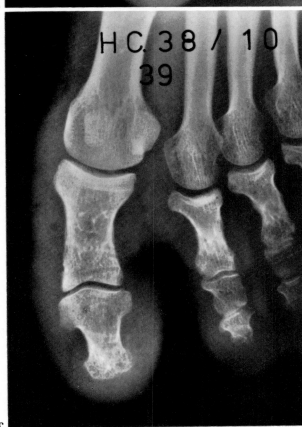

a

b

c

359

Fig. 204a–d. Clinical example: Pseudarthrosis at the base of the fifth metatarsal

A., Santolo, a 36-year-old building labourer. The lateral margin of the foot had been injured by a stone. He had continued to have moderate symptoms and had received no treatment

a Pseudarthrosis was diagnosed at 8 months

b Rigid internal fixation with a small cancellous screw and without bone graft.
Postoperatively a complete plaster cast was applied and worn for 3 months. Progressive consolidation of the pseudarthrosis

c Review at 10 months: full function, mild symptoms related to change in the weather. Full working ability. The pseudarthrosis has consolidated

d Removal of the metal at 17 months: On removal of the screw the threaded part broke off and was left behind. A further review was impossible because the patient left the country

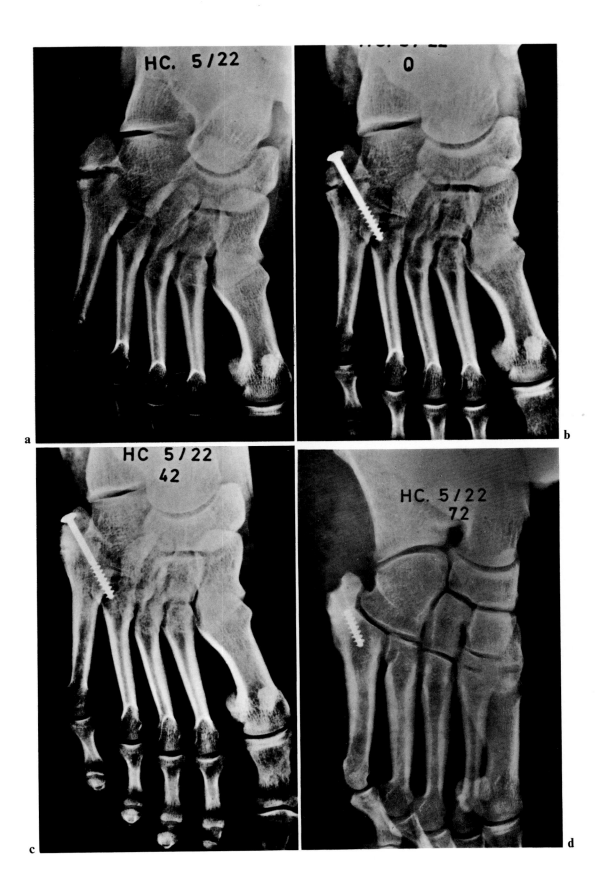

Fig. 205a–d. Clinical example: Delayed fracture healing at the neck of the 5th metatarsal

S., Danté, a 47-year-old interior decorator who had fallen off a ladder. He had a fracture of the neck of the fifth metatarsal in satisfactory position. Treatment with plaster cast

a Non-union at 8 weeks and progressive osteoporosis at the periphery

b Internal fixation at 2 months: Intramedullary, corticocancellous bone peg from the iliac crest, finger L-plate and additional lag screws.
No complications. Postoperative treatment without plaster, no weight bearing for 10 weeks. The fracture had united at 10 weeks. Full weight bearing at the end of 12 weeks. Removal of metal at 5 months

c, d see page 364f

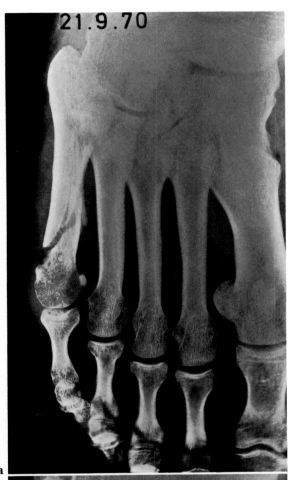

a

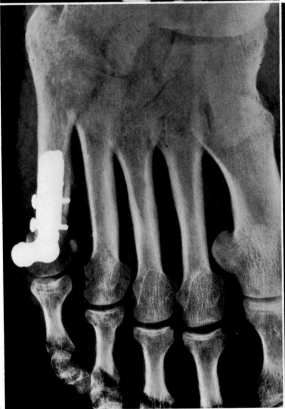

b

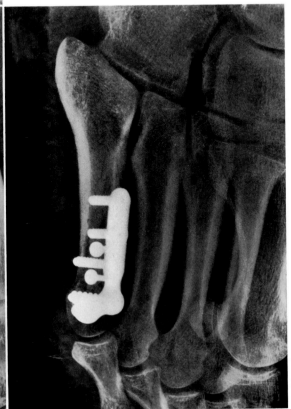

Fig. 205c, d

c Review at 9 months: no complaints, full function, still some osteoporosis

d Review at 10 years: Some local pain is probably due to primary chronic arthritis, which developed in the meantime. Full function, no muscular atrophy, normal radiographs

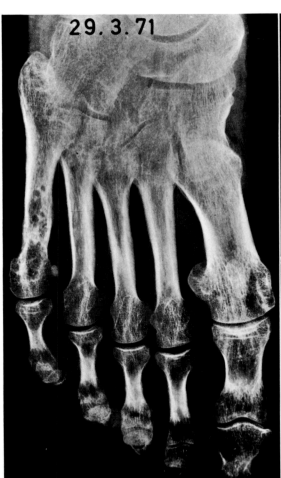
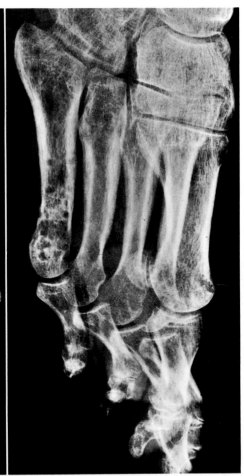

c

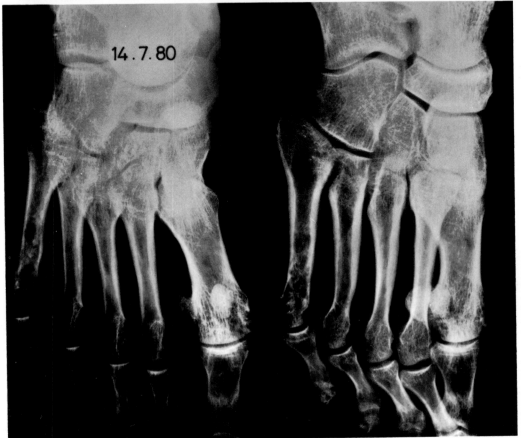

d

Fig. 206 a–c. Clinical example: Arthrodesis of the interphalangeal joint of the big toe with a screw

D., José Luis, a 27-year-old building worker who had an impacted articular fracture of the proximal phalanx of his big right toe, as well as a fracture of the shaft of the third metatarsal. Pain persisted in the interphalangeal joint of the big toe

a Post-traumatic arthrosis of the interphalangeal joint of the big toe

b Typical retrograde arthrodesis of the joint with 3.5-mm cortical screw at 3 months.
No complications, functional postoperative treatment. Full walking ability at the end of 8 weeks

c Removal of the screw at 4 months: the arthrodesis has consolidated

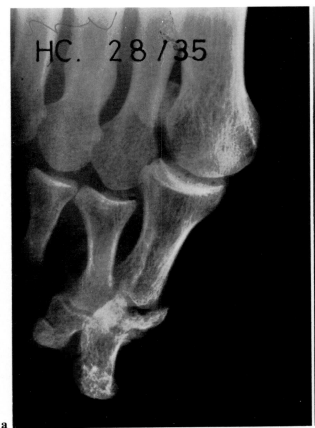

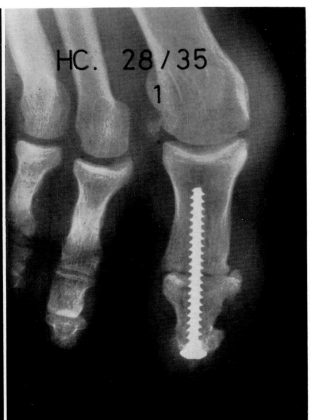

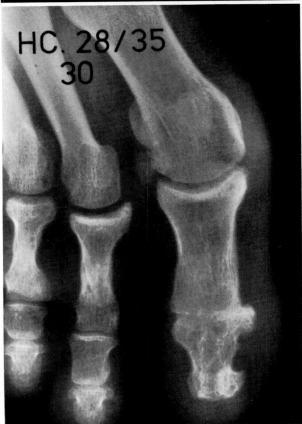

XVIII. Special Indications

Besides the classic and less common sites for use of small implants, two special indications may be discussed: fractures in children and reconstructive surgery in rheumatic disease. The latter has become of increasing interest in recent years.

1. Internal Fixation in Children

In the rare cases where internal fixation is indicated in children, epiphyseal fractures and traumatic epiphysiolysis are usually involved. However, it may also be considered in open fractures, in some types of irreducible or unstable shaft fractures and in avulsion fractures of the insertion of ligaments which include avulsion of the epicondyles (Figs. 207–209).

As there is scarcely any danger of post-traumatic ankylosis in children, external splints can be used with impunity, and these operations are more in the nature of accurate open reduction. Nevertheless, biomechanical relationships between implant and bone must be carefully considered. The delicate implants of the SFS are especially appropriate for the use in children. The one-third tubular plate is usually employed for the forearm and tibia, but recently the 3.5-mm screw DCP has also been used. In order to avoid growth disturbance, screws should never cross the epiphyseal and apophyseal lines. Washers must be applied when using screws independently, as the screw heads may otherwise sink into the soft young bone.

In children the implants are rapidly covered by exuberant callus masses, and early removal of the implants is recommended as it may become impossible later.

Transverse fractures in children always produce accelerated growth in the length of the bone affected, especially after internal fixation. This problem must be given careful consideration, particularly in the lower limbs.

2. The Use of the SFS in Surgery of Rheumatoid Disease

Here the metal implants are especially used for arthrodesis, following the techniques described in the general section. The brittle and delicate bones of the rheumatoid patient often require especially thin implants. In contrast the risk of infection is not increased in these patients, even when they have been treated with steroids for several years. The quality of the scars is surprisingly good. As in the childhood skeleton, the SFS offers various possibilities of stabilization with limited external support, which provides much relief for the patients.

3. Clinical X-ray Examples
(Figs. 210–215)

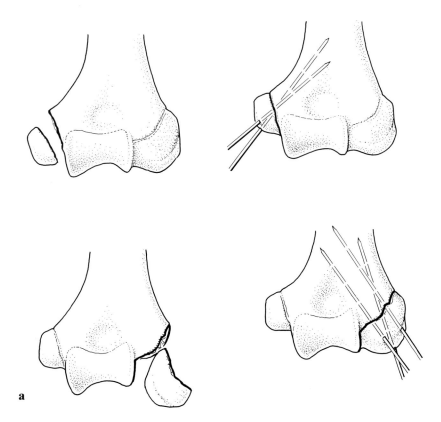

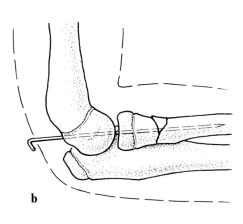

Fig. 207a, b. Internal fixation of elbow fractures in children

a Condylar and epicondylar fractures are fixed with Kirschner wires. At the medial side the ulnar nerve must be exposed and protected

b Fractures of the neck of the radius, which are reduced by closed manipulation, may be stabilized by medullary wiring through the humerus. Bending or breaking of the Kirschner wire must be avoided by fixing the position of the elbow with a plaster cast

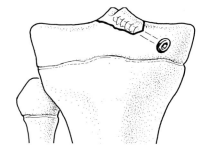

Fig. 208. Avulsion of the intercondylar spine of the tibia in children

Fixation with a small cancellous screw which avoids the epiphyseal line

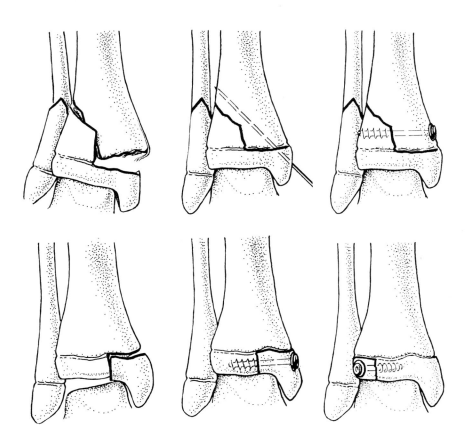

Fig. 209. Internal fixation of epiphyseal fractures of the lower tibia in children

Examples of screw fixation of epiphyseal fractures as an alternative to open reduction and fixation with Kirschner wires

Fig. 210a–c. Clinical example: Instable fracture of the proximal humerus of a child

F., Werner, a 14-year-old schoolboy who had a skiing accident

a Very unstable and displaced fracture of the proximal shaft of the humerus. Closed reduction failed. He was referred to hospital after 3 days

b Internal fixation with a 3.5-mm T-plate. Uncomplicated course. Functional treatment. Full weight bearing after 6 weeks

c Review and removal of the implants at 6 months: no complaints, full function, no muscular atrophy

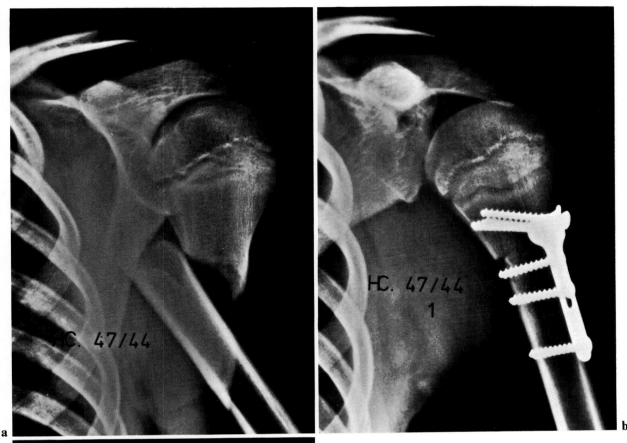

a

b

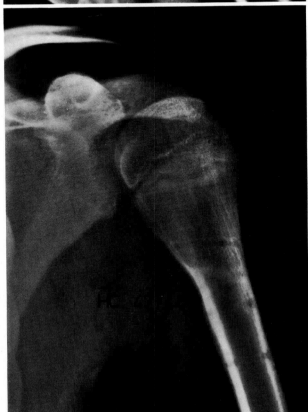

c

Fig. 211a–c. Clinical example: Screw fixation of an oblique fracture of olecranon in a child

J., Bernhard, a 15-year-old schoolboy who had a skiing accident

a Displaced fracture of the olecranon far from the epiphyseal line

b Emergency internal fixation with two screws and washers.
No complications. Discharge with a circular plaster cast for 4 weeks. Full use after 6 weeks

c Review and removal of the implants at 5 months: no symptoms, full function, the fracture is healed

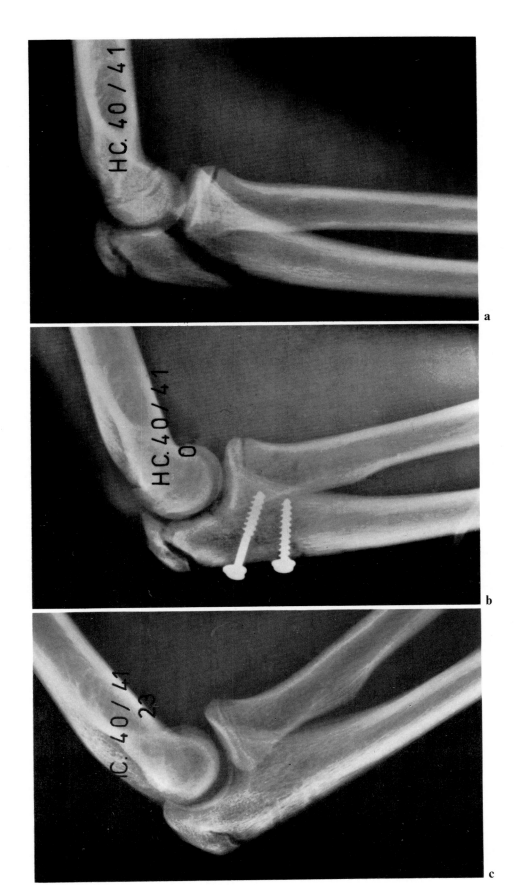

Fig. 212a–c. Clinical example: Internal fixation with plates in an open fracture of the forearm of a child

G., B., a 10-year-old schoolboy

a Open fracture of the distal forearm. Closed reduction failed because of interposition of the soft tissues

b Internal fixation with two 2.7-mm DCPs. Removable plaster slab for the wrist joint for 4 weeks. He is back to apparatus gymnastics after 2 months. Removal of implants at 4 months

c Review at 13 months: no complaints, full range of movements, equal strength of both hands, equal length of both forearms

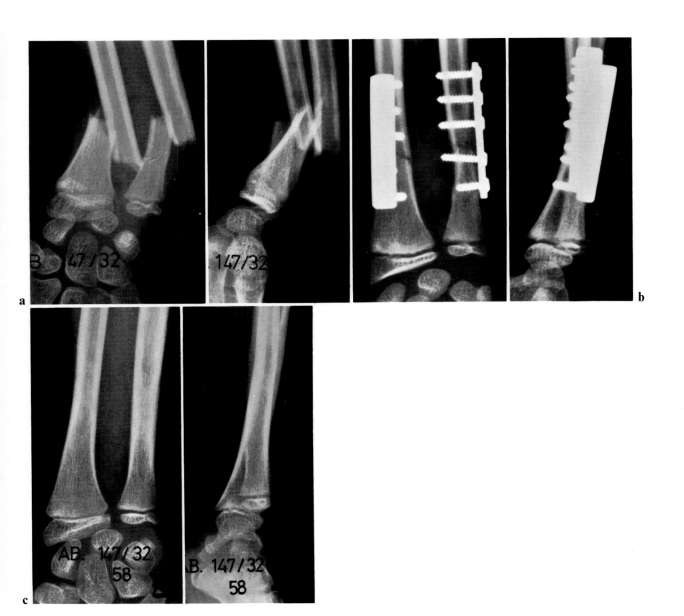

a

b

c

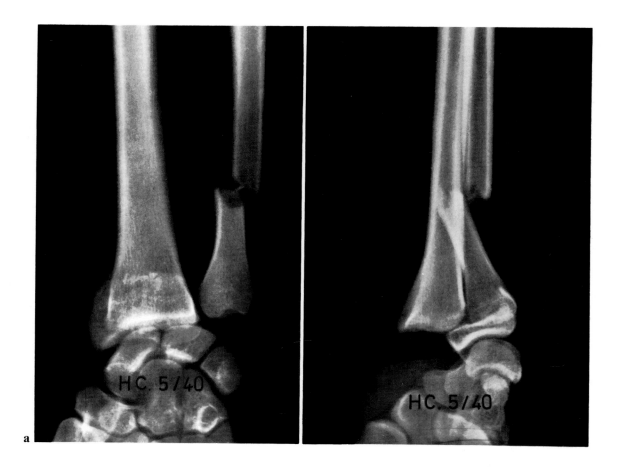

Fig. 213a–c. Clinical example: Displaced epiphyseal fracture of the distal radius

B., Hansjörg, a 16-year-old schoolboy who fell from a fence onto his left hand

a Displaced epiphyseal fracture of the distal radius of Aitken type I with fracture of the distal shaft of the ulna. Unsuccessful closed reduction

b Emergency internal fixation: open reduction of the radius and fixation with two parallel Kirschner wires. Fixation of the ulna with a one-third tubular plate.

No complications. A plaster slab is applied for discharge. The Kirschner wires are removed after 4 weeks, the plate from the ulna at 4 months

c Review after 9 years: full function. The X-ray shows a regular joint surface, non-union of the avulsed ulnar styloid process. A slight irregularity may be seen on the cortex of the ulnar shaft

378

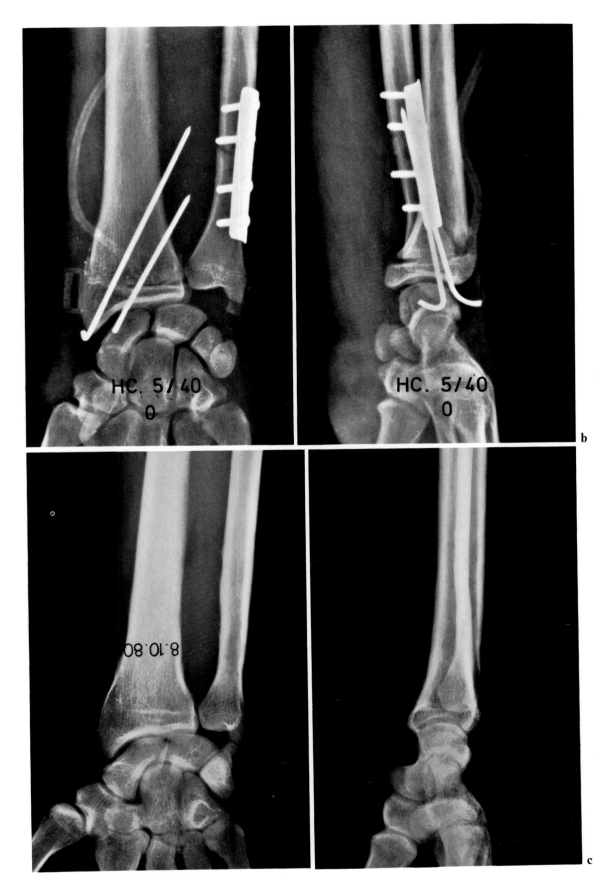

HC. 5/40
0

HC. 5/40
0

b

8.10.80

c

379

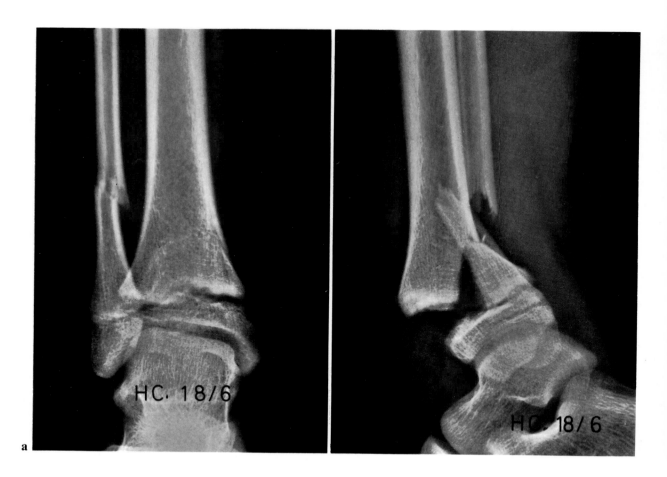

Fig. 214a–c. Clinical example: Epiphyseal fracture of the distal tibia

Sch., Thomas, an 11-year-old schoolboy who had a fall while skiing

a Distal epiphyseal fracture Aitken type I of the right tibia with fracture of the fibula. Closed reduction was not successful

b Emergency internal fixation: Removal of interposed soft tissues medially, fixation of the reduced fracture with small cancellous screws. Open reduc-tion of the fibula, which did not set by closed manipulation and fixation with an oblique Kirschner wire.
Uneventful course. Plaster cast on discharge. Removal of the implants elsewhere after 6 weeks

c An X-ray film taken after $4^1/_2$ months shows healing of the fractures and regular epiphyseal lines

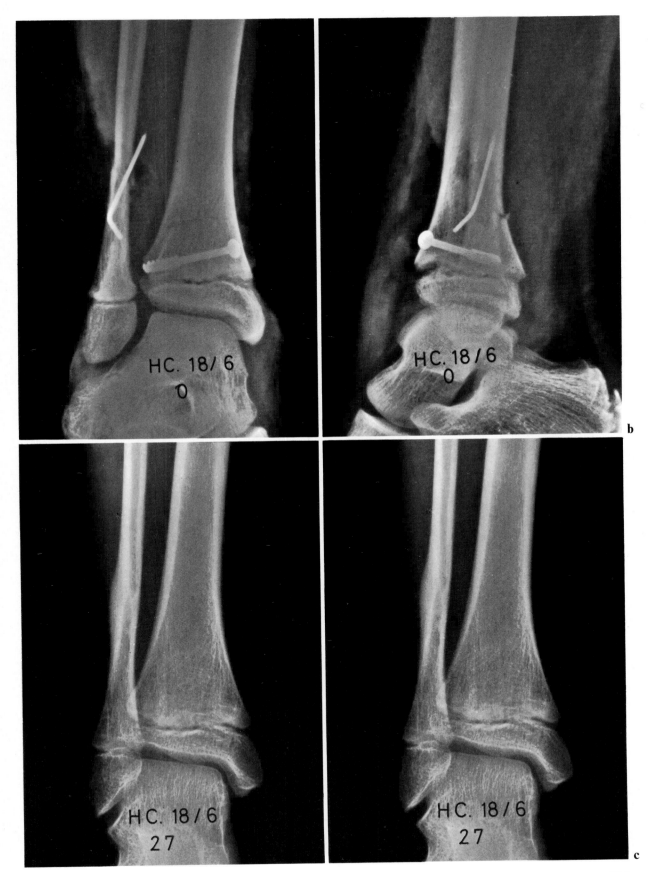

HC. 18 / 6
0

HC. 18 / 6
0

b

HC. 18 / 6
27

HC. 18 / 6
27

c

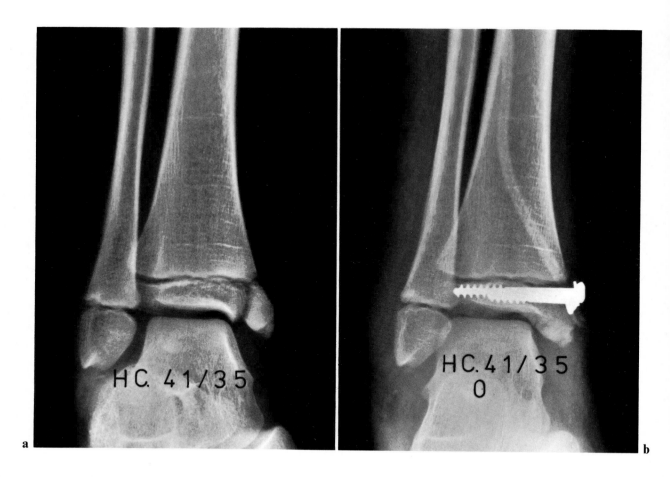

a   b

Fig. 215a–d. Clinical example: Distal epiphyseal fracture of the tibia

K., Dagmar, a child of 8 years

a The patient was hit by a bicycle. Fracture of the epiphysis of the medial malleolus Aitken type II

b Emergency internal fixation: Reduction and fixation with two small cancellous screws and washers parallel to the epiphyseal line and the joint surface. No complications. Plaster cast on discharge. Weight bearing at the end of 5 weeks. Removal of the metal at 8 weeks

c Review at $2^{1}/_{2}$ years: No complaints. The scar is somewhat hypertrophic. Full function. Little changes of the epiphyseal lines in the fracture area. A small avulsed fragment at the tip of the fibula, which was overlooked in the initial X-rays has grown to a large osteophyte and proves that an additional lateral injury of the fibulotalar or the fibulocalcanear ligament was present

382

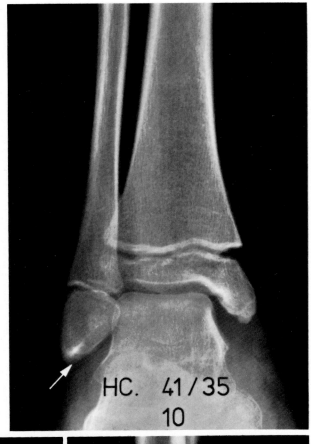

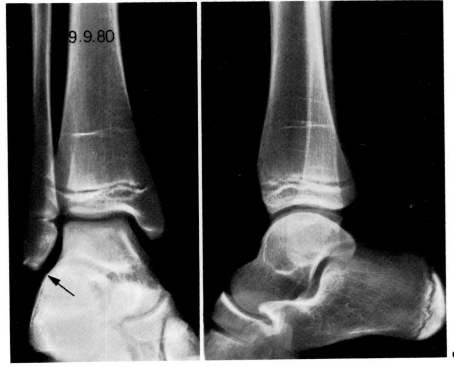

References

Ali Khan MA, Lucas HK (1978) Plating of fractures of the middle third of the clavicle. Injury 9:263–267

Allgöwer M (1973) Luxationsfrakturen im Ellbogenbereich. Z Unfallmed Berufskr 2:71–74

Allgöwer M, Scharplatz D (1976) Fracture-dislocation of the elbow. Injury 7:143–159

Allgöwer M, Huggler A, Segmüller G (1967) Innere Fixation bei Achsenkorrektur am unteren Tibiaende. In: Müller ME (ed) Posttraumatische Achsenfehlstellungen an der unteren Extremität. Huber, Bern Stuttgart, p 137

Allgöwer M, Rüedi T, Kolbow H (1975) Erfahrungen mit der dynamischen Kompressionsplatte (DCP) bei 418 frischen Unterschenkelschaftbrüchen. Arch Orthop Unfallchir 82:247–256

Allgöwer M, Kinzl L, Matter P, Perren SM, Rüedi T (1977) The dynamic compression plate. Springer, Berlin Heidelberg New York

Almquist E (1973) Compression plate fixation for Barton's or Smith Type II fractures. Handchirurgie 5:29

Angehrn R (1980) Resultate der operativen Knochenbruchbehandlung am Handskelett. Analyse von 570 Fällen der AO-Dokumentation. Inauguraldissertation, Basel

Bandi W (1964) Indikation und Technik der Osteosynthese am Humerus. Helv Chir Acta 31:89–100

Bandi W (1969) Die gelenknahen Frakturen des Oberarmes. Chirurg 40:193–198

Bandi W (1970) Zur Mechanik der supramalleolären, intraarticulären Schienbeinbrüche des Skifahrers. In: Heinkelein J, Lechner F (eds) Kongr. Ber. 9. Internat. Kongress für Skitraumatologie und Wintersportmedizin. Nebel-Verlag, Garmisch-Partenkirchen, p 74

Bandi W (1972) Chondromalacia patellae und femoropatellare Arthrose. Helv Chir Acta [Suppl] 11

Bandi W (1972) Die Arthrose des femoro-patellaren Gelenkes und ihre Therapie. Hefte Unfallheilkd 110:181–186

Bandi W (1974) Die distalen, intraartikulären Schienbeinbrüche des Skifahrers. Aktuel Traumatol 4:1–6

Bandi W (1977) Die retropatellaren Kniegelenkschäden. Pathomechanik und pathologische Anatomie, Klinik und Therapie. Huber, Bern Stuttgart Wien

Barac M, Stare J, Ranic V, Hranilovic B (1979) Unsere Erfahrungen bei der Behandlung des Sprungbeinbruches. Hefte Unfallheilkd 133:33–36

Barton NJ (1979) Fractures of the shafts of the phalanges of the hand. Hand 11:119–133

Baumann H (1965) Ellbogen. In: Nigst H (ed) Spezielle Frakturen- und Luxationslehre, vol II/1. Thieme, Stuttgart

Beck E (1972) Radiusköpfchenfrakturen. Hefte Unfallheilkd 114:69–76

Beck E (1974) Osteosynthese von Speichenköpfchenbrüchen. Aktuel Chir 9:23–28

Bernett P, Krueger P, Proschka G, Wiendl HJ (1970) Ergebnisse konservativer und operativer Behandlung distaler, intraartikulärer Tibiafrakturen. In: Heinkelein J, Lechner F (eds) Kongr. Ber. 9. Internat. Kongress für Ski-Traumatologie u. Wintersportmedizin. Nebel-Verlag, Garmisch-Partenkirchen, p 108

Blömer J (1975) Nachuntersuchung operativ und konservativ behandelter Schlüsselbeinbrüche. Internat. Kongreß f. Notfallchirurgie

Blömer J (1977) Ergebnisse operativ und konservativ behandelter Schlüsselbeinbrüche. Unfallheilkunde 80:237

Böhler J (1969) Gelenknahe Frakturen des Unterarmes. Chirurg 40:198–203

Böhler J (1977) Die Komplexverletzungen der Hand; Taktik der Sofortversorgung frischer Verletzungen. Unfallheilkunde 80:39–42

Bonnin JG (1950) Injuries to the ankle. Heinemann, London

Buch J (1979) Die operierten Talusfrakturen. Hefte Unfallheilkd 133:37–41

Burri C (1971) Zur operativen Behandlung der acromeoclaviculären Luxationen. Aktuel Traumatol 4:245

Burri C (1972) Ergebnisse nach operativer und

konservativer Behandlung der acromeoclaviculären Luxation. Hefte Unfallheilkd 110:295

Burri C (1973) Ellbogenfrakturen beim Erwachsenen. Hefte Unfallheilkd 114:32

Burri C (1978a) Frakturen des Pilon tibial. Springer, Berlin Heidelberg New York

Burri C (1978b) Die Behandlung schwerster Ellbo-
gengelenksverletzungen. Aktuel Traumatol
8:127

Burri C, Rüter A (1978) Verletzungen des oberen
Sprunggelenkes. Hefte Unfallheilkd 131. Springer, Berlin Heidelberg New York

Burri C, Rüedi T, Matter P, Pfeiffer KM, Pusterla
C (1969) Stabile Osteosynthese: Frakturen im
Handbereich. Aktuel Chir 4:305

Danis R (1949) Théorie et pratique de l'ostéosynthèse. Masson, Paris

Danis R (1956) Le vrai but et les dangers de l'ostéosynthèse. Lyon Chir 51:740

Decoulx P, Razemon JP, Rouselle Y (1961) Fractures du pilon tibial. Rev Chir Orthop 47:563

Doliveux P (1972) Table ronde sur les fractures
des métacarpiens et des phalanges. Bull Soc Orthop Quest

Dorfmann GR (1978) Determination of treatment
in fractures of the fifth metatarsal shaft. J Foot
Surg 17:16–21

Durband MA (1969) Metacarpalefrakturen unter
besonderer Berücksichtigung der therapeu-
tischen Möglichkeiten aus neuester Sicht. Inauguraldissertation, Zürich

Eitemüller JP, Haas HG (1978) Behandlungsergebnisse bei 258 Kahnbeinverletzungen an der
Hand. Arch Orthop Trauma Surg 91:45–51

Engert J, Klumpp H, Simon G (1979) Schlüssel-
beinpseudarthrosen im Kindesalter. Chirurg
50:631–635

Fambrough RA, Green DP (1979) Tendon rupture
as a complication of screw fixation in fractures
in the hand. A case report. J Bone Joint Surg
61-A:781–782

Flemming F (1962) Versorgung komplizierter Mittelhandfrakturen mittels Pull-out-wire-Technik.
Monatsschr Unfallheilkd 65:112

Fyfe IS, Mason S (1979) The mechanical stability
of internal fixation of fractured phalanges. Hand
11:50–54

Galeazzi R (1935) Über ein besonderes Syndrom
bei Verletzungen im Bereich der Unterarmkno-
chen. Arch Orthop Unfallchir 35:557

Gamstätter G (1977) Spätkomplikationen am Ell-
bogen- und Handgelenk nach Radiusköpfchenresektion. 120. Tagung der Vereinigung Nord-
westdeutscher Chirurgen

Ganz R (1971) Isolierte traumatische Knorpellä-
sion am Kniegelenk. Hefte Unfallheilkd 110:146

Ganz R (1976) Isolierte Knorpelabscherungen am
Kniegelenk. Hefte Unfallheilkd 127:79

Gasser H (1965) Delayed union and pseudarthrosis
of the carpal navicular: treatment by compres-
sion-screw osteosynthesis. J Bone Joint Surg
47-A:249

Gay R, Evard J (1963) Les fractures récentes du
pilon tibial chez l'adulte. Rev Chir Orthop
49:397

Gedda KO, Moberg E (1953) Open reduction and
osteosynthesis of socalled Bennett's fracture in
the carpometacarpal joint of the thumb. Acta
Orthop Scand 22:249

Geiser M (1970) Erfahrungen mit der Arthrodese
des Großzehengrundgelenkes. In: Scholder P
(ed) Der Vorfuß. Huber, Bern Stuttgart Wien,
p 110

Hackenbruch W (1979) Differential diagnosis of
ruptures of the lateral ligamants of the ankle
joint. Arch Orthop Trauma Surg 93:293–301

Hamas RS, Horrell ED, Pierret GP (1978) Treatment of mallet finger due to intraarticular fracture of the distal phalanx. J Hand Surg
3:361–363

Heim D (1980) Die Peronealsehnenluxation. Inauguraldissertation, Basel

Heim U (1969) Die Technik der operativen Behandlung der Metacarpalfrakturen. Helv Chir
Acta 36:619

Heim U (1970a) Zur operativen Technik der dista-
len, intraartikulären Tibiaimpressionsfrakturen.
In: Heinkelein J, Lechner F (eds) Kongr. Ber.
9. Internat. Kongress für Ski-Traumatologie und
Wintersportmedizin. Nebel-Verlag, Garmisch-
Partenkirchen, p 91

Heim U (1970b) Die Behandlung von Frakturen
der Metatarsalia und Zehen unter besonderer
Berücksichtigung der Osteosynthese. Z Unfallmed Berufskr 63:305

Heim U (1971) Le matérériel AO dans le traitement chirurgical des fractures des phalanges et
métacarpiens. Chirurgie 32:3

Heim U (1972a) Traitement des fractures de la
phalange proximale et des métacarpiens par la
technique AO. Ann Orthop Ouest 4:80

Heim U (1972b) Le traitement chirurgical des fractures du pilon tibial. J Chir (Paris) 104:307

Heim U (1973a) Indications et technique de l'ostéosynthèse AO dans le traitement des fractures
de la main. Arch Orthop Belg 39:957

Heim U (1973b) L'ostéosynthèse rigide dans le
traitement des fractures de la base du premier
métacarpien. Acta Orthop Belg 39:1073

Heim U (1973c) Indication et technique des sutures ligamentaires dans les fractures malléolaires.
Rev Chir Orthop 59 [Suppl 1]:270

Heim U (1973 d) Die Schraubenosteosynthese des Radiusköpfchens, Indikation und Technik. Z Unfallmed Berufskr 66:11

Heim U (1974a) Periphere Osteosynthesen. Indikation und Technik. Zentralbl Chir 99:1319

Heim U (1974b) Osteosynthesen am distalen Radius. Z Unfallmed Berufskr 67:31–34

Heim U (1977) Stabilisation des ostéotomies de l'extrémité inférieure du radius par petit plaque et T. Ann Chir 31:313

Heim U (1978a) Zur Verschraubung der Navikularefraktur nach der AO-Technik. Therapiewoche 28:4459–4465

Heim U (1978b) Grundlagen zur operativen Stabilisierung der Mittelhandfrakturen II–V. In: Segmüller G (ed) Das Mittelhandskelett in der Klinik. Huber, Bern Stuttgart Wien, pp 38–43

Heim U (1978c) Die Behandlung der frischen intraartikulären Brüche der MP- und PIP-Gelenke. Hefte Unfallheilkd 141:65

Heim U (1979a) Die operative Behandlung der gelenknahen Speichenbrüche des Erwachsenen. Hefte Unfallheilkd 82:15–22

Heim U (1979b) The treatment of nonunion in the bones of the hand. In: Chapchal G (ed) Pseudarthroses and their treatment. Thieme, Stuttgart, pp 168–169

Heim U, Damur-Thür F (1977) Spongiosa aus dem Tibiakopf als autologes Transplantationsmaterial. Arch Orthop Unfallchir 89:211

Heim U, Näser M (1976) Die operative Behandlung der Pilon tibialfraktur. Technik der Osteosynthese und Resultate bei 128 Patienten. Arch Orthop Unfallchir 86:341

Heim U, Näser M (1977) Fractures du pilon tibial. Résultats de 128 ostéosynthèses. Rev Chir Orthop 63:5

Heim U, Osterwalder M (1977) Arthrodèse de l'interphalagienne distale (et de l'interphalangienne du pouce) par vissage. Ann Chir 31:291

Heim U, Pfeiffer KM (1972) Periphere Osteosynthesen unter Verwendung des Kleinfragmente-Instrumentariums der AO. Springer, Berlin Heidelberg New York

Heim U, Pfeiffer KM (1974) Small fragment set manual. Springer, Berlin Heidelberg New York

Heim U, Pfeiffer KM (1975a) Ostéosynthèses périphériques. Masson, Paris

Heim U, Pfeiffer KM (1975b) Osteosintesis periferica. Editorial Cientifico-Medica, Barcelona

Heim U, Trüb HJ (1978) Erfahrungen mit der primären Osteosynthese von Radiusköpfchenfrakturen. Helv Chir Acta 45:63

Heim U, Pfeiffer KM, Meuli HC (1973) Resultate von 332 AO-Osteosynthesen des Handskelettes. Handchirurgie 5:71

Heiss J, Prokscha GW, Wagner T (1979) Konservative und operative Behandlung von Talusfrakturen. – Indikation, Technik und Behandlungsergebnisse. Hefte Unfallheilkd 133:67–71

Huene DR (1979) Primary internal fixation of carpal navicular fractures in the athlete. Am J Sports Med 7:175–177

Huffaker WH, Wray RC Jr, Weeks PM (1979) Factors influencing final range of motion in the fingers after fractures of the hand. J Plast Reconstr Surg 63:82–87

Hunter JM, Cowen NJ (1970) Fifth metacarpal fractures in a compensation clinic population. J Bone Joint Surg 52-A:1159

Iselin M, Iselin F (1967) Traité de chirurgie de la main. Flamarion, Paris

Iselin M, Blanguernon S, Benoist D (1965) Fractures de la base du 1er métacarpien. Mem Acad Chir 82:771

Jahna H (1954) Behandlung und Behandlungsergebnisse von 734 frischen, einfachen Brüchen des Kahnbeinkörpers der Hand. Wien Med Wochenschr 104:1023

Jahna H (1965) Erfahrungen und Nachuntersuchungsergebnisse von 47 De Quervain'schen Verrenkungsbrüchen. Arch Orthop Unfallchir 57:51

Kavanaugh JH, Brower TD, Mann RV (1978) The Jones fracture revisited. J Bone Joint Surg 60-A:776–782

Kehr H, Hierholzer G, Kraus J, Konold P, Ecke H, Pannike A (1979) Zur operativen Behandlung der Talusfrakturen. Hefte Unfallheilkd 133:30–32

Kempf I, Touzard RC (1978) Les fractures du calcaneum. J Chir (Paris) 115:377–386

Kilbourne B, Paul EG (1958) The use of small bone screws in the treatment of metacarpal, metatarsal and phalangeal fractures. J Bone Joint Surg 40-A:375

Kirschner P (1977) Veränderungen am Ellbogen- und Handgelenk nach Radiusköpfchenresektion. Vereinigung Mittelrheinischer Chirurgen

Knofler EW (1978) Ein Beitrag zur operativen Behandlung des Schulterblatthalsbruches. Beitr Orthop Traumatol 25:54–56

Koch F (1971) Die Claviculapseudarthrose; ihre Entstehung und Behandlung. Monatsschr Unfallheilkd 74:330

Koob E (1967) Die Verschraubung der Kahnbeinpseudarthrose der Hand. Hefte Unfallheilkd 91:190

Koob E (1972) Möglichkeiten der Fehler bei der Verschraubung des Kahnbeinbruches der Hand. Handchirurgie 4:67

Koob E, Goymann V, Haas HG (1971) Ergebnisse

nach Verschraubung der Kahnbeinpseudarthrose der Hand. Handchirurgie 2:205

Kraumann H, Kafka I, Slegl O, Vokoun Z (1979) Spätergebnisse der operativen Behandlung des Fersenbeinbruches. Hefte Unfallheilkd 133:217–219

Kuner EH, Müller T, Lindenmaier HL (1978) Einteilung und Behandlung der Talusfrakturen. Hefte Unfallheilkd 131:197–211

Kurock W (1978) Therapeutisches Vorgehen bei 49 zentralen Talusverletzungen. 95. Tagung der Deutschen Gesellschaft für Chirurgie

Labitzke R, Kehr H, Rehn J (1972) Zur Behandlung von Olecranon-Frakturen und Olecranon-Pseudarthrosen. Arch Orthop Unfallchir 74:247

Leach RE, Bolton PE (1968) Arthritis of the carpometacarpal joint of the thumb; results of arthrodesis. J Bone Joint Surg 50-A:1171

Lindemaier HL (1976) Bandverletzungen bei der Luxationsfraktur des oberen Sprunggelenkes. Unfallchirurgie 2:28

Lister G (1978) Intraosseous wiring of the distal skeleton. J Hand Surg 3:427–435

Massengill JB, Alexander H, Parson JR (1979) Mechanical analysis of Kirschner wire fixation in a phalangeal model. J Hand Surg 4:351–356

Matter P, Rittmann WW (1978) The open fracture. Assessment, surgical treatment and results. Huber, Bern Stuttgart Wien

Matti H (1936) Technik und Resultate meiner Pseudarthroseoperation. Zentralbl Chir 63:1442

Matti H (1937) Über die Behandlung der Navicularefraktur und der Refractura patellae durch Plombierung mit Spongiosa. Zentralbl Chir 64:2353

Matzen PF (1978) Indikation der operativen Therapie bei Frakturen und Luxationen im Schulterbereich. Beitr Orthop Traumatol 25:44–52

Maudsley RH, Chen SC (1972) Screw fixation in the management of the fractured carpal scaphoid. J Bone Joint Surg 54-B:432

Maurer G, Lechner F (1965) Konservative und operative Behandlungsmöglichkeiten bei Stauchungsbrüchen des distalen Unterschenkels. Unfallheilkunde 68:207

McLaughlin HL (1954) Fracture of the carpal navicular (scaphoid) bone. Some observations based on treatment by open reduction and internal fixation. J Bone Joint Surg 36-A:765

McLaughlin HL, Perkes JC (1969) Fracture of the carpal navicular (scaphoid) bone: gradations in therapy based upon pathology. J Trauma 9:311

Meuli HC, Meyer V, Segmüller G (1978) Stabilization of bone in replantation surgery of the upper limb. Clin Orthop 133:179–183

Mitchell WG, Shaftan GW, Sclafani SJ (1979) Mandatory open reduction: its role in displaced ankle fractures. J Trauma 19:602–615

Moberg E (1967) Aspetische Knochennekrosen. Langenbecks Arch Klin Chir 319:429

Moberg E, Henricksson B (1960) Technique for digital arthrodesis. A study of 150 cases. Acta Chir Scand 118:331

Mockwitz J (1979) Ergebnisse nach konservativer und nach operativer Behandlung von Sprungbeinbrüchen. Hefte Unfallheilkd 133:51–55

Mohr KU (1970) Indikation und Methode der operativen Wiederherstellung der Klavikula. Med Welt 21:557

Morscher E (1973) Posttraumatische Fehlstellungen und Pseudarthrosen am Ellbogen beim Erwachsenen. Hefte Unfallheilkd 114:76–84

Müller J (1977) Plastic reconstruction of the talofibular ligament by autologous, skin graft. In: Willenegger H (ed) Reconstruction in ligamentous lesions. Thieme, Stuttgart

Müller J (1978a) Ergebnisse verschiedener Operationsmethoden bei Kahnbeinpseudarthrosen der Hand. Unfallheilkunde 80:345–352

Müller J (1978b) Über die Indikation zur konservativen oder operativen Behandlung der Scapulafrakturen. Aktuel Traumatol 8:139–142

Müller J, Plaas U, Willenegger H (1971) Spätergebnisse nach operativ behandelten Malleolarfrakturen. Helv Chir Acta 38:329–337

Müller ME (1964) Les fractures du pilon tibial. Rev Chir Orthop 50:557

Müller ME (1966) Treatment of non-unions by compression. Clin Orthop 43:83–92

Müller ME (1967) Posttraumatische Fehlstellungen an der unteren Extremität. Huber, Bern Stuttgart

Müller ME (1977) Zur Einteilung und Reposition von Kinderfrakturen. Unfallheilkunde 80:187–190

Müller ME, Allgöwer M, Willenegger H (1963) Technik der operativen Frakturbehandlung. Springer, Berlin Heidelberg New York

Müller ME, Allgöwer M, Willenegger H (1969) Manual der Osteosynthese. Springer, Berlin Heidelberg New York

Müller ME, Allgöwer M, Schneider R, Willenegger H (1977) Manual der Osteosynthese, 2. Aufl. Springer, Berlin Heidelberg New York

Müller ME, Allgöwer M, Schneider R, Willenegger H (1979) Manual of internal fixation, 2nd. edn. Springer, Berlin Heidelberg New York

Mumenthaler M (1961) Die Ulnarisparesen. Thieme, Stuttgart

Naett R, Bacha AL (1973) Die AO-Plattenosteosynthese am Handskelett. Handchirurgie 5:79

Odenheimer K, Harvey JP Jr (1979) Internal fixation of fracture of the head of the radius. Two case reports. J Bone Joint Surg 61-A:785–787

Pannike A (1970) Zur Behandlung der offenen, schweren Kombinationsverletzungen an Unterarm und Hand. Therapiewoche 20:1926

Pannike A (1972a) Osteosynthesen in der Handchirurgie. Springer, Berlin Heidelberg New York

Pannike A (1972b) Die nicht reponierbare, transnavikuläre Verrenkung der Hand. Therapiewoche 22:4026–4027

Pannike A (1973) Finger- und Mittelhandverletzungen. Therapiewoche 23:1831

Pannike A (1977a) Die Behandlung der frischen Frakturen des Handskelettes. Unfallheilkunde 80:51–56

Pannike A (1977b) Korrektureingriffe nach Verletzungen des Handskelettes. Orthopaede 6:100–112

Pannike A, Meyer J (1969) A new method of bone stabilization in reconstructive surgery of the hand. Excerpta Med Int Congr Ser 174:946

Pauwels F (1965) Gesammelte Abhandlungen zur funktionellen Anatomie des Bewegungsapparates. Springer, Berlin Heidelberg New York

Pearson JR (1961) Combined fracture of the base of the fifth metatarsal and the lateral malleolus. J Bone Joint Surg 43-A:513

Perren SM, Allgöwer M (1976) Biomechanik der Frakturheilung nach Osteosynthesen. Nova Acta Leopold 44, 223:61–84

Perren SM, Allgöwer M, Mathys R, Schenk R, Willenegger H, Müller ME (1969) The reaction of cortical bone to compression. Acta Orthop Scand [Suppl] 125:19

Perren SM, Huggler A, Russenberger M, Allgöwer M, Mathys R, Schenk RK, Willenegger H, Müller ME (1969) The reaction of cortical bone to compression. Acta Orthop Scand [Suppl] 125:19

Perren SM, Matter P, Rüedi T, Allgöwer M (1975) Biomechanics of fracture healing after internal fixation. Surg Annu 361–390

Pfeiffer KM (1972a) Zur Frage der primären Schraubenosteosynthese von Navikularefrakturen. Helv Chir Acta 39:111–122

Pfeiffer KM (1972b) Der Platz der stabilen Osteosynthese in der Behandlung von Frakturen der Hand. Ther Umsch 29:679–685

Pfeiffer KM (1975) Radiusfrakturen loco classico. Ther Umsch 32:788–799

Pfeiffer KM (1976) Fortschritte in der Osteosynthese von Handfrakturen. Handchirurgie 8:17–22

Pfeiffer KM (1978a) Perilunäre, transskaphoidale, transkapitale, transstyloidale Handgelenks-Luxationsfraktur. Operative Rekonstruktion. Handchirurgie 10:39–40

Pfeiffer KM (1978b) Luxationsfrakturen an der Basis des Metacarpale I (Sattelgelenk). Typus Bennett und Typus Rolando. In: Segmüller G (ed) Das Mittelhandskelett in der Klinik. Huber, Bern Stuttgart Wien, pp 50–58

Pfeiffer KM, Nigst H (1970) Schraubenarthrodese von Fingergelenken. Handchirurgie 2:149–151

Pyper JB (1978) Non-union of fractures of the clavicle. Injury 9:268–270

Rahmenzadeh R (1969) Die funktionelle Behandlung der Frakturen im Bereich des Talus und Calcaneus. 46. Tagung der Bayrischen Chir. Verh.

Ricklin P (1960) Entbehrliche Knochen. Helv Chir Acta 27:397

Riedeberger J (1972) Operative und konservative Behandlung der schweren Fersenbeinfrakturen. Zentralbl Chir 97:625

Rittmann WW, Matter P (1977) Die offene Fraktur. Beurteilung, operative Behandlung und Resultate. Huber, Bern Stuttgart Wien

Rittmann WW, Perren SM (1974a) Corticale Knochenheilung nach Osteosynthese und Infektion. Springer, Berlin Heidelberg New York

Rittmann WW, Perren SM (1974b) Cortical bone healing after internal fixation and infection; biomechanics and biology. Springer, Berlin Heidelberg New York

Rüedi T (1973) Frakturen des Pilon tibial: Ergebnisse nach 9 Jahren. Arch Orthop Unfallchir 76:248–254

Rüedi T (1978) Spätresultate nach operativer Behandlung der Gelenkbrüche am distalen Tibiaende. Unfallheilkunde 81:319–323

Rüedi T, Wolff G (1975) Vermeidung posttraumatischer Komplikationen durch frühe definitive Versorgung von Polytraumatisierten mit Frakturen des Bewegungsapparates. Helv Chir Acta 42:507–512

Rüedi T, Matter P, Allgöwer M (1968) Die intraarticulären Frakturen des distalen Unterschenkelendes. Helv Chir Acta 35:556

Rüedi T, Burri C, Matter P, Allgöwer M (1970) Operationsstatistik bei Frakturen des Pilon tibial. In: Heinkelein J, Lechner F (eds) Kongr. Bericht 9. Internat. Kongreß für Skitraumatologie u. Wintersportmedizin. Nebel-Verlag, Garmisch-Partenkirchen, p 87

Rüedi T, Burri C, Pfeiffer KM (1971) Stable internal fixation of fractures of the hand. J Trauma 11:381

Rüedi T, Moshfegh A, Pfeiffer KM, Allgöwer M (1974) Fresh fractures of the shaft of the humerus. Conservative or operative treatment? Reconstr Surg Trauma 14:65–74

Rüedi T, Stadler J, Gauer E (1975) Operativ versorgte Malleolarfrakturen. Ergebnisse nach 3–4 Jahren mit besonderer Berücksichtigung des Talusprofils. Arch Orthop Unfallchir 82:311–323

Rüedi T, Webb JK, Allgöwer M (1976) Experience with the dynamic compression plate (DCP) in 418 recent fractures of the tibial shaft. Injury 7:252–257

Rueff FL, Wilhelm K, Hauer G (1973) Fehlergebnisse nach Osteosynthesen von Unterarmschaftfrakturen. Monatsschr Unfallheilkd 76:1

Russe O (1954) Erfahrungen und Ergebnisse bei der Spongiosafüllung der veralteten Brüche und Pseudarthrosen des Kahnbeines der Hand. Wiederherstellungschir Traumatol 2:175

Russe O (1960a) Nachuntersuchungsergebnisse von 22 Fällen operierter, veralteter Brüche und Pseudarthrosen des Kahnbeines der Hand. Z Orthop 93:5

Russe O (1960b) Fracture of the carpal navicular. Diagnosis, non-operative treatment and operative treatment. J Bone Joint Surg 42-A:759

Sander K (1972) Frakturen und Luxationen im Bereich des proximalen Radius. Beitr Orthop 19:519

Schärli AF (1980) Osteosynthese kindlicher Hand- und Fußfrakturen nach dem Zuggurtungsprinzip. Unfallchirurgie 6:24–27

Scharf W (1979) Ergebnisse konservativ behandelter Schlüsselbeinbrüche. Unfallchirurgie 5:141–145

Schenk R, Willenegger H (1967) Morphologic findings in primary fracture healing. Symp Biol Hung 7:75

Scheuer I (1978) Konservative und operative Behandlung von Radiusköpfchenbrüchen und deren Ergebnisse. Aktuel Traumatol 8:119–121

Schweiberer L (1971) Der heutige Stand der Knochentransplantation. Chirurg 42:252

Schweiberer L (1976a) Theoretisch-experimentelle Grundlagen der autologen Spongiosatransplantation im Infekt. Unfallheilkunde 79:151

Schweiberer L (1976b) Bedeutung der autologen Spongiosatransplantation sowie Fragen der Vaskularisation von Transplantaten. Nova Acta Leopold 223, 44:371

Schweiberer L, Hertel P (1974) Die Ergebnisse nach operativer Behandlung von 48 frischen Monteggia-Verletzungen. Aktuel Traumatologie 4:147

Segmüller G (1973) Operative Stabilisierung am Handskelett. Huber, Bern Stuttgart Wien

Segmüller G (ed) (1978) Das Mittelhandskelett in der Klinik. Biomechanik, Verletzungen, Anomalien: Diagnostik und Therapie. Huber, Bern Stuttgart Wien

Segmüller G, Schönenberger F (1971) Technik der Kompressionsarthrodese am Finger mittels Zugschraube. Handchirurgie 2:218

Siegling CW (1978) Erfahrungen mit der operativen Versorgung der Akromioklavikularluxation nach Trauma. Beitr Orthop Traumatol 25:660

Simonetta C (1970) The use of AO plates in the hand. Hand 2:43

Smillie IS (1960) Osteochondritis dissecans. Livingstone, Edinburgh London

Smillie IS (1967) Treatment of osteochondritis dissecans. J Bone Joint Surg 39-B:248

Spiessl B, Schargus G, Schroll K (1971) Die stabile Osteosynthese bei Frakturen des unbezahnten Unterkiefers. Schweiz Monatsschr Zahnheilkd 81:39

Stauffer UG (1978) Indications for operative treatment of fractures in childhood. Prog Pediatr Surg 12:187–208

Steel WM (1978) The AO small fragment set in hand fractures. Hand 10:246–253

Steffelaar H, Heim U (1974) Sekundäre Plattenosteosynthese an der Clavicula. Arch Orthop Unfallchir 79:75

Swanson AB (1968) Silicone-rubber implants for replacement of arthritic or destroyed joints in hand. Surg Clin North Am 48:1113

Szyszkowitz R, Marti R, Wilde CD, Reschauer R, Schloffmann W (1979) Die offene Reposition und Verschraubung der Talusfrakturen. Hefte Unfallheilkd 133:41–48

Terbrüggen D (1975) Die Osteosynthese der Scapulafraktur im Rahmen der Schultergürtel-Mehrfachverletzung. Hefte Unfallheilkd 126:62

Tetering JP Van, Bloem J (1978) Über Arthrodesen kleiner Fingergelenke. Klinische Untersuchung und Resultate von Kirschnerdraht- und Zuggurtungsarthrodesen. Handchirurgie 10:127–129

Thelen E (1976) Acromioclavicular-Sprengungen. – Ergebnisse nach operativer und konservativer Versorgung in 162 Fällen. Unfallheilkunde 79:417–422

Titze A (1979) Indikationen zur Osteosynthese an der Hand und an den Fingern. Unfallchirurgie 5:146–149

Trojan E (1955) Die operative Behandlung des veralteten Kahnbeinbruches der Hand. Verh Dtsch Orthop Ges 43:160

Truchet P (1970) Fractures du pilon tibial. In: Heinkelein J, Lechner F (eds) Kongr. Bericht 9. Internat. Kongreß für Skitraumatologie u. Wintersportmedizin. Nebel-Verlag, Garmisch-Partenkirchen, p 69

Tscherne H (1973) Luxationsfrakturen im Ellbogenbereich. Hefte Unfallheilkd 114:59

Tscherne H (1976) Konservative und operative Therapie der Schulterblattbrüche. Hefte Unfallheilkd 126:52

Wagner H (1964) Operative Behandlung der Osteochondritis dissecans des Kniegelenkes. Z Orthop 98:333

Weber BG (1965) Behandlung der Sprunggelenks-Stauchungsbrüche nach biomechanischen Gesichtspunkten. Hefte Unfallheilkd 81:176

Weber BG (1969) Zur Behandlung der frischen fibularen Bandruptur und der chronischen, fibularen Bandinsuffizienz. Arch Orthop Unfallchir 65:251–257

Weber BG (1972) Die Verletzungen des oberen Sprunggelenkes. 2nd edn. Huber, Bern Stuttgart Wien

Weber BG, Cech O (1976) Pseudarthrosis. Pathophysiology, Biomechanics, Therapy, Results. Huber, Bern Stuttgart Wien

Weber BG, Süssenbach F (1970) Epiphysenfugenverletzungen am distalen Unterschenkel. Huber, Bern Stuttgart Wien

Weber BG, Brunner C, Freuler F (1978) Die Frakturbehandlung bei Kindern und Jugendlichen. Springer, Berlin Heidelberg New York

Weber BG, Brunner C, Freuler F (1980) Treatment of fractures in children and adolescents. Springer, Berlin Heidelberg New York

Weber M (1970) Operative Behandlung der Navicularepseudarthrosen der Hand. Erfahrungen der Schweizerischen Unfallversicherungsanstalt aufgrund von 345 Fällen. Inauguraldissertation, Zürich

Weller S (1960) Zur Behandlung von frischen Kahnbeinbrüchen der Hand. Dtsch Med Wochenschr 14:544–546

Weller S (1974) Konservative und operative Behandlung von supracondylären Oberarmfrakturen. Aktuel Traumatologe 4:79–83

Welz K (1974) Zweitosteosynthesen an der Clavicula. Zentralbl Chir 99:1485–1487

Weyand F (1976) Zur Behandlung der distalen, intraartikulären Humerusfrakturen. Unfallchirurgie 2:166

Wilhelm K (1971a) Die stabile Osteosynthese bei Frakturen des Handskelettes. Arch Orthop Unfallchir 70:275

Wilhelm K (1971b) Ein Beitrag zur Behandlung der Ellenbogengelenksfrakturen. Monatsschr Unfallheilkd 74:422

Wilhelm K (1971c) Die stabile Osteosynthese bei offenen Handskelettfrakturen. Arch Orthop Unfallchir 71:6

Wilhelm K (1975) Luxationen und Frakturen im Handbereich. Chirurg 46:313

Willenegger H (1961) Die Behandlung der Luxationsfrakturen des oberen Sprunggelenkes nach biomechanischen Gesichtspunkten. Helv Chir Acta 28:225

Willenegger H (1967) Plastischer Ersatz der Kniebänder mit autologer Cutis. Helv Chir Acta 34:75

Willenegger H (1969) Problems and results in the treatment of comminuted fractures of the elbow. Reconstr Surg Trauma 11:118

Willenegger H (1971) Spätergebnisse nach konservativ und operativ behandelten Malleolarfrakturen. Helv Chir Acta 38:321

Willenegger H (1977) Reconstruction in ligamentous lesions. Thieme, Stuttgart

Willenegger H, Guggenbühl A (1959) Zur operativen Behandlung bestimmter Fälle von distalen Radiusfrakturen. Helv Chir Acta 26:81

Willenegger H, Terbrüggen D (1973) Die operative Versorgung des Außenknöchels bei Malleolarfrakturen. Med Techn (Berlin) 93:80

Willenegger H, Weber BG (1965) Malleolarfrakturen. Langenbecks Arch Klin Chir 318:489

Willenegger H, Riede U, Schenk R (1969) Experimenteller Beitrag zur Erklärung der sekundären Arthrose bei Frakturen des oberen Sprunggelenkes. Helv Chir Acta 36:343

Willenegger H, Riede UH, Schenk R (1971) Gelenkmechanische Untersuchungen zum Problem der posttraumatischen Arthrosen im oberen Sprunggelenk. I. Die intraartikuläre Modellfraktur. Langenbecks Arch Klin Chir 328:258

Willenegger H, Riede UH, Schweizer G, Marti J (1973) Gelenkmechanische Untersuchungen zum Problem der posttraumatischen Arthrosen im oberen Sprunggelenk. III. Funktionell-morphometrische Analyse des Gelenkknorpels. Langenbecks Arch Klin Chir 333:91

Willenegger H, Ledermann M, Burckhardt A (1974) Zur Indikation der Navicularverschraubung an Hand von Nachkontrollen. Helv Chir Acta 41:239

Wondrak E (1979) Über die Indikation zur Operation von Fersenbeinbrüchen. Hefte Unfallheilkd 133:224–225

Zimmermann H (1970) Frakturen des Vorfußes. In: Scholder P (ed) Der Vorfuß. Huber, Bern Stuttgart Wien, p 204

Zwank L, Schweiberer L (1979) Abgewandelte Spickdrahtosteosynthese bei mikorchirurgischen Fingerreplantationen. Chirurg 50:264–266

Subject Index

Slide series to supplement the book

Small Fragment Set Manual

Technique Recommended by the ASIF-Group
By U. Heim, K. M. Pfeiffer
1975. 144 slides with legends in four languages
(English, German, French, Spanish). This
collection comprises 157 illustrations from the
book "Small Fragment Set Manual". The slides
will be supplied in a ring binder together with
the text. Order No. 92104-4

C. F. Brunner, B. G. Weber

Special Techniques in Internal Fixation

Translated from the German by T. C. Telger
1981. 91 figures. X, 198 pages
ISBN 3-540-11056-9

Current Concepts of Internal Fixation of Fractures

Editor: H. K. Uhthoff
Associate Editor: E. Stahl
1980. 287 figures, 51 tables. IX, 452 pages
ISBN 3-540-09846-1

F. Freuler, U. Wiedmer, D. Bianchini

Cast Manual for Adults and Children

Forewords by A. Sarmiento, B. G. Weber
Translated from the German by P. A. Casey
1979. 121 figures in 352 separate illustrations,
2 tables. XII, 248 pages
ISBN 3-540-09590-X

Springer-Verlag
Berlin
Heidelberg
New York

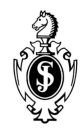

E. Letournel, R. Judet

Fractures of the Acetabulum

Translated from the French by R. A. Elson
1981. 289 figures in 980 separate illustrations.
XXI, 428 pages
ISBN 3-540-09875-5

Manual of Internal Fixation

Techniques Recommended by the AO Group
by M. E. Müller, M. Allgöwer, R. Schneider,
H. Willenegger
In collaboration with numerous experts
Translated from the German by J. Schatzker
2nd, expanded and revised edition. 1979. 345 figures
in color, 2 Templates for Preoperative Planning.
X, 409 pages
ISBN 3-540-09227-7

A. Sarmiento, L. L. Latta

Closed Functional Treatment of Fractures

1981. 545 figures, 85 tables. XII, 608 pages
ISBN 3-540-10384-8
Distribution rights for Japan: Igaku Shoin Ltd.,
Tokyo

F. Séquin, R. Texhammar

AO/ASIF Instrumentation Manual of Use and Care

Introduction and Scientific Aspects
by H. Willenegger
Translated from the German by T. Telger
1981. Approx. 1300 figures, 17 separate Checklists.
XVI, 306 pages
ISBN 3-540-10337-6

Treatment of Fractures in Children and Adolescents

Editors: B. G. Weber, C. Brunner, F. Freuler
With contributions by numerous experts
1980. 462 figures, 31 tables. XII, 408 pages
ISBN 3-540-09313-3
Distribution rights for Japan: Igaku Shoin, Ltd.,
Tokyo

Springer AV Instruction Programme

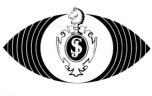

Springer-Verlag
Berlin
Heidelberg
New York

Films/ Videocassettes:

Theoretical and practical bases of internal fixation, results of experimental research

Internal Fixation – Basic Principles and Modern Means

The Biomechanics of Internal Fixation

The Ligaments of the Knee Joint. Pathophysiology

Internal fixation of fractures and in reconstructive bone surgery

Internal Fixation of Forearm Fractures

Internal Fixation of Noninfected Diaphyseal Pseudoarthroses

Internal Fixation of Malleolar Fractures

Internal Fixation of Patella Fractures

Medullary Nailing

Internal Fixation of the Distal End of the Humerus

Internal Fixation of Mandibular Fractures

Corrective Osteotomy of the Distal Tibia

Internal Fixation of Tibial Head Fractures
(available in German)

Joint replacement

Total Hip Prosteses
(3 parts)
Part 1: Instruments, Operation on Model
Part 2: Operative Technique
Part 3: Complications. Special Cases

Elbow-Arthrosplasty with the New GSB-Prosthesis

Total Wrist Joint Replacement

Replantation surgery:

Microsurgery for Accidents

Slide Series:

ASIF-Technique for Internal Fixation of Fractures

Manual of Internal Fixation

Small Fragment Set Manual

Internal Fixation of Patella and Malleolar Fractures

Total Hip Prostheses
Operation on Model and in vivo, Complications and Special Cases

Further films and slide series in preparation

Please ask for information material
Springer-Verlag
Heidelberger Platz 3,
D-1000 Berlin 33, or
Springer-Verlag New York Inc.,
175 Fifth Avenue,
New York, NY 10010